Medical Manpower in Britain

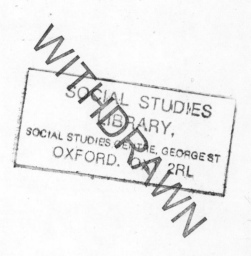
Thurs 27th week
Thurs 3rd Fed - dinner

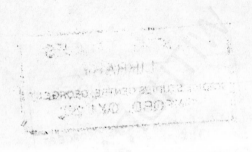

Medical Manpower in Britain

James Parkhouse, M.A., M.D., F.F.A.R.C.S.
Professor of Anaesthetics, University of Manchester

CHURCHILL LIVINGSTONE
EDINBURGH LONDON AND NEW YORK 1979

CHURCHILL LIVINGSTONE

Medical Division of Longman Group Limited

Distributed in the United States of America by Longman Inc., 19 West 44th Street, New York, N.Y. 10036, and by associated companies, branches and representatives throughout the world.

© Longman Group Limited, 1979

First published 1979

ISBN 0 443 01780 8

British Library Cataloguing in Publication Data

Parkhouse, James
  Medical manpower in Britain.
  1. Medical personnel - Great Britain - Supply and
  demand
  I. Title
  331.1'1   RA410.9.G7   78-40728

Printed in Singapore by
Multiprint Services

Preface

This book is the result of a number of years of amateur interest in medical manpower. During this time the Nuffield Provincial Hospitals Trust have given financial help and encouragement which I am glad to have the chance of acknowledging. Much of the present text, in a slightly different form, has appeared in a series of articles in the journal 'Medical Education' and I am grateful to the Editor and to the publishers, Blackwell Scientific Publications, for permission to reproduce the material as part of this book.

It would be impossible to give due thanks to everyone whose writings, public utterances and informal conversation have helped me. Many organisations have given generously of their time and information, including the Department of Health and Social Security, the Scottish Home and Health Department, the General Medical Council and the University Grants Committee. I have received nothing but kindness and courtesy in the course of my sometimes tiresome enquiries and my ignorance has always occasioned patient, and often enthusiastic explanation. This pleasant impression perhaps measures a national asset in relation to medical manpower that should not be underestimated.

My wife, Hilda, was entirely responsible for the preparatory work and drafting of Chapters 5, 6 and 7, and for a great deal of constructive comment on the remainder of the text. I should also like to record my thanks to my former Research Assistant, Mr. Robin Darton, for his meticulous reading and criticism, particularly of the numerical sections.

Most of the statements in the text describing 'the present' situation, and most of the 'current' manpower figures refer to 1975. This was the latest date for which all the necessary figures were available at the time of writing. The reader will appreciate that in some matters there will have been appreciable changes in the meantime. I have tried, wherever possible, to give the precise date to which facts and figures refer but on behalf of the various bodies who supplied these figures I should like to emphasise the point that what was true at the time of writing is not necessarily true at the time of reading. Practically everything in the book is based on information which is made public, and I hope that the reader may be stimulated to seek more up to date data for himself.

Finally, I should like to thank my secretary, Mrs. Pat Coventry, and Mrs. Janet Black for so much perfect typing, and to the publishers for producing the text so quickly.

Manchester, 1978   J.P.

Contents

1. The Background

The story of medical manpower forecasting, and planning, in Britain
begins for all practical purposes after the Second World War. The names
of some of the major reports, such as those of Willink and Todd, have become household words, yet most indiscriminate critics have probably never
read the original papers and scant acknowledgement is given to the reservations that all responsible authors have expressed on their own behal-
ves. Medical manpower planning is not easy; the reports of the past are
milestones on the hard road towards understanding, not mere gravestones
to their hapless originators, and their important place needs to be seen
in relation to the evolution of post-war medicine in Britain as a whole.

THE GOODENOUGH REPORT

The first attempt to estimate medical manpower requirements in the
post-war period was made by the Inter-Departmental Committee on Medical
Schools (The Goodenough Report, 1944). In general terms, this report included a number of important observations and recommendations relevant to
medical manpower and the career structure. For example, the interdepen-
dence of medical education and the National Health Service was stressed:
'the spirit of education must permeate the whole of the Health Service,
and that Service must be so defined and conducted that, among other
things, it secures for medical education the necessary staff, accommo-
dation, equipment and facilities. Medical education cannot be regarded
as merely incidental to the hospital service'. The dangers of neglecting the promotion of health, as an integral part of medical education
were stressed, with particular reference to the need for better teaching
of social medicine, child health and the psychological aspects of disease. The increasing role of women in medicine was clearly foreseen, and
the report established a fundamental principle of far-reaching consequence in recommending 'that the payment to any school of capital ex-
chequer grants in aid of medical education should be conditional upon the
school being co-educational and admitting a reasonable proportion of
women students'. With regard to distribution, the great preponderance of
medical graduates in London, Edinburgh and Glasgow, with a lack of undergraduate facilities in East Anglia and the South West was noted.
More specifically in regard to the need for doctors, the report was
cautious: 'future policy must be largely determined by the demand for and
supply of medical practitioners in the future. The question of demand is

1

one upon which at the present time there can be much speculation but no authoritative pronouncement. It has been assumed that more doctors will be needed'. As an appendix to the report, however, a memorandum on medical manpower was supplied by the Government Actuary, and signed G. S. W. Epps. Almost the first point made in this memorandum was the inadequacy of available published statistics, and the consequent difficulty in making good estimates. Concerning future requirements, estimates were made on three bases, a) that the pattern of retirement of doctors would continue as before. This was felt to be a highly unlikely assumption, since many civilian doctors during the later years of the war were remaining in practice beyond the normal retirement age, b) that the future would see an increasing tendency towards retirement after the age of 60 and c) that there would be a drastic change in the pattern of retirement above the age of 60. Next, an estimate was made of the number of practising doctors from the current stock who would 'survive' for successive five year periods up to 1963. To these estimates were added new entrants to the profession at the rate of 1,650 a year (based on the medical school output at the time). This calculation showed that, on assumption (b) above, the estimated number of doctors in active practice would be expected to rise from 45,413 in 1943 to 54,380 in 1963. The estimate was based on available data, which suggested that 81.5% of British graduates remained in civilian practice in the United Kingdom, and that these British graduates constituted 91.5% of the total stock of doctors practising in the United Kingdom. These assumptions would thus account for emigration and immigration, loss of women doctors from active practice and all other gains and losses. The assumptions were based on pre-war information and the comment was made that if 'these totals were to change substantially from past levels, the same percentages might not apply'. In order to derive estimates for the number of undergraduate places required - i.e. the requisite entry to the medical schools - it was assumed (on evidence available at the time) that 87.5% of students would eventually qualify. The sequence of events could altogether be envisaged, therefore, as follows: if 2,000 students were admitted to the medical schools, about 1,750 would become doctors. Of these, 81.5%, or 1,425, would remain to practise in Great Britain. They would enter the total pool of practising doctors, of which British graduates would make up 91.5%. Conceptually, therefore, by the time incoming doctors from Ireland and elsewhere were allowed for, a medical school intake of 2,000 might be expected to result in an addition of 1,560 doctors to the active stock.

The final step in the Actuary's calculations was to estimate the medical school inputs that would be needed, a) to maintain a minimum stock of 45,400 doctors in active practice, b) to achieve a minimum stock of 50,000 doctors and c) to achieve a minimum stock of 55,000 doctors. In each of the latter two cases alternative estimates were given according to whether the target figure was to be arrived at within 10 or 15 years. On this basis it was shown that, 'for example, if it were desired to achieve increases in the existing number of 45,400 practising doctors so as to reach 50,000 in 10 years' time and 55,000 in a further five years, assuming the less stringent retirement conditions of basis (b) during that period, the number of new doctors starting practice in Great Britain would have to be about 1,850 a year during the five years 1949-1953, and about 2,050 a year during the subsequent five years. The related annual numbers of qualified practitioners emerging from the British medical schools would be about 2,070 and 2,300 respectively. The corresponding annual numbers of new students who should start their training in these schools (say) six years earlier would have to be about 2,370 and

2

2,630'.

The general conclusion was that in order to meet such targets there would have to be an increase over the existing quota of 2,300 annual entrants to the British medical schools. It is interesting to note, however, that according to the figures given in the Actuary's tables, the required number of entrants to the medical schools showed a striking _fall_ in the more distant future. For instance, although the required number of new entrants to medical practice to achieve a stock of 55,000 doctors within 10 years (retirement basis b) was shown as 2,859 for the years 1949-53, it fell to 1,062 for the years 1954-58 and only rose to 1,210 for the years 1959-63. The latter figures would imply a required medical school intake of about 1,300-1,400 a year, although they were actually too low to be shown in the relevant table (p.255 of the report). No comment was made upon this in the text of the appendix, or of the report itself, but two points are clear. First, that the concept of time-limited medical school expansion is clearly not new, since it was implicit in the Goodenough figures, even if not explicitly stated in the text, that although the size of the medical schools may need to rise in the immediate future it would have to fall again later. Second, that the further into the future projections are made, the more difficult it is to guarantee their reliability. In some respects the Government Actuary's attempts, in 1944, to estimate the 'survival' of existing doctors after a lapse of 20 years or more, and his attempts to calculate required input in order to maintain a given stock at such long range, bear a striking resemblance to the recent attempts of the B.M.A.'s Hospital Junior Staffs Committee to estimate medical school requirements on the basis of what the manpower stock will be in 2013.

EVENTS FOLLOWING GOODENOUGH

During the late 1950s there began to be some concern about a possible over-production of doctors. The report of the Committee on General Practice within the National Health Service (The Cohen Report, 1955), foresaw that if entry into general practice continued at the current rate there would 'come a time in the not too distant future when the general medical service may be unable to continue to support this expansion'. This comment, of course, related specifically to general practice and did not discuss the possibility that in future years a greater proportion of medical graduates might enter other fields of work. Nevertheless there were statements in the medical journals, as recalled by Abel-Smith and Gales (1964) that, 'the profession is probably becoming overcrowded' and that, 'perhaps too many doctors were being trained for too few openings in the future, and that a surplus during the next few years was inevitable'. These anxieties were later recalled by Lord Cohen of Birkenhead in a House of Lords Debate (1961) after publication and discussion of the Willink Report.

THE WILLINK REPORT

In 1955 the Willink Committee was set up 'to consider the future numbers of medical practitioners and the appropriate intake of medical students'. Its report was published in 1957 (The Willink Report, 1957). Once again, the point was almost immediately made that adequate statistical information relating to numbers of doctors in practice, age and sex distribution and particulars of retired doctors was not readily available, 'thus at the very outset of our enquiry we were confronted with an awkward statistical problem'. Use was made of the Central Medical Recruitment Committee's Index (see Chapter 4), and in addition the Willink Committee made its own estimate of the numbers of doctors in active practise. They arrived at an approximate total of 44,960 active men, and a total of 11,400 women, of whom 8,300 were active and 3,100 'retired'. This gave an overall active stock of 53,260, compared to the total active figure of 55,600 supplied by the B.M.A, as a result of a count of the C.M.R.C. Index. The difficulties of arriving at an accurate figure were discussed. As in the Goodenough Report, the question of retirement arose. It was noted that in 1955 many elderly doctors were still practising; it was not anticipated that eligibility for superannuation (as from 1958) would cause an immediate large flood of retirements, and for the purpose of the calculations it was assumed that the proportions of doctors who remained active in various age groups would remain the same in future years as in 1955.

The Government Actuary's Department was once more asked to estimate the numbers of doctors required to enter the profession in Great Britain in order to maintain the stock at the 1955 figure (Appendix 3 of the report). The approach was much the same as that of the Government Actuary in 1944, and it is interesting to note that the estimated required annual average intake for the period 1960-65 was 1,180, to maintain a stock of 53,260 doctors, compared to Mr. Epps's estimate of 1,210 for the period 1959-63 to maintain a stock of 55,000. The final three sentences of the Willink Appendix are of interest: 'an extension of the calculations indicates that after 1975 the average annual intake requirements will, in fact, for a time increase very rapidly: they are estimated at about 1,480 in 1975-80, 1,670 in 1980-85 and 1,710 in 1985-90. Thereafter they may begin to decline, but considerable fluctuations are still to be expected. It will be realised that these long-term estimates are not put forward as forecasts, they merely give the arithmetical result of extending calculations based on the assumptions employed in dealing with a shorter period'.

Having looked at the requirements for maintaining an existing stock, the Willink Report next considered expansion. Estimates for general practice were based on the criterion that the average number of patients treated by a general practitioner (the average list size) should be 2,500 in non-rural areas and 2,000 in rural areas. It was estimated that the achievement of this target would require about 625 additional principals for England, Scotland and Wales. Increase in population size, and a rise in the proportion of old people, were thought likely to require an additional annual increase of 75 in the number of general practitioners for the country as a whole. For the hospital service, an average annual expansion of 160 trained specialists was envisaged until about 1965, after which 'expansion of the specialist services will have slowed down' so that the required annual increase might be about halved. No reason was given for this assumption. It was envisaged that 'hospitals will increase their junior staff by about the same amount as their specialist staff'. It was said that this increase in junior hospital staff would be achieved partly by some younger doctors staying longer in the hospital service and partly by the increasing involvement of general practitioners in hospital work, although it is not clear how these trends were taken into account in the numerical estimates that were derived. Further sections of the report dealt with local authority medical staff, doctors employed in Universities and by the Medical Research Council, in factory and industrial medical services, the pharmaceutical industry and Government departments. The Committee went into a good deal of detail about small sectors of the medical profession, for instance doctors employed in mines and quarries, ordnance factories, the gas industry, etc. With regard to university-employed doctors, a distinction was drawn between those with N.H.S. contracts and those without so that, by implication, allowance was made for the staffing of pre-clinical departments by medically qualified staff.

The medical staffing of the Armed Forces was next considered separately, and the point was made that with the ending of National Service a reduced number of doctors would suffice to meet the requirements of the Armed Forces. With a given medical school output, a greater number of doctors would then be available for civilian need, but not with any great precision. The general point is important, since doctors working in the Armed Forces are clearly caring for a section of the population which must otherwise be catered for by an increased number of civilian doctors (see pages 6-7).

The international movement of doctors was discussed in some detail, although the predictions make curious reading in the light of subsequent events. The loss of British graduates overseas, in particular to Commonwealth countries, was expected to decline as local medical schools increased their output towards self-sufficiency. No mention whatsoever was made of the movement of British graduates to the United States, Scandinavia or other parts of the world outside the British Commonwealth and Colonies. Incoming doctors, apart from those from Northern Ireland and the Irish Republic, were classified as Commonwealth or foreign. The general conclusion was that 'since about 1950 the number of foreign trained doctors admitted to the Foreign List[†] and taking up residence here, has been insignificant and it is probable that most of that small number come only for postgraduate study and experience and will in due course return to their own countries'. With regard to the Commonwealth, the report 'estimated that the number of doctors from the Commonwealth at present settling here each year is about 75'. Taking all the evidence and the estimates together, the conclusion was that the net 'export' of doctors from Great Britain was likely to be about 160 a year during 1955-60, progressively falling to 50 a year in 1970-71. It should be noted that this figure was a net figure for the loss of all doctors from Britain, not merely British graduates.

On the evidence of Deans of Medical Schools, it was estimated that 'wastage' of medical undergraduates during training was 4.78% (sic) for men and 8.45% (sic) for women. It was assumed that the proportion of women students in medical schools would be about one-fifth.

A balance sheet could now be drawn up along the following lines:

Existing deficiency of doctors:

General Practice	625
Local Authority	125
Doctors in Government Departments	40
	790 (780)[*]

(* figure given in Paragraphs 75, 107, 110 of the report)

---

† of the General Medical Council

Annual requirement for expansion:

General Practice	75
Consultants	160
Junior hospital staff	160
University (whole-time)	12
Industry	45
Pharmaceutical Industry	10
	462 (465)*

Armed Forces (annual requirement)	55
'Export' (annual loss)	160 (falling to 50 by 1970)

(* figure given in Paragraphs 75, 107, 110 of the report)

The anticipated future stock of doctors in 16 years' time (1971) was derived as follows:

Active Civilian doctors in 1955   53,260

Expansion:

1955-1960 (465/year)	2,325
1960-1965 (440/year)	2,200
1965-1971 (280/year)	1,680
Deficiency in 1955 to be made up	780
	60,245
Wastage from death and premature retirement (Paragraph 110)	200
	60,045 (60,000)**

(** figure given in Paragraph 110 of the report)

In addition, there would be 1,800 doctors in the Armed Forces.

The required intake of medical students was then stated as being, from 1957 onwards or as soon as practicable thereafter, about 1,760. This figure was derived from a table given in paragraph 107 of the report, showing the 'average annual requirements' for successive five-year periods. This table made no specific allowance for the make-up of the existing deficiency of 780 doctors, but it was suggested that some excess output until 1962 would make up about a third of this deficiency. The remainder of the deficiency would, it was thought, be met by the reduced need for doctors in the Armed Forces, 'even after allowance is made for

6

any increase in civilian medical services required to meet the increase in civilian population consequent upon the decrease in size of the Armed Forces'. The table in paragraph 107 showed the required average numbers of doctors for five year periods up to 1970 and for 1970-71, from which the average annual need was calculated (paragraph 108) as 1,655 (allowing for an entry of 70 a year from Northern Ireland). Assuming a 6% wastage during the undergraduate course this presupposed an entry requirement of 1,760.

The general conclusions of the Willink Report were that up to that time the medical schools had not been producing too many doctors; that the output of the medical schools was already determined up to 1961 but that after that year a reduced output would suffice. It was suggested that the student intake could be reduced by about one-tenth from as early a date as practicable. It was, however, envisaged that student intake would need to be raised again from about 1970, in order to ensure an increased output in 1975. The final sentence read, 'this forecast is, however, so speculative that it would seem prudent for there to be another review of the situation in about 10 years' time'.

EVENTS FOLLOWING WILLINK

The Royal Commission on the remuneration of doctors and dentists, 1957-60 (The Pilkington Report, 1960) accepted the Willink conclusion that the supply of potential doctors was reasonably close to requirements, and felt that the question of using remuneration as an instrument either for encouraging a greater flow of potential doctors, or reducing the present flow, did not arise. In a notable Memorandum of Dissent, however, Professor John Jewkes wrote as follows: 'I have stressed earlier that there is, in the long run, no sound way of determining the earnings of doctors and dentists except that of searching for levels which will result in rates of recruitment adequate to meet the requirements, however those requirements may be fixed. Earnings, recruitment and requirements must be looked at together, not sporadically but as part of an unceasing scrutiny designed to avoid the kind of maladjustments which have occurred since 1948. The surplus of senior registrars; the shortage of dentists; the assertions that there is a shortage of consultants; the dispute as to whether a surplus or a shortage of registrars is threatened; these are all cases of a breakdown or a possible breakdown of balance with which the rate of earnings is inevitably and intimately associated. Somewhere within the National Health Service there should be an organ for research and planning which would concern itself with the facts of supply and demand and with speculations about probable future changes and which, at the shortest notice, could set forth an up-to-the-moment assessment of recruitment and requirements. So far in the history of the service these broad assessments have been entrusted to ad hoc committees which, however vigorously they may have carried through their tasks, have been able to report only after a relatively long period of work, partly because they have come new to their tasks but mainly because they have been compelled to start from scratch in the collection of the kind of statistics and information which constitute the vital raw material of their studies.' The two significant statements in this paragraph, namely the interrelationship of earnings, recruitment and requirement in various branches of the profession and at various places of work, and the need for an efficient body to oversee planning and research on medical manpower, reverberate with undiminished insistence almost 20 years later.

The basis of current medical manpower policy was challenged in an article by Lafitte and Squire (1960), who set out to show that some of Willink Committee's calculations had been falsified by events. In the first place, they contended that it was unsafe to assume anything less than an 8% population increase over the period 1955-70, whereas Willink had accepted an official projection of an approximately 4½% increase. they disputed the Willink projections for 'export' of doctors, although they based their doubts upon the needs of the Commonwealth and Developing Countries, rather than the desires and ambitions of the doctors themselves, and again the United States was not mentioned. Lafitte and Squire also felt that the tendency for doctors to retire earlier had been substantially underestimated and, with regard to expansion, commented that it was 'far from clear why the Committee should have arbitrarily halved its estimates for the period after 1965'. On the basis of their own 'admittedly amateurish' estimates the authors concluded that, although the medical schools had already reduced their intake by 10% at the time of the Willink Committee, urgent consideration should be given to raising the numbers of students in the medical schools. Their estimate for the required average annual output of doctors between 1955 and 1960 was 2,100 and they argued that if the actual numbers were to come down in accordance with the Willink recommendations then by 1965 there would be a shortfall requiring, from 1965-70 an annual output of 2,470 to redress the balance. Although Lafitte and Squire touched upon the expectations of the affluent society, and the increasing demand for 'middle class' standard of medical care they did not attempt to develop this theme in a quantitative manner.

The British Government announced in February, 1961 that it had decided to review the conclusions of the Willink Report in the light of new data (Abel-Smith and Gales, 1964). In November of the same year the House of Lords debated the growing shortage of doctors. Lord Taylor raised the problems of staffing in provincial non-teaching hospitals, and observed that the Health Service would have collapsed if it had not been for the enormous influx of junior doctors from such countries as India and Pakistan. A new factor in the manpower equation - the dependence of the National Health Service on overseas doctors - thus became a subject for active discussion. It was conceded that population estimates, retirement patterns of doctors and the needs of the Armed Forces might require revision, and it was announced that the Government felt that 'the prospective demand for medical services would justify a rise in the University intake of pre-clinical students from Great Britain of 10% above the level recommended by the Willink Committee'.

The question of emigration also aroused controversy during the early 1960s. Davison (1961, 1962) obtained figures for numbers of doctors from the United Kingdom settling in North America, which cast serious doubt on the Willink assumptions. Seale (1961, 1962) produced data purporting to show that the numbers of medical graduates from Great Britain and Ireland registering in Australia, New Zealand, U.S.A., Canada, South Africa and Rhodesia accounted for a third of the annual output of the British and Irish medical schools. Seale's observations were challenged by Mr. Enoch Powell (then Minister of Health) and even criticised by President Kennedy. The more detailed history of the controversy is reviewed by Abel-Smith and Gales (1964) who made a careful study of their own which will be referred to in relation to the general question of emigration and immigration (Chapter 6). Thus, within five years of the publication of the Willink Report the tide had turned against reduction in the medical school output. The feeling was reinforced by important estimates of required expansion in higher education as a whole: the Report of the Committee on Higher Education (The Robbins Report, 1963) envisaged that the number of students taking medical subjects would rise from 16,500 in 1961-62 to 21,000 in 1980-81.

Mr. Anthony Barber (1963) acknowledged in the House of Commons that the country was short of doctors, and the Government asked the medical schools to increase their intake by 15%, over and above the 10% increase already requested in order to restore the Willink cut. Hill (1964) argued further, that the Robbins estimates, which were based on the demand for higher education places rather than the need for doctors, were inadequate. He derived an annual 'wastage' figure of over 2,000 a year, which included an estimated 400 British doctors a year permanently emigrating and 190 women doctors not working. Thus a medical school output of over 2,000 a year would be needed merely to replace losses, regardless of any contemplated expansion. He did not attempt an analysis of the annual gains and losses of overseas doctors, although the point was made that to replace the 3,500 foreign doctors in Britain at that time would require the entire output of all the British medical schools for two years; but a supplementary comment, not unfamiliar to present-day ears, was that 'there are indications that the "brain-drain" to this country, especially from India, may soon cease'. Hill's paper was more of a shotgun assault than a closely argued, constructive series of alternative proposals, but the sentiments must have been echoed by many people at the time. The decision to establish a new medical school at Nottingham had already been announced by September 1964, but Hill made further proposals for a rapid increase in the output of graduates, including a scheme for affiliating regional clinical centres with local Universities or Polytechnics, in a manner not unlike the recent proposals put forward by advocates of medicine in the Open University.

In 1966 Paige and Jones published 'Health and Welfare Services in Britain in 1975'. This was a comprehensive review financed by the Department of Economic Affairs in relation to a general study of the British economy supported by a grant from the Treasury. It attempted to look 10 years ahead to the likely health and welfare situation in 1975. Appendix A dealt with 'The Future Supply of Doctors'. In fact, some attempt was made to relate supply to demand, although many aspects of the latter which received consideration in the text of the report, such as care of the aged and handicapped and the mental health services, were not analysed quantitatively in terms of manpower. Some of the figures were surprisingly unreliable; for example, only estimates were given (Table A2) for numbers of senior and junior hospital staff in 1962 (four years before publication) and these were misleadingly different from reality, especially in regard to the ratio between grades (12,000 senior and 10,700 junior staff quoted, compared to actual totals of 11,091 and 12,576). Forecasts were based on doctor/population ratios, the need to reduce G.P. list sizes and the assumption that the numbers of hospital doctors would continue to rise more or less according to the recommendations of The Platt Report (1961), (see Chapter 2). The estimate for 1980 was that over 82,000 active doctors might be needed: a shortage in 1975 was considered unavoidable and it would be 'a very long time before there is an over-supply of doctors'.

Shortly before the publication of the Todd Report in 1968, Peacock and Shannon (1968), in the Lloyds Bank Review, looked at the question of medical manpower forecasting from the economic point of view. This was an important contribution, in that it introduced a number of highly relevant concepts of an essentially non-medical nature which had been given

9

little consideration in the manpower planning estimates hitherto discussed. The authors commented on the difficulty of defining 'good health'
and the problem of reaching any satisfactory index of how many doctors
are 'needed'. In discussing the market forces which operate, they commented that 'if advertised posts in the N.H.S. for doctors are to be
filled, the salaries must be tempting enough to offset the attractions,
in the short run, of private practice or of employment abroad and, in the
long run of alternative employment'. A strong plea was made for the provision of alternative assumptions for measures of output, and for the
possible combinations of different types of manpower (doctors, nurses,
etc.) and of capital investment which might be capable of achieving stated objectives with different degrees of efficiency and at different
costs. The authors made the important point that it is not sufficient
merely to criticise reports such as Willink on the basis that they should
have made better population estimates, since all such estimates are inherently unreliable: 'what should be done is to incorporate into this
sort of exercise a much greater flexibility, offering, instead of single
forecasts with their spurious air of precision, a range of forecasts for
the different variables concerned, with some sort of probabilities attached to them wherever possible'. The possibilities of substitution of
alternative forms of health manpower for fully trained doctors were developed to some extent, and thus yet another important factor in the manpower
debate may be said to have come into play. Finally, the paper served as
a valuable reminder, along with Mr. Enoch Powell's book (1966), that in a
situation where the demand for better health care and more medical staff
is potentially unlimited, the determining factor is likely to be what the
nation can afford. As we have subsequently learned, the question of priorities, both within the Health Service and in relation to the national
economy as a whole, is often more important than an isolated estimate of
the likely supply of doctors, or an assessment, however idealistically
derived, of the demand for their services.

THE TODD REPORT

The Royal Commission on Medical Education (The Todd Report, 1968)
was not specifically charged with the responsibility of assessing medical
manpower needs, but it nevertheless felt so strongly about the necessity
for additional medical school places that it produced an interim report
on this subject. The short-term assessments of medical manpower requirements were set out in an annex to Appendix 12 of the Report. Wastage
from death and retirement was considered to need 1,350 replacements a
year. This estimate was about 100 higher than the Willink estimate, due
to the greater anticipated loss of working capacity for women doctors as
part of the increasing stock of younger medical graduates. Permanent
emigration to developed countries, of graduates of British medical schools
and of those qualifying abroad who had been in Britain long enough to be
regarded as part of the permanent stock of doctors in Britain, was estimated at at least 300 a year, largely on the evidence of Abel-Smith and
Gales (1964). General practice was assessed as requiring an extra 5,000
doctors by 1975, in order to maintain the ratio of principals to population which had obtained in 1961 and to restore the relationship between
numbers of assistants and trainees and of principals which had existed in
1953-55. It was estimated that this combined increase of trainees and
principals would enable a better distribution of practice sizes to be
achieved and to ensure that, except in special circumstances, no list
would be greater than 2,500 or 2,000 in rural areas (i.e. these were upper

10

limits, as compared to the <u>average</u> practice sizes recommended by Willink).
Hospital service requirements were derived from the studies of the Joint
Working Party on Medical Staffing Structure in the Hospital Service (The
Platt Report, 1961) and of the Wright Committee in Scotland (The Wright
Report, 1964). Essentially, this was an estimate of the numbers of hospital doctors required by various Regions to ensure that there was no
understaffing in relation to 'the norm'. Allowance was also made for
population growth up to 1975, and the annual needs over the 10 year period 1965-75 were given as 830. Further allowances were made of 130 a
year for doctors serving in underdeveloped territories, and of 210 a year
for the needs of other fields of practice. The balance sheet thus read
as follows:

Requirements to provide adequate medical services:

(Average annual numbers 1966-75)

Wastage from death and retirement	1,350
Permanent emigration to developed countries	300
General Practice	500
Hospital Service	830
Service in underdeveloped territories	130
Needs of other fields of practice	210
	3,320

Supply:

British Medical Schools	2,070
Immigration	250
	2,320
Deficit per year	1,000
Deficit in 10 year period	10,000

With regard to migration, the overall estimate was that 'over the
next 10 years' there would be an annual outflow of 300 doctors to developed countries and 130 to raise the numbers temporarily serving in developed countries, and an annual intake of 250 doctors from permanent or
semi-permanent immigration. The annual <u>net</u> loss would thus be 180. How
much this estimate was belied by events between 1965 and 1975, particularly in regard to the annual inflow of overseas doctors, is sufficiently
obvious. Indeed, the Todd Committee, once again, was constrained to re-
mark that 'the aim is to provide a broad assessment, and not to specify
the exact requirements that could be calculated from detailed projections
of the component elements according to present and predicted trends. Much
of the statistical information which would form the basis for such a procedure is lacking; even if it were available, an attempt to be over-
precise could be misleading since several of the factors in the calculation will depend on future decisions rather than follow from events al-

11

ready passed'. It should be noted, however, that the Todd recommendations were intended as estimates of the true need for British graduates
in order to provide a self-sufficient Health Service, rather than merely
a passive forecast of what was likely to occur. In this sense, acknowledgement of the fact that the National Health Service would continue to
depend upon acquiring 250 overseas doctors each year for the succeeding
10 years was an admission of defeat, and insofar as this is true the
Commission's assessments of the need for medical school places in the
immediate future were an underestimate. In fact, it was assumed 'that
most of these immigrants would be from Ireland and the older Commonwealth
countries'.

The Todd Report also made long-term estimates of need (Chapter 6).
These were based on population estimates, and a population growth rate up
to 1975 of 0.8% was accepted from the Government Actuary's Department.
The Commission found that observed values for the doctor-population quo-
tient in Britain from 1911 to 1961 lay close to a smooth curve representing a constant annual rate of increase of 1.25% and passing through the
point representing the estimate already derived for required numbers of
doctors in 1971. Various factors determining the future demand for doctors were discussed, including progress in medical treatment and preventive medicine, changes in the structure and organisation of the Health
Services and the likely age structure of the population. The appropriately modified estimates of future need were 'related not directly to the
size of the population but to the requirements of the population for medical care; an important consequence of this is that the estimates are
likely to be less influenced by errors in the population forecasts'. Probable future developments in other countries were considered, and space
was devoted to discussion of possible future trends in losses and gains
from various sources. The reservations expressed in the annex to Appendix 12 were, however, reiterated in Chapter 6: 'our forecasts should be
taken as only very rough indications of future requirements; they should
be reviewed continuously and amended to take account of new information
and developments'.

Taking all factors into account, the future needs for medical graduates were estimated as follows:

1965-74	3,100
1975-79	3,500
1980-84	3,850
1985-89	4,250
1990-94	4,550

In the light of these estimates the report (Table 5, page 148) gave
the average annual intake to the medical schools required 'to give as
rapid a build up as we think practicable towards the annual number of
graduates needed'. It was pointed out that this build up would 'gradually
reduce the deficit'. It is important to appreciate that the recommended
intake figures of the Todd Commission were based on what was considered
to be feasible, and fell short of the actual estimated requirement. The
4,300 places a year recommended for 1975-79 would produce an estimated
3,850 graduates a year for 1980-84, but the shortfall for previous years
would not have been made good. The total requirement between 1965 and
1994 (Table 4 of the report) was 111,750, and the estimated output, given
the recommended annual intakes, was 99,650, leaving a gap of 12,100. It

12

should further be noted that in the annex to Appendix 12 of the report the table showing estimates of the students normally resident in Britain who would graduate from medical schools in England, Wales and Scotland actually showed a lower average annual number for the years 1970-74 than the number shown in Table 5 of the report.

A general resume of the Todd Commission's assumptions and proposals has more recently been given by Ellis (1975).

EVENTS FOLLOWING TODD

Although most of the recommendations of the Todd Commission concerning its main theme of medical education proved controversial, the interim report on manpower requirements was rapidly accepted. Plans were put into operation for the immediate expansion of the existing medical schools, wherever possible, and for the establishment of new medical schools in Southampton and, at a slighly later stage, Leicester. Although precise details may have been open to question there was for several years no serious argument with the broad principles of the Todd recommendations in regard to the urgent need for more doctors.

Within the fabric of the Todd Report were far-reaching recommendations regarding the career structure and the organisation of training. Apart from the macro-planning aspects of medical manpower in general - that is, the overall need for a given number of doctors - there were clearly micro-manpower planning implications. For example, there was the important question of whether enough junior hospital posts would be available to implement the training schemes envisaged by the Commission, including vocational training for general practice, and what impact the introduction of these schemes would have on hospital staffing. Feasibility studies were carried out (Parkhouse and McLaughlin, 1975) and altogether a good deal of interest was generated, from the manpower planning point of view, in the inner workings of the system. Such factors as rate of movement through training grades, probability of achieving 'success' as defined by obtaining a consultant post rather than 'falling off the ladder', availability of residual training capacity for overseas postgraduate students, the dynamics of exchange of doctors at various levels between the National Health Service and the Universities, and many other practically important aspects of manpower planning had not seriously been considered in any of the reports devoted to estimates of overall numbers. Likewise there remained the vital questions of proper distribution of doctors - between grades, regions and specialties. Much work had by this time begun on the application of statistical techniques to manpower planning problems in other fields (see, for example, Bartholomew: 'Stochastic Models for Social Processes', 1967). The Institute of Mathematics and its Applications organised a symposium in 1974 on manpower planning, at which medical manpower planning was discussed (Parkhouse and McLaughlin, 1976). Further manpower planning studies continue to be reported (e.g. Bartholomew, 1976) and the potential applicability of the mathematical techniques that are available to medical problems will become increasingly evident. It remains true to say, however, that, as with statistics in general, no technique will compensate for inadequacy in the original data. Perhaps one of the most useful effects of the mathematical approach to medical manpower planning is that when attempts are made to test statistical models against real-life situations the inadequacy of the available data is clearly revealed.

In 'The Practice of Manpower Forecasting' (1973) Ahamad and Blaug included a case study on doctors in the United States, Britain and Canada

by Ahamad which included some comments on Goodenough, Willink and Todd.
The Todd estimates for future requirements in general practice were criticised on the basis that in advocating a substantial increase in the number of assistants and trainees no account had been taken of the effect
that these trainees would have on the need for principals. Although, as
already indicated (page 10), this specific criticism is probably unfoun-
ded, it did emphasise the important role of substitution, and raised considerations of some consequence in regard to the hospital service. For
example, reduction in the number of junior staff must be compensated for
by increase in the consultant establishment in order to maintain the size
of the total available workforce, or alternatively an intermediate career
grade must be established. It is in working out the implications of
transitional arrangements of this kind that micro-planning is important.
Ahamad also commented on the Todd Commission's long-term projections,
pointing out that no attempt had been made to test the goodness of fit of
the projection curve by statistical methods. Although it was true that a
calculation showing a growth rate of 1.25% a year drove the curve through
the projection for 1975, the best statistical estimate of the slope of
the relevant log-linear regression equation was 1.24% a year. A linear
regression equation, which implied a declining rate of growth, showed no
less good a fit and yielded an estimated number of doctors in 1975 of
71,100 compared to the Royal Commission's 78,100. The criticism served
as a useful reminder of the wide margin of error that should be accepted
for projections such as those of Todd. In summing up, Ahamad commented
on the need to supply alternative projections of requirements by making
different assumptions about the relevant parameters, in order to illustrate the range of possible outcomes as an aid to policy making: 'cur-
iously few attempts were made to investigate the effects of alternative
assumptions on the projected stock; for this reason methods of altering
the future stock of doctors by means other than the student intake - for
example, through retirement rates, or immigration - have not been properly
investigated'. Noting the crudeness of the models currently used for
medical manpower forecasting Ahamad made pertinent comment in relation to
the micro-planning aspect, 'it is obvious that we know very little about
the utilisation of doctors and that there may be wide disparities in the
provision of care between rich and poor, between ethnic groups, between
areas, and so on: in this sense, shortages of doctors seem to exist, but
these shortages will not necessarily be eliminated by simply increasing
the supply of doctors. Any extra doctors who become available may move
to the already well-stocked areas or may treat the already well-treated
groups of the population. In such a case, adjustment of supply and demand may take place through the elimination of queues, or through an increase in the time spent per patient, or by a reduction of hours worked,
or by an increase in the price of care, and so on. Thus we cannot solve
the existing problems in the provision of health services by simply increasing the supply of doctors'. In relation to the queueing problem, it
is interesting to note that a number of operational studies have been
undertaken of medical staff requirements in relation to workloads, particularly those involving emergency cases requiring treatment with various
degrees of urgency as in the provision of an anaesthetic service (Taylor
et al, 1970; Jennings, 1975).

In 1972, the Central Manpower Committee was set up to advise the
D.H.S.S. on manpower policy. A paper from the Department of Health and
Social Security on medical manpower planning (Shore, 1974) noted that
manpower planning 'mistakes' could be either quantitative (in the macro-
planning sense) or qualitative, in terms of the way in which medical

students are selected and trained and in which various types of medical work are presented. In the micro-planning context, Shore referred to the possible control of medical manpower, firstly by choice - picking the most appropriate applicant for the job - which is likely to break down in a shortage situation; secondly by price - arranging for certain groups of doctors to receive larger increases in remuneration than others as an incentive - as in the case of general practitioners since the 'G.P. Charter'; thirdly by control of posts - the identification of designated areas in general practice and the adjustment of the number of senior registrar posts in the hospital service according to anticipated vacancies.

In view of the several different strands of thought that were being woven around the question of medical manpower during the few years after the publication of the Todd Report, it is not surprising that sooner or later the Commission's basic assumptions should come to be questioned. Fry (1975) posed the question 'How many doctors?' and made the point that 'a major deficiency in all the work, analysis and planning for medical manpower requirements is the lack of reliable information on what the doctor does and what he should be doing that is useful and productive and what may be shared and passed on to his paramedical colleagues or even placed as the responsibility of the consumer, the patient'. He referred to many other imponderables in the balance of manpower and attempted to make a case that too many doctors were being produced in the United Kingdom. His calculations failed to take adequate account of the major contribution to the hospital workforce of large numbers of overseas doctors. It had, in fact, by this time become increasingly clear that the question of whether Britain was producing 'enough doctors', without entering into any discussion of how they should be deployed, could be answered in two ways: if we were to produce enough doctors to fill future career vacancies in the consultant and general practitioner grades there would still be large deficiencies in the numbers of junior hospital staff, but if we were to produce enough doctors to fill the junior hospital posts promotion prospects for many of these graduates would be non-existent (Parkhouse and McLaughlin, 1975a).

This issue has come to preoccupy, to an increasing extent, those concerned with manpower planning since Fry's article was published. A more rigorous analysis of the ways in which the future needs for doctors can be assessed (Parkhouse, 1976) indicated the wide range of possible developments over the next few years and tried to emphasise that, in the present state of knowledge, it is unrealistic to expect any single estimate, however derived, to be a reliable guide to policy. If the National Health Service continued to grow and thus to demand more and more doctors, and if the inflow of overseas graduates were to cease dramatically, we might well not be producing enough doctors even on the Todd estimates. On the other hand, if for economic reasons the stock of doctors were to remain constant, and overseas graduates were to continue to come, we might be producing far too many doctors. The same type of plea was made by Maynard (1976) in a review of the literature: 'the fact that the previous forecasts have borne little relation to outcome is not surprising, generally the planning procedures have involved point estimates and not ranges, or a variety of estimates each conditional upon a particular state of the world'. The need is clearly for a dynamic, rather than a static manpower analysis and for continuous collection of the necessary background data.

The Todd recommendations with regard to future numbers in medical schools were revised in 1970, when the target figure agreed between the D.H.S.S. and the University Grants Committee for medical student intake in 1979 was 4,100. Officially, this remains the target, while controversy

continues about over-production and possible future unemployment of doctors. It is relevant to note that population estimates have been substantially revised since the Todd Report, the current trends and predictions being reviewed by Maclure (1977) and by the D.H.S.S. (The Way
Forward, 1977). There is more than one parallel, in terms of manpower
planning, between the doctors' dilemma and the teachers' dilemma; in
both cases population trends are likely to make a significant difference
to manpower requirements - and in the case of teachers have already done
so. But also in both cases the number of career posts is likely to depend at least as much on the national economy as on any other factor.
There would arguably be no surplus of teachers if we could afford to reduce class sizes and introduce other desirable improvements in our educational system. Likewise as Klein (1977) has pointed out, 'if there is
now anxiety about a surplus of doctors, it is largely because views about
Britain's economic prospects have changed since the present training programmes were drawn up'.

The principal anxieties and uncertainties of the last few years have
concerned (i) dependence on overseas doctors: the extent to which this
should be allowed to continue and the period of time over which it might
reasonably·be eliminated. Allied with this is the question of whether
manpower planning should make allowance, in the future, for the elective
admission of quotas of overseas trainees in various specialties for specific periods of postgraduate training before returning home; (ii) the
fact that such policy decisions may be overtaken by a dramatic fall in
the inflow of overseas doctors as a result of the TRAB test and other factors; (iii) the extent to which the proportion of women graduates will
increase and the effect that this will have on the composition and productivity of the medical workforce; (iv) the unpredictability of the future trend in emigration, bearing in mind on the one hand the current disillusionment with the National Health Service and its financial unattrac-
tiveness compared to medical employment elsewhere, and on the other hand
the increasing restrictiveness of immigration regulations in other countries; (v) the possible effect of free movement within the E.E.C. on
medical manpower; (vi) anxiety about unemployment of doctors in Britain
if medical school output continues to increase (Bell, 1976). It is possible to advance a number of arguments in favour of increased production
of doctors: the fact that the demand for medical services will inevitably
increase and that current economic restrictions will be temporary, the
fact that losses through emigration are likely to continue, that early
retirement will become common and that the future will see many women
graduates who are not able to work full-time throughout their professional
lives and, perhaps most important of all, that the silent stealing away of
overseas doctors, without continual replacement, will leave large defec-
iencies to be made up. The advocates of reduced medical school output,
on the other hand, point to the closing down of career opportunities
abroad and the massive over-production of doctors, with consequent unemployment, in European countries, the trend towards re-definition of the
doctor's function and substitution of other forms of health manpower (less
expensive to train and less demanding in terms of resources) and the increasing tendency of women doctors to work full-time. Inevitably, there
are suggestions that there is a deliberate policy of the D.H.S.S. 'to
create a glut of doctors so that they can direct labour, so that doctors
will all become members of multi-disciplinary teams with no authority but
with total responsibility' (Greenwood, 1977) and that, 'if supply out-
stripped demand the profession's negotiating position would become untenable' (Ford, 1976). At the other extreme there is the more down-to-earth

view that 'when recruitment to general practice was such that the number
of U.K. graduates actually fell last year and 16,000 overseas graduates
were required to prop up the Health Service, it was difficult to convince
people that there were sufficient medical graduates in this country'
(Wilson, 1977).

Doran (1976) attempted a stocktaking analysis of the future situation from which he concluded that by 1995, on certain assumptions, there
would be a surplus of about 15,000 fully trained general practitioners.
One assumption appeared to be, however, that a fixed proportion of the
output of the medical schools would enter general practice and, although
the methods of calculation were not entirely clear, criticism could be
made on the grounds that 'survival' estimates of successive cohorts of
doctors already in practice appeared to be based on fixed percentages of
loss rather than age distributions. Likewise, the Hospital Junior Staffs
Committee of the B.M.A. (H.J.S.C., 1977) argued that if the medical school
output were kept level after 1981 the country would 'end up' with over
80% more economically active British doctors than at present. The calculation was made on a very long-term basis, to the year 2013 by which
time, according to the assumptions made, all doctors who graduated before
1981 would have left the system. The process of estimation, therefore,
was essentially a very simple one of building up an imaginary model from
a 'clean' starting point at which the output of graduates could be regulated. Unfortunately, no alternative calculations were made to show what
the effect of such regulation would be, and the exercise had virtually no
relevance for the immediate future.

The initial assumptions made by the H.J.S.C. were different in several respects from those in the main evidence on manpower of the British
Medical Association to the Royal Commission on the National Health Service (B.M.A., 1977). Medical school output figures were taken from the
Church House Conference (Report, 1976), 'wastage' rates were looked at
differently, the average working life of doctors was assessed at a lower
figure and the starting-point was from supposed 1975 numbers of doctors
which were actually often lower than the actual figures quoted by the
B.M.A. for 1974. Within a matter of weeks the H.J.S.C. (1977a) had revised its calculations, thus openly acknowledging the need, which all
workers in the field will recognise, for both honesty and continuing
thought.

The British Medical Association, in the body of its own draft evidence (B.M.A., 1977) commented once again on the imponderables, and noted
that even reliable figures for the actual projected numbers of medical
graduates were hard to come by: 'the discrepancy once again highlights
the need for manpower statistics to be subject to greater scrutiny'. Two
separate assumptions were made - firstly nil growth in total medical manpower and secondly an expansion of 4% a year in the number of consultants
and a substantial increase in the number of G.P.s to secure an average
list size of about 1,600 - 1,700. It was further assumed that 50% of medical graduates would be women, who would contribute a 60% work schedule,
and that the average length of service for all doctors would be 35 years.
On this basis it was calculated that, with a wastage rate of 9% during the
undergraduate course, the number of medical school places needed to maintain a 'nil growth' situation would be 2,823. Allowing for expansion,
according to the second assumption, the number of medical school places
would need to reach 4,697 by 1980. These estimates made no allowance for
postgraduate wastage (apart from relative underemployment of women doctors
as referred to above); a 20% allowance for wastage (for example through
emigration) would require a medical school intake in 1980 of 5,636 to

permit expansion, and 3,388 to maintain a 'nil growth' position. These figures should be compared to the actual medical school intake estimate of the University Grants Committee for 1979, of 3,275. Although the B.M.A. commented that they were 'extremely concerned' about the possibility of unemployment it is hard to understand why this anxiety should exist on the basis of the figures produced, unless there should be a rigid insistence upon further medical school expansion after 1979 in the face of a known and implacable policy of no N.H.S. expansion.

The British Medical Association's 1977 Annual Conference (Editorial, 1977) included an extended debate on medical manpower, in which anxieties were reiterated, both about future unemployment and about continuing shortages. The Secretary of State for Health and Social Security, Mr. David Ennals, announced in Parliament in July 1977 (News and Notes, 1977) that he did not expect a surplus of doctors by 1980 and that there had been 'no change in the Government's aim to reduce our dependence on overseas doctors, to remove the disparities between regions of the country, and to overcome shortages in certain specialties. I see no possibility of achieving these objectives as soon as 1980'. Further debate took place at the British Medical Association's Council meeting in October 1977 (Scrutator, 1977), when particular emphasis was placed on the urgent need to ensure sufficient posts for newly qualified doctors in the pre-registration (intern) year. Although it had been recognised for at least 10 years that the increasing output of the medical schools could lead to difficulties at this stage unless effective action was taken, a situation was reached in 1977 where almost no margin existed. This is a further sharp reminder of the importance of micro-planning and the vital role of the career structure (see Chapter 2). If medical manpower planning is to make any sense at all, the output of the medical schools must ultimately be related to the staffing of the career grades, that is the numbers of trained general practitioners, hospital doctors and others. The numbers of training posts must then be arranged accordingly. The worst possible situation is to allow anxiety to build up over avoidable 'tight spots', such as the pre-registration year, in a way that might seriously influence the broader view of health needs.

Whether or not there will ever be an absolute 'freeze' on the total numbers of doctors in the country is, of course, an open question. Its fundamental influence on the medical manpower requirement is well illustrated by the B.M.A.'s projections. Faced with continuing economic difficulties there must be a continual search for alternative means of delivering something like an equivalent service to the public at lower cost, for example by substitution of non-medical manpower. An alternative suggestion, at least in theory, was that proposed by Rudolph Klein (1977) when he wrote, 'one answer to a threatened surplus of professionals is to reduce their relative earnings so as to make it possible to employ more of them'. This point of view, from an economist, presents a striking contrast to the contention of Peacock and Shannon (1968) that the viability of N.H.S. employment for doctors must in the long run depend on its competitiveness, in financial and other terms, with the alternatives that are available at home and abroad. From within the medical profession, this view was well expressed by Mortimer (1977) in response to Rudolph Klein: 'the relative earnings of senior doctors, and particularly of consultants have been falling sharply for several years. The consequence has been an equally sharp decline in the numbers of suitably qualified medical graduates coming forward for specialist training, which is most serious in those specialties least favoured in economic terms. Mr. Klein.... should not underestimate the erosion of goodwill and the accretion of cynicism and disaffection that have already taken place. In other words, the choice is not between relatively few highly paid doctors and more doctors earning less, but between a number of doctors well paid and a smaller number paid less'.

Possible future policy choices were again discussed largely from the economic point of view by Maynard and Walker (1977) and suggestions were made for improving the efficiency of manpower forecasting: providing ranges of estimates rather than single figures, increasing the flexibility of undergraduate training to allow application of 'medical science' degrees in various ways, modelling of future trends, examining different possible relationships between numbers of doctors and 'production of health care', and realistic acceptance of budgetary restraints. There was little novelty in this mixture of suggestions, which were actually aimed more at examining the structure of the system than at improving the quality of forecasting as an art in itself. Furthermore, the basis of the article was an unconvincing critique of the Todd estimates, in which the relationship between the medical schools and the non-university qualifying diplomas (e.g. the M.R.C.S., L.R.C.P., or 'Conjoint' Diploma) did not appear to be fully understood.

Virtually all people who have tried to make estimates and forecasts, or who have commented on the medical manpower situation, have stressed the need not so much for yet another major review as for the setting up of a body which can maintain continual surveillance of the position and make frequent, well-informed estimates, each based on the latest available information and each analysing the consequences of a wide range of possible future developments and policy decisions. Although strong representations had been made about the urgent need to clarify the medical manpower position, the Royal Commission on the National Health Service announced in October 1977 (Scrutator, 1977) that, in the interests of completing its tasks in the allotted time, it had decided against producing an interim report on manpower. In April 1977, the Secretary of the British Medical Association wrote to the Chief Medical Officer at the Department of Health and Social Security concerning the B.M.A. Council's recommendation that the Department should now set up a body to undertake a fact-finding enquiry into the likely future needs for medical manpower and the appropriate numbers for medical school intakes. The Chief Medical Officer, in his reply (C.M.O., 1977) expressed concern that 'yet another body should start looking at the medical manpower field at this stage'. He referred to the recent re-constitution of the Central Manpower Committee (see Chapter 4) and the channels for exchange of information and identification of problems and difficulties, commenting that 'this machinery already exists and we could build on it in some way or another, if this seems desirable. If we were jointly to contemplate setting up another body, would it differ very greatly from what we already have?'. The Chief Medical Officer acknowledged the need for continuing research and monitoring, and stated that the D.H.S.S. now had a 'model' with which the likely outcomes of various assumptions could be tested.

The effectiveness of the new-style Central Manpower Committee and the existing 'machinery' as a means of manpower forecasting and as an advisory system on long-term policy must remain in doubt, but it is unlikely that the Chief Medical Officer's view will assuage all the anxieties that exist. Much might depend, for example, on the extent to which the D.H.S.S. is willing to publish details of its 'model' and the conclusions derived from its use. There can be no doubt, however, that some lessons have been learned from past experience; the progressive improvement in the quality and speed of production of manpower data (see Chapter 4), the

19

increasing insistence on joint discussion, the very existence of 'models' and, above all, the medical profession's own awareness of the importance of the problem, are all hopeful signs. They are the new milestones showing us the road ahead; they cannot tell us how far we still have to go, until we can see where lies the end of the journey.

REFERENCES

Abel-Smith, B. & Gales, K. (1964) *British Doctors at Home and Abroad.* London: Bell.

Ahamad, B. & Blaug, M. (1973) *The Practice of Manpower Forecasting.* San Francisco: Jossey-Bass Inc.

Barber, A. (1963) *Hansard* (House of Commons) No. 28, Col. 686.

Bartholomew, D.J. (1967) *Stochastic Models for Social Processes.* London: Wiley.

Bartholomew, D.J. (1976) *Manpower Planning.* Middlesex: Penguin Books.

Bell, D. (1976) Medical manpower: My Crystal Ball is clouded. *British Medical Journal,* 2, 1401-1402.

B.M.A. (1977) Submission of evidence to the Royal Commission on the National Health Service. *British Medical Journal,* 1, 299-334.

C.M.O. (1977) Letter from the Chief Medical Officer. *British Medical Journal,* 2, 208.

Cohen Report (1955) *Report of the Committee on General Practice within the National Health Service.* London: H.M.S.O.

Cohen (Lord) of Birkenhead (1961) *Hansard* (House of Lords) 5th Series, 235, Col. 1171.

Davison, R.H. (1961) Medical emigration. Second thoughts on the Royal Commission. *Lancet,* 1, 1107-1108.

Davison, R.H. (1962) Medical emigration to North America. *British Medical Journal,* 1, 786-787.

D.H.S.S. (1977) *The Way Forward.* London: H.M.S.O.

Doran, F.S.A. (1976) Expansion of the medical schools. *British Medical Journal,* 2, 1272-1274.

Editorial (1977) Difficult questions at Glasgow. *British Medical Journal,* 2, 349.

Ellis, J. (1975) The Todd Commission's assumptions and proposals. *Proceedings of the Royal Society of Medicine,* 68, 495-499.

Ford, J.A. (1976) Forthright evidence on manpower. *British Medical Journal,* 2, 1152.

Fry, J. (1975) How many doctors? The dangers of possible medical unemployment. *Update,* August, 263-273.

Goodenough Report (1944) *Report of the Inter-Departmental Committee on Medical Schools.* London: H.M.S.O.

Greenwood, R.K. (1977) Manpower. *British Medical Journal,* 1, 854.

Hill, K.R. (1964) The need for more medical schools. *Lancet,* 2, 517-519.

Hospital Junior Staffs Committee (1977) Present and projected numbers of medical students and doctors. *British Medical Journal,* 1, 659-660.

Hospital Junior Staffs Committee (1977a) *British Medical Journal,* 1, 854.

Jennings, A.M.C. (1975) The provision of an anaesthetic service. *British Journal of Hospital Medicine,* 13, 404-414.

Klein, R. (1977) Doctors and the economy. *The Times,* 24 March.

Lafitte, F. & Squire, J.R. (1960) Second thoughts on the Willink Report. *Lancet,* 2, 538-542.

Maclure, S. (1977) Manpower planning - the teachers' tale. *British Medical Journal,* 1, 498-500.

Maynard, A. (1976) Medical manpower planning in Britain: a critical appraisal. Unpublished working paper.

Maynard, A. & Walker, A. (1977) Too many doctors? *Lloyds Bank Review,* July, 24-36.

Mortimer, T.F. (1977) Doctors and the economy. *The Times,* 29 March.

News and Notes (1977) Recent questions in the Commons. *British Medical Journal,* 2, 584.

Paige, D. & Jones, K. (1966) *Health and Welfare Services in Britain in 1975.* Cambridge: University Press.

Parkhouse, J. (1976) Do we need more doctors or not? *Proceedings of the Royal Society of Medicine,* 69, 815-821.

Parkhouse, J. & McLaughlin, C. (1975) *Feasibility Study on Postgraduate Medical Education.* London: The Institute of Mathematics and its Applications.

Parkhouse, J. & McLaughlin, C. (1975a) Future prospects for British graduates and the Health Service. *Lancet,* 1, 211-214.

Parkhouse, J. & McLaughlin, C. (1976) Medical manpower planning. In *Manpower Planning.* Symposium Proceedings Series No. 8. London: The Institute of Mathematics and its Applications.

Peacock, A. & Shannon, R. (1968) The new doctors' dilemma. *Lloyds Bank Review,* January, 26-38.

Pilkington Report (1960) *Doctors' and Dentists' Remuneration 1957-60.* Cmnd. 939. London: H.M.S.O.

Platt Report (1961) *Medical Staffing Structure in the Hospital Service.* London: H.M.S.O.

Powell, E. (1966) *A New Look at Medicine and Politics.* London: Pitman.

Report (1976) *Report of a meeting to discuss pre-registration house officer posts* (the Church House Conference), 4 May. London: D.H.S.S.

Robbins Report (1963) *Report of the Committee on Higher Education.* Cmnd. 2154. London: H.M.S.O.

Scrutator (1977) The Week. *British Medical Journal,* 2, 1095.

Seale, J.R. (1961) Supply of doctors. *British Medical Journal,* 2, 1554-1555.

Seale, J.R. (1962) Medical emigration from Britain, 1930-61. *British Medical Journal,* 1, 782-786.

Shore, E. (1974) Medical manpower planning. *Health Trends,* 6, 32-35.

Taylor, T.H., Jennings, A.M.C., Nightingale, D.A., Barber, B., Leivers, D., Styles, M. & Magner, J. (1970) A study of anaesthetic work. *British Journal of Anaesthesia,* 42, 70, 76, 167, 357, 362.

Todd Report (1968) *Royal Commission on Medical Education.* Cmnd. 3569. London: H.M.S.O.

Willink Report (1957) *Report of the Committee to Consider the Future Numbers of Medical Practitioners and the appropriate intake of Medical Students.* London: H.M.S.O.

Wilson, M.A. (1977) Manpower planning. *British Medical Journal,* 1, 854-855.

Wright Report (1964) *Report of the Committee on the Medical Staffing Structure in Scottish Hospitals.* London: H.M.S.O.

2. The Career Structure

The broad principles of the career structure for doctors in the
National Health Service were laid down at its inception, and for many
years the hospital-based specialties were the focus of attention. The
Report of the Interdepartmental Committee on the Remuneration of Consultants and Specialists (The Spens Report, 1948) recommended that after
the pre-registration period had been completed there should be three
grades for doctors in training for the special branches of medicine.
Passage through these grades, which would be of limited tenure, would
lead to a permanent post in the consultant grade. Originally, posts in
the training grades were designated as junior registrar, normally of one
year's tenure, middle grade registrar, normally held for two years and
senior registrar, normally held for three years. The Spens Committee
took the view that occupants of posts at all three grades were potential
aspirants to consultant appointments, and should therefore be regarded as
trainees, but it was accepted that at each stage some would not achieve
promotion. It was regarded as inadvisable to enable trainees easily to
prolong their tenure in the junior registrar and registrar grades beyond
the normal time, but it was recognised that 'some' specialties demanded
lengthy periods of training and therefore the position of the senior
registrar awaiting a consultant appointment should be safeguarded by the
possibility of extended tenure. Nevertheless, 'all possible steps should
be taken by encouraging the interchange of specialists between hospitals
to minimise and equalise this unavoidable waiting period'.

The Spens recommendations were adopted, but after discussions
between the Health Departments and representatives of the medical profession, two additional grades were introduced. These were not training
grades, and were of unlimited tenure: the junior hospital medical officer
and senior hospital medical officer grades. The S.H.M.O. grade was felt
to be needed for two reasons, to find an appropriate position in the
N.H.S. for doctors who were no longer trainees but who had neither the
training nor the qualifications to justify consultant status (e.g. local
authority hospital doctors, tuberculosis specialists and general practitioners with local hospital appointments) and to satisfy a more permanent need for doctors to carry out work requiring less skill and responsibility than that of consultants. The full particulars of the S.H.M.O.
grade were set out in a Ministry of Health Circular in 1950; some
specialties were designated as unsuitable for S.H.M.O. appointments,
except in special circumstances while others were regarded as suitable

(e.g. blood transfusion, diseases of the chest, geriatrics, infectious diseases, obstetrics (antenatal and postnatal clinics and work under supervision) ophthalmology (non-operative), orthopaedics, paediatrics (child welfare), physical medicine, venereal disease and some aspects of psychiatry and mental deficiency). There was also a category of specialties in which establishments could provide for 'assistantships to consultants', remunerated on the S.H.M.O. scale; these were anaesthetics, pathology, radiology and radiotherapy. The J.H.M.O. grade was intended to provide a place in the new N.H.S. structure for non-trainee doctors fulfilling a function at a lower level. At the time of the Platt Report (1961) it was noted that J.H.M.O. appointments were no longer always of unlimited tenure. It was also agreed during the 1950s by the Ministry of Health and the Joint Consultants Committee that, pending the outcome of general discussions on staffing structure, hospitals with large casualty departments might be authorised to appoint 'senior casualty officers' for a period of four years on the S.H.M.O. salary scale.

The Spens Committee also recommended the establishment of the distinction award system for consultants. The employment of general practitioners in hospitals was provided for from the start of the N.H.S. - either as part-time clinical assistants or medical officers, as members of the staffs of cottage hospitals or, with appropriate training and qualifications, as part-time consultants or S.H.M.O.s.

The Report of the Royal Commission on Doctors and Dentists' Remuneration, 1957-60, the Pilkington Report, (1960) regarded the Spens recommendation about distinction awards as 'a practical and imaginative way of securing a reasonable differentiation of income and providing relatively high earnings' for a significant minority of consultants. It is interesting to note that suggestions had been received that a preferable alternative to the distinction award system would be to designate certain consultant posts, with special responsibility, as commanding higher remuneration. Although the Pilkington Commission did feel that the range of work and responsibility could vary considerably within the same grade, and was concerned about the lack of clear definition of these responsibilities, it nevertheless felt that the establishment of a hierarchy of consultants would present too many problems.

The Report of the Joint Working Party on Medical Staffing Structure in the Hospital Service (The Platt Report, 1961) pointed out that the National Health Service had not been in existence very long before the strict concept of S.H.O. and registrar posts being primarily training posts for consultant appointments had to be abandoned. The first, and perhaps most important departure came as early as 1950, when the name junior registrar was changed to senior house officer and hospital authorities were instructed that this grade should not be regarded primarily as a training grade for future consultants. The next year, following discussions between the Health Departments and the Joint Consultants Committee, the registrar grade also ceased to be regarded primarily as a training grade.

The Platt Report itself reviewed the general experience since 1948 with particular reference to the problem of the S.H.M.O. grade, by then widely regarded as unsatisfactory, and the increasing difficulty arising from excessive numbers of senior registrars in relation to career vacancies. The Committee asked for a census of junior medical staff. It noted that over the 10 year period 1949-59 the total number of doctors in the hospital service had increased by about 30%; the senior registrar grade in England, Scotland and Wales had grown to 1,600 by 1951, by which time some reduction was obviously necessary and was implemented. The

23

total was about 1,200 by the end of 1953, and 1,248 in 1960. The Platt Report contained a number of important comments; for example, on the undesirability of assuming that the N.H.S. could continue to depend so heavily on overseas doctors, and the need for adequate career prospects from the junior grades: 'on one point there can be no doubt: the hospital service cannot hope to have an adequate and efficient staff of fully registered housemen and registrars unless reasonable prospects of a good career in some branch of medicine can be seen by the doctors who stay in the service to work in these capacities'. There was considerable discussion of the 'necessary staffing assistance to consultants' and throughout the report it seemed that all assumptions concerning the 'right' number of junior staff were based on consultant preferences and market forces. The registrar grade as a training grade received its final death blow; only the name was retained, but any implication that it denoted a doctor in training for the consultant grade 'should finally be effaced by this report'. Thus, the senior registrar was established as the only clearly defined trainee; it was recommended that Joint Advisory Committees, with membership from the local University, the Board of Governors and the Regional Hospital Board, be set up in each Region to supervise the progress and attend to the welfare of senior registrars and these Committees, in various forms, still exist. The report did not recognise the existence of any category of work which could specifically be designated as 'senior registrar work' but did recognise a need to bridge the gap, in non-teaching hospitals (which would usually not have senior registrars), between the consultant and the registrar or S.H.O. Hence was proposed the establishment of a sub-consultant grade, the medical assistant grade, as an alternative to the S.H.M.O. as a means of providing 'the necessary staffing assistance to the consultants'. Problems were clearly envisaged, and it was admitted that 'most of the professional bodies see objection to a sub-consultant grade.... whose status would be near to that of consultant posts'. In fact, the function of the proposed medical assistant grade was not clearly defined; it was offered as a means of providing an opportunity for some registrars to remain in the hospital service 'on a satisfactory basis', to provide a career for senior registrars (sic) and other doctors 'who do not eventually secure consultant posts' and of providing a doctor to undertake 'some routine duties' and 'to deputise for the consultant during off-duty periods and holidays'. It would seem unlikely that the legitimate career aspirations of junior doctors, already referred to in the report, would be adequately met by this means, especially as some senior registrars would apparently be included, and it is hard to imagine that a grade so described would not be too close to the consultant's status for comfort. Furthermore, there was a somewhat pseudo-naive failure, throughout the report, to refer in any way to the relationship between medical assistant appointments and higher specialist qualifications.

Nothing specific was offered to S.H.O.s or registrars in terms of any form of organised training: 'though the doctors in the house and registrar grades are there to work as pairs of hands,* they are also there as part of the process of preparing themselves for their ultimate career for which study is still essential. The duties of those engaged in postgraduate study should allow time for it'. The main preoccupation, though, was with securing an adequate number of doctors for the hospital

---

* A phrase which came to be as fimiliar and as opprobriously construed as
  Lord Moran's 'falling off the ladder'.

service, to provide consultant support; the two main suggestions for achieving this were an echo of the Willink Report of 1957: encouragement of young doctors to remain longer in the hospital service, particularly those intending to enter general practice, and the increased involvement of general practitioners themselves in hospital work. It was in fact recommended that new entrants to general practice should ideally have spent at least two years in the hospital service after becoming fully registered, and this may be regarded as the first tentative step towards the introduction of vocational training for general practice.

Altogether, it might perhaps be said of the Platt Report that it presented a remarkably lucid account of the current situation and its problems, while at the same time offering a set of solutions which were equally remarkable for their ineffectiveness. There remained the outstanding difficulty of reconciling the proper career ambitions of trainees with the need to provide a sufficient work force. Should all those other than trainees be consultants, and if so on what terms? The question was looked at again in the Report, 'The Responsibilities of the Consultant Grade' in 1969, but in the meantime the Royal Commission on Medical Education had produced its Report (The Todd Report, 1968).

One of the most important recommendations of the Todd Report related to the period between the completion of the pre-registration year and entry into general practice or a senior registrarship - in other words, the S.H.O. are registrar grades which had been left very largely in limbo since the Platt Report. The Todd Committee recommended that this period should constitute a three year phase of 'general professional training' for all graduates. Intending general practitioners would spend two years of this G.P.T. in appropriate hospital appointments, and one year as a trainee in general practice, while aspirants to a career in a hospital specialty would normally spend the full three years of G.P.T. in suitable hospital appointments (although for some specialties a period of time spent in general practice would be appropriate). The emphasis was intended to be upon 'general' training, so that the graduate would have every opportunity to provide himself with a broad foundation for his future career, and to delay his final, definitive career choice for as long as appropriate. At the conclusion of G.P.T., trainees would either enter higher professional training (the equivalent of a senior registrarship) in order to proceed directly and rapidly to a consultant appointment, or would receive, as 'junior specialists', a 'less demanding' form of further training en route to the 'Hospital Specialist' grade, in which they might remain permanently or from which they might achieve promotion to a consultant post at a later stage. The concept of a 'sub-consultant grade' was thus revived in a different form and on a much more flexible basis. Furthermore, since the hospital specialist grade was intended to be a career grade carrying a substantial degree of clinical responsibility for the care of patients, it was implied that the Platt definition of the consultant as the only person in the hospital service with independent clinical responsibility would change.

The Todd proposals were extensively debated and discussed, but the details are only relevant to the present theme insofar as they concern manpower and the career structure. On the whole the reception of these recommendations was unenthusiastic. The annual representative meeting of the British Medical Association in July 1969 resolved, 'that the period of postgraduate training envisaged in the Todd Report is excessive' and 'that the Todd Report on Medical Education should not be implemented until its effect on the staffing of regional hospitals be fully investigated' (B.M.A., 1970). There was also considerable misgiving about the establishment of a permanent sub-consultant grade. Although the Todd recommendations had a good deal to say, under the name of General Professional Training, about the S.H.O. and registrar grades they did not really provide a clearly defined postgraduate training pattern at this stage. Many critics were still left with the feeling that between the pre-registration year and acceptance within the senior registrar fold, as a future consultant in one of the specialties, there remained an ill-defined period during which the graduate must necessarily float about, largely at the dictates of fortune and his own initiative, acquiring 'general' training with no specific purpose in view. The proposals seemed to do little for the enthusiastic young graduate anxious to get ahead with his career as soon as possible. Likewise they seem to do little to bring British postgraduate training into accord with that of other countries, although it was evident that the prospective entry of Britain into the E.E.C. was very much in the minds of the Todd Commission. The arrangement of postgraduate training in Western Europe, almost always over a considerably shorter time-scale than in Britain, was much more in accord with the residency programmes of North America into which graduates, at the completion of internship, could enter directly into a career-orientated and efficiently planned specialty training. Presumably something of the kind would need to evolve in Britain in order to attain equivalence with the E.E.C.; yet the Todd 'General Professional Training' seemed to be no more than a loose preparation for a senior registrarship or a career in general practice.

The general tenor of the Todd Report, however, and many of its administrative recommendations, provided a powerful stimulus to the Royal Colleges and their Faculties with a result that the criteria for training at the S.H.O. and registrar levels were vigorously overhauled. It thus came about that the term 'general professional training' was taken over by the Colleges as a means of describing the early stages of graduate training in their own special fields. This represented, of course, a drastic modification of the original concept, but without abolishing the rather arbitrary 'bar' between general professional training and higher specialist training (the 'bar', in practice, often being the acquisition of a higher diploma). One important element in the Todd G.P.T. proposals, from the manpower point of view, would have been the provision for trainees to obtain experience outside their own specialties. It is important to develop the distinction between training in a specialty and training for a specialty. Many foreign graduate training programmes, for instance in Scandinavia, stipulate how much time should be spent in the specialty itself and how much in other relevant fields of work. The obstetrician, for example, might benefit from a year's general surgery and the anaesthetist from a year of internal medicine. In the competitive and unco-ordinated environment of the British hospital scene such arrangements had always been difficult and in many cases remain so to the present time. The development of vocational training programmes for general practice, which was given great impetus by Todd, has achieved remarkable results along these lines, largely by making use of S.H.O. posts in under-subscribed specialties such as E.N.T. surgery, geriatrics and psychiatry which would otherwise be short of good applicants. However, for the hospital specialties the virtual abandonment of G.P.T. proper in favour of the Colleges' interpretation of it did nothing for the trainee in this respect.

The feasibility of the Todd recommendations was examined (Parkhouse and McLaughlin, 1975) and with few exceptions it may be said that there would have been sufficient S.H.O. and registrar posts in the National

Health Service to implement 'general professional training'. In fact, in some specialties the existing number of posts was far more than required. Hence, there was no real possibility of using the Todd proposals, as some had imagined might happen, as a subtle means of directing graduates into the training paths appropriate for the future needs of the Health Service. It could safely be assumed that as long as the popular specialties had jobs to offer graduates would seek to fill them, to the detriment of the less popular and more needy disciplines. Unless drastic modifications could be made in the numbers of available junior posts in different specialties the Todd scheme would never act as a means of directing labour. On the other hand, the general philosophy of the Todd Report, as of the subsequent J.C.C. Sub-Committee Report on Hospital Staffing Structure, (see below) was that numbers of training posts should be directly related to the specific needs of training, and it became clear that an implementation of this concept might have curious consequences. With the introduction of vocational training, general practice would account for a very large number of junior trainees in hospital posts of certain kinds. The need for general medicine posts at S.H.O. level, for example, might well be two or three times as great as the need for general surgery posts, in order to accommodate trainee general practitioners as well as trainee physicians. The number of junior posts in E.N.T. surgery or accident and emergency might, in fact, need to be greater than the number in general surgery itself. Thus, there would be major consequences in terms of hospital staffing and the whole balance of medical manpower.

In 1969 a sub-committee on hospital staffing structure of the Joint Consultants Committee submitted a Report (1969) which was accepted by the Joint Consultants Committee and by the Central Committee for Hospital Medical Services as a basis for discussion with the Health Departments as follows:

'It is suggested that a new career structure could be based on the following propositions:

    (a) The postgraduate training of doctors should take only as long as the needs of training require and should lead without undue delay to a permanent post in a specialty. The length of training would be decided by professional opinion, but in general it is thought that training for a hospital specialty would be completed in about eight years after qualification and for general practice in a somewhat shorter period. There would no doubt be some variation in the length of time required for training in different specialties. The training programmes would be flexible enough to allow individuals reasonable freedom to alter their preferences during training and to take account of variations in rate of progress.

    (b) There should be no permanent sub-consultant grade.

    (c) A balance should be attained between the number of career vacancies anticipated in each specialty and the number in training for career posts in that specialty, taking into account entrance to the consultant grade from other fields of work such as university posts. This would require an expansion of the consultant grade, control of the number of training posts in the various specialties, and limitation of tenure of those posts.

    (d) There should be a special grade (to be called the hospital practitioner grade) in the hospital career structure for general practitioners.'

It was pointed out that a growth rate of hospital medical manpower of at least 3% a year was likely to continue. In recent previous years the growth had been much greater at junior level than at consultant level; application of the above propositions would require a more rapid increase in the growth at consultant level until the desired balance had been achieved. The training grades would continue to expand, although more slowly. It was estimated that annual growth rates of 4% in the consultant grade and 2.5% in the training grades would produce, by about 1978, the 'balance at present lacking'. In fact, this 'balance' meant a change from a ratio of 1.5 training posts to each consultant post to a ratio of 1.3, the latter ratio having been estimated 'on the basis of a staffing projection which took into account the known manpower factors which would affect the level of hospital staffing over the next decade'. Assumptions were also made about population changes, medical migration, number entering general practice and length of training in different specialties. Making due allowance for the various factors, it was believed that 'implementation of the propositions would be feasible' and that the effect should be to substantially reduce the average length of time spent by doctors between qualification and obtaining a hospital career post. The detailed basis of the calculations was not shown, but it is clear that very considerable 'wastage' was assumed from the training grades in order to sustain a ratio of 1.3 trainees to every consultant without considerable delay and frustration in achieving promotion. The main recommendations were accepted by the Health Departments, and became the target figures for the differential growth of the hospital grades over the next few years.

The feasibility of implementing the recommendations of this report in regard to a large consultant expansion as opposed to the setting up of a sub-consultant grade, was in fact dubious. The British Medical Journal (Editorial, 1969) pointed out that it was only the graduates of 1969 and 1970 who would be available to fill consultant appointments in 1977 and 1978 and that it might be unrealistic to expect the proposed increase of over 4,000 consultants by that time. It was, incidentally, anticipated by the British Medical Journal at that time that by 1978 'the 6,500 foreign graduates in the hospital service will have been reduced to 4,000'. Doubt was also expressed about the ability to maintain quality in the consultant grade which must depend essentially on an element of competition for posts, in the face of such a massive expansion. While much of the opposition to a 'sub-consultant grade' had been based on fears that it would imply a lowering of standards, insufficient weight had perhaps been given to the contrary argument that when the only available career grade is that of consultant, and the inscrutable demands of the hospital service require increasing numbers of people, it is almost inevitable that the quality of the consultant grade itself will be in jeopardy when recruitment is difficult (Parkhouse and McLaughlin, 1975).

Freeman (1969) examined some of the implications of an altered career structure in which the number of junior posts would be strictly related to training requirements and the number of consultant appointments would rise. He made allowance in his calculations for the use of residual training capacity to accept 'non-U.K. Nationals' as postgraduate trainees. On this basis, the re-arrangements, although requiring increases in the consultant grade did not imply more than a trivial reduction in the numbers of junior staff; he concluded that the net increase was needed 'to improve the working conditions of both consultant and junior staff alike'. He did discuss, however, the altered consultant life-style that would result from an expansion of the grade and felt that 'many consultants would object to the changes implied'. Against the

28

possibility that expansion of the consultant grade would lead to reduced
income, Freeman proposed an item of service type of contract and an increase in the amount of private practice commensurate with the increase
in the number of consultant surgeons seeking that practice.

The Report of the Working Party on the Responsibilities of the Consultant Grade, 1969 (under the chairmanship of Sir George Godber and including Mr. Freeman as a member) reiterated the fact that 'since the
Platt Working Party's report there has been considerable dissatisfaction
both with the lack of a planned training programme - causing unnecessary
delays before appointment to a consultant vacancy - and with the medical
assistant grade'. It attempted to re-establish the principle that in-
depentent clinical responsibility for the care of patients should be
exercised at consultant level only, and that this should therefore be the
only permanent career grade in the hospital service. The report gave its
view that delegation of routine service work to a permanent sub-consultant grade and to well supervised junior doctors would cause discontent,
since young men and women 'rightly expect to apply the full range of
skills and judgment which they have acquired'. The only practicable
alternative form of hospital staffing was seen by the report in the
following terms: 'medical work in hospitals could be so arranged that the
nature of the service contribution of junior doctors is appropriate to
the requirements of their training. Consultants would be supported by an
increased number of general practitioners and others working part-time in
hospital, and by juniors but only to the extent dictated primarily by
training programmes which would lead these juniors in due course to consultant or general practice. Each individual consultant following an increase in the number of consultants would be enabled to carry out more
items of care himself for any individual patient than is at present
possible'. The report was absolutely clear in its recommendation of this
type of solution. It also proposed the introduction of a system of
vocational or specialist registration, as had been envisaged by Todd.
However, this was clearly seen as relating exclusively to consultant
status: 'vocational registration should be preceded by a designated
training programme ordinarily lasting for approximately eight years'.
Clearly such a specialist registration would bear no relationship whatever to specialist registers in other countries. Movement from one consultant post to another was encouraged by the report, and the 'proleptic'
appointment of senior registrars to consultant posts during the last year
of their training period, on the understanding that they would take up
the post on completing their training, was advocated.

The recommendations of the Godber Report were received with no more
enthusiasm than the Todd proposals for a sub-consultant grade. The statement that the consultant 'would be enabled to carry out more items of care
himself' was generally regarded as a euphemism for acting as his own
S.H.O. and dealing with his own emergencies in the middle of the night.
In other words, the suggestion that consultants might to some extent do
in H.N.S. hospitals what they normally do in private practice, and what
many specialists routinely do in the hospitals of other countries, was
not well received.

In the light of his earlier thoughts, and the reception given to the
J.C.C. Progress Report and 'The Responsibilities of the Consultant Grade',
Freeman (1970) proposed new contractual arrangements for hospital medical
staff. He suggested four grades: Grade 1 would be a training contract
for one year (the pre-registration year). Grade 2 would be an appointment on a yearly basis renewable for up to three years (not necessarily
consecutively) for training, or indefinitely for service. The existing

structure of S.H.O. and registrar appointments would thus be merged, but posts would be offered on two different bases, either for training or for service. Grade 3, the counterpart of the existing senior registrar grade, would again be available either for training or for service, and permanent tenure would only be granted after careful consideration of individual cases. Grade 4 would be a service grade at consultant level. Freeman gave much thought to the numerical balance between grades in order to maintain a suitable work force. The great importance of his proposals lay in their separation of training and service employment below consultant level and the very large degree of flexibility that was envisaged.

The Hospital Consultants and Specialists Association published a 'Survey of Hospital Staffing' in 1974 (H.C.S.A., 1974). This was based on a questionnaire sent to 'about 8,000' consultants of whom 2,378 replied; from these unopened replies a 10% sample of all consultants in the Regional Hospitals of England and Wales was, according to the report, selected in order to be representative. The opinions expressed, perhaps not surprisingly, indicated considerable staff deficiencies in relation to 'notional work loads'. The precise basis on which the evidence was assessed is not always clear; in the words of the report itself: 'This deficiency amounts to nearly 3,000 consultants, 10,000 in the grades of intermediate grade, and 14,000 in the junior grade. We estimate that the total requirement of doctors in the intermediate grade is approximately 18,000 and in the junior grade approximately 21,000. Overall our recommendation is for the hospital doctors in the ratio of 1 consultant to 1.3 doctors of intermediate grade, and 1.6 doctors of junior grade. This provides an average of three assistants for each consultant, although the numbers show variation from one specialty to another'. The figures are worthless in themselves, but the conclusion is an interesting comment on the view of the H.C.S.A. at the time about the career structure is hospital medicine. It was noted in Appendix D of the report that two-thirds of the respondents favoured the type of career structure proposed by Freeman (1970).

The Report of the Committee of Inquiry into the Regulation of the Medical Profession, The Merrison Committee, (1975) was indirectly concerned with the career structure on account of its views about the stages of medical education and the appropriate forms of registration. One recommendation was that the undergraduate course should be followed by a period of 'Graduate Clinical Training' the nature of which would 'not greatly differ from the nature of the pre-registration year or of general professional training'. This phase might, 'last something like two years' and, 'would be achievable were the undergraduate course to be correspondingly reduced in length'. It would thus seem to have been intended to carry the graduate to about the point at which full (general) registration is granted - the end of the present pre-registration year - but by means of a more variegated and extended diet of post-graduation experience. Thereafter would follow 'specialist education' which would embrace the present S.H.O., registrar and senior registrar grades. Very little was said about the way these combined stages should be controlled, although the problems of reconciling the various interests were recognised and the importance of better arrangements was stressed: 'We can only hope that our report... will persuade the profession of the desirability of tackling resolutely the task of organising specialist education'.

The Merrison Report advocated the introduction of specialist registration but this was conceptually related to 'accreditation', as understood by the Royal Colleges, and to the existing system of N.H.S. de facto 'specialist registration' through the process of appointment to career-grade posts. It was therefore to be understood as signifying eligibility for a consultant appointment and, as with the Godber report proposal, this would not imply comparability with the specialist registration criteria of other countries. The Committee felt no doubt that specialist education and registration should apply to general practice as well as to the hospital specialties.

During the 1970s very little actual progress has been made towards resolving any of the outstanding problems of the career structure. It is widely recognised that there is gross imbalance between the number of junior posts and the number of consultants, and that this disparity is by no means wholly accounted for by the needs of vocational training for general practice. Too many alternative opinions, and perhaps too many vested interests, have prevented the making of any clear policy decisions. Meanwhile, dependence on overseas doctors in the junior hospital grades has continued to increase until the present time; but major changes in the balance between immigrant doctors and British graduates seeking junior hospital posts are occurring. Much of the inherent difficulty, and indeed sheer impracticability of the existing hospital career structure has up to now been masked by the presence of large numbers of compliant and relatively uncommitted overseas doctors who have filled the gaps in the service, conveniently moving from region to region and even from specialty to specialty where vacancies have occurred. This 'cushion' of supporting staff has given enormous flexibility and has concealed the difficulty of providing an adequate manpower structure for the hospital service purely on the basis of well organised training programmes and fully rewarding specialist practice. The time may rapidly be coming when the problem needs to be faced in earnest. The growth in numbers of junior staff has coincided with a progressive blurring of many of the traditional distinctions between teaching and non-teaching hospitals. This has been beneficial in many ways, but has led to an implicit assumption that the staffing structure of the great teaching institutions should be mirrored in every hospital of the land. The tradition of consultant dependency on supporting junior staff has grown out of this. But a staffing structure ideal for teaching, at various levels, is by no means necessarily ideal for providing an efficient service to patients.

If, purely for domestic training purposes, it is necessary to have large numbers of S.H.O.s and registrars then they must be distributed throughout teaching and non-teaching hospitals alike, as is beginning to happen with medical students. But if, as is truly the case, we need far fewer S.H.O.s and registrars pruely for training purposes, then where should they be? If we are to organise University-based training programmes in the major teaching centres, is this to deny the role of the regional hospital in teaching altogether, and deprive its consultants of the satisfaction of having juniors to train? If we are to identify our residual capacity to train (Parkhouse, 1972), over and above our domestic requirements, and offer this on a properly organised basis to overseas trainees, are they to be placed in regional hospitals or teaching centres? Is it not better to work out the appropriate combinations of 'teaching' and 'non-teaching' experience for both British and foreign trainees? All of these are fundamental questions which still await coherent answers. The same may be said of the arguments surrounding the career grades. The 'sub-consultant grade' continues to have its advocates (Helsby and Wright, 1976; Clarke, 1977) and its vociferous opponents (Wigfield, 1977). Eight years ago the British Medical Journal (Editorial, 1969) returned to the idea rejected by the Pilkington Committee (1960) of a hierarchical system for consultants, 'which might provide an answer to the distribution of the routine work between senior and junior consultants. In such a system differential payments could displace the existing secret merit awards. Surely a hospital service of this nature could provide better opportunities and incentives for satisfying work in all provincial hospitals'. Certainly the term 'sub-consultant' was hideously inept. Perhaps too much significance has come to be attached to the connotations of the word 'consultant' and perhaps the establishment of two career grades of specialist and senior specialist would attract greater support.

The career structure now clearly emerges as the crucial problem for the immediate future. The rapidly increasing flow of high-calibre British medical graduates can eventually provide a fully-staffed, self-sufficient health service of magnificent quality, providing that a proper career structure is worked out. Otherwise a great disaster may be in store, and only a few years are available to make and implement the necessary plans.

UNIVERSITY MEDICAL STAFF

The existence of a salaried service for the N.H.S. hospital staff has made it possible to achieve a great measure of equivalence between N.H.S. and university appointments in the clinical specialties. University posts exist for medically qualified staff at lecturer, senior lecturer and professorial level, and there are less permanent posts for tutors and research assistants. There is no fixed linkage between N.H.S. grade and university status; most lecturers have honorary senior registrar grading but some are graded as registrar and some as consultant. Although the majority of senior lecturers have honorary consultant grading this is not invariably the case. Once a candidate has been offered an academic post, the question of his N.H.S. grading should be discussed as a separate matter. This arrangement enables the maximum degree of flexibility to be achieved; a lecturer may progress, for example, from registrar to senior registrar and even to consultant status (in an honorary capacity) while occupying the same academic post. He may at any stage revert to an N.H.S. post of appropriate grade, in competition with other applicants, and experience gained in a university department is recognised by the Royal Colleges and their Faculties as contributing towards specialist training.

From the manpower point of view, the university career structure is pyramidal, with relatively few posts at professorial level. Although it is regarded as perfectly acceptable for an academic to remain as a senior lecturer permanently, on a salary scale equivalent to that of an N.H.S. consultant, it is the case that many doctors occupy university posts only temporarily, and eventually compete for N.H.S. career posts. The D.H.S.S. tables of hospital staff include occupants of university posts who have honorary N.H.S. contracts.

As far as clinical work is concerned, it is usual to designate the notional number of 'sessions' that a university doctor will undertake. It is clear that difficulties might conceivably arise if consultant responsibilities had to be met but the best candidate for a senior lecturer post was not sufficiently experienced clinically to merit consultant grading. It is also true that part of the funding of university posts is sometimes provided by the N.H.S., on the general understanding that a particular type of clinical work will be covered. In practice, this has not so far presented a serious threat to university independence, but has on the whole enabled academic and clinical interests to be reconciled to the best advantage of both sides.

Salary scales of medically qualified staff in clinical university de-

partments are the same as equivalent N.H.S. scales, and university doctors
are eligible for distinction awards, but a full-time university post does
not carry the entitlement to personal payment for private practice. Although the clinical senior lecture or professor has parity with his whole-
time N.H.S. colleagues, therefore, he is at a financial disadvantage compared to many part-time consultants who engage in private practice. Furthermore, medically qualified staff in non-clinical university departments
are paid on lower salary scales than clinical staff - in fact, on the same
scales as university staff in other faculties. This has been a long-standing problem, obviously hard to resolve and making for great difficulty in
recruitment. The great majority of the teaching staff in departments of
anatomy, physiology and biochemistry are now, in fact, not medically qualified.

Further difficulties arose with the introduction of a new contract
for N.H.S. junior hospital staff, which enabled many registrars and senior
registrars to earn a great deal more money than a salaried university
lectureship, even on the clinical scale, could provide. After considerable discussion of the possible solutions to this problem, it was agreed
that university staff with honorary N.H.S. grading below that of consultant should be entitled to extra duty payment in respect of the relevant
components of their clinical work, in broadly the same way as their N.H.S.
counterparts. The Medical Research Council agreed that doctors engaged in
research under their sponsorship should also be entitled to extra duty payments where appropriate, many such doctors being attached to university departments. Although this arrangement avoided a catastrophic collapse in
academic recruitment at the more junior levels, it was not a happy resol-
ution in the long term.

The question that must be asked is what would happen to senior academic posts if a new N.H.S. consultant contract were negotiated, providing
an itemised form of remuneration rather than a fixed salary. There would
seem to be a limited number of options for the comparable remuneration of
academic posts in this situation. One solution would be for clinical
academic staff to receive payment from both the university, on the standard non-clinical scale, and from the N.H.S. in respect of the clinical
commitments undertaken. This would abolish the anomaly of clinical scales,
and provide a single salary structure for academic staff throughout the
university; but it is quite contrary to the purpose of academic posts that
their occupants should be paid according to the amount and kind of clinical
work that they do; and in the case of doctors undertaking large amounts of
clinical work the question would arise of whether they were full-time or
only part-time university employees. Double appointments are feasible, as
with the 'A plus B' posts of a few years ago in which defined numbers of
sessions were financed by the N.H.S. and the university, and it may be that
reconsideration of these rather inflexible arrangements becomes necessary.
Secondly, as with junior posts, it would simply be possible to permit payment for some N.H.S. work over and above the present clinical university
salary. The objections to this in principle have been stated; in practice
it would result in higher rewards in some specialties than others, and in
a general atmosphere unlikely to appeal to doctors with a genuine desire
for an academic career, as distinct from a clinical appointment with a
little extra prestige.

It would perhaps be possible, although not easy, to negotiate a new
salary scale for clinical academic staff that would bear a reasonable relationship to average N.H.S. consultant earnings, exclusive of private
practice; or, as a variant of this, to provide additional or more generous
'distinction' awards of some kind for academic staff. Neither course would

be likely to appeal to N.H.S. negotiators since an 'across the board' payment, or an arbitrary allocation of special awards, would be inconsistent
with the principle of payment for actual work done, and seen to be done.
This principle, on which a 'closed' contract is necessarily based, illustrates the difficulties of the problem; who is to decide, and on what
basis, whether an academic employee - or for that matter an N.H.S. consultant - is at any particular moment 'doing' something which merits payment?
What of the many hours spent reading journals, preparing tutorials, mark-
ing examination papers, analysing research data and - most important of
all - thinking? There are great dangers here of degrading not only the
work of the universities but of the N.H.S. itself.

It is vital that the universities should be able to attract their
fair share of the best people, in both clinical and pre-clinical departments. The suggestion has been made, not unreasonably, that all medically
qualified staff in pre-clinical departments should have some form of clinical involvement, not only to get the benefit of a more favourable salary
scale, but to bring a wider perspective to the teaching of their subjects.
On the more purely clinical level it is to be hoped that some lessons have
been learned from the consequences of introducing a 'closed' contract for
junior hospital staff.

REFERENCES

B.M.A. (1970) Report of the Royal Commission on Medical Education and
     subsequent developments. *British Medical Journal (Supplement)*, 1, 95.
Clarke, C.A. (1977) Wrong ways to choose right medics. *The Times Higher
     Education Supplement*, 21 January.
Editorial (1969) Progress Report on hospital staffing. *British Medical
     Journal*, 4, 573-574.
Freeman, M.A.R. (1969) Possible future trends of medical staffing in the
     hospitals of England and Wales. *British Medical Journal*, 4, 612-615.
Freeman, M.A.R. (1970) A new deal. *British Journal of Hospital Medicine*,
     May, 761-765.
Godber Report (1969) *The Responsibilities of the Consultant Grade*. London:
     H.M.S.O.
Helsby, R.C. & Wright, R.B. (1976) Hospital medical staff: A time for
     reappraisal. *Lancet*, 1, 631-632.
Hospital Consultants & Specialists Association (1974) *Hospital Medical
     Staffing*.
Merrison Report (1975) *Report of the Committee of Inquiry into the Regul-
     ations of the Medical Profession*. Cmnd. 6018. London: H.M.S.O.
Parkhouse, J. (1972) The economics of medical education - National and
     International. *British Journal of Medical Education*, 6, 84-86.
Parkhouse, J. & McLaughlin, C. (1975) *Feasibility Study on Postgraduate
     Medical Education*. London: The Institute of Mathematics and its
     Application.
Pilkington Report (1960) *Doctors' and Dentists' Remuneration 1957-60*.
     Cmnd. 939. London: H.M.S.O.
Platt Report (1961) *Medical Staffing Structure in the Hospital Service*.
     London: H.M.S.O.
Report (1969) Hospital staffing structure (medical and dental). Progress
     Report on discussions between representatives of the Health Depart-
     ments and the Joint Consultants Committee. *British Medical Journal
     (Supplement)*, 4, 53-54.

Spens Report (1948) *Remuneration of Consultants and Specialists*. London: H.M.S.O.

Todd Report (1968) *Royal Commission on Medical Education.* Cmnd. 3569. London: H.M.S.O.

Wigfield, A.S. (1977) "Specialist" and hospital practitioner grades. *British Medical Journal*, 1, 842.

3. Actual Manpower Developments in relation to Predictions and Recommendations

NUMBERS OF MEDICAL GRADUATES

The numbers of British doctors qualifying from medical schools in Great Britain during the 1950s and 1960s can be seen from the following table:

1953	1,910
1955	1,800
1957	1,782
1959	1,707
1961	1,690
1963	1,643
1965	1,618
1967	1,810

The additional number of non-British-based students in each year was relatively small (e.g. 100 in 1955 and 146 in 1959).

The lowest output was actually in 1964, when the number of graduates fell to 1,511. The upward turn continued into the 1970s and some current figures and projections are given in Table 3.1, in which an allowance of 6% has been made for 'wastage' during the undergraduate curriculum. The number of doctors expected to enter the pre-registration year is slightly less than the number of graduates and the figures in the last column are very rough approximations.

TOTAL NUMBERS OF DOCTORS

The Goodenough Report (1944) made its maximum estimates on the basis that we should require an increase in the stock of active doctors to 55,000 in 10 years time - i.e. by 1954. In fact, the Willink (1957) estimate showed an active stock of 53,260 civilian doctors in 1955. Thus the maximum estimate of the Goodenough Committee was almost fulfilled, but detailed information for the intervening years, for example concerning immigration and emigration, is sparse.

The Willink Committee estimated that the stock of active doctors

Table 3.1. *Great Britain based on U.G.C. data at 25.10.76.*

Year	UGC Input Estimate	Output Estimate (Intake - 6%)	Approx. input to pre-reg. year
1972		2,343[A]	
1973		2,289[A]	
1974	3,275[D]	2,594[A]	2,575
1975	3,459[D]	2,644[A]	2,620
1976	3,686[D]	2,760[B]	2,740
1977	3,723[D]	3,025[BC]	3,005
1978	3,747[D]	2,980[B]	2,960
1979	3,921[D]	3,178[E]	3,155
1980	3,945[D]	3,251	3,225
1981		3,465	3,440
1982		3,500	3,475
1983		3,522	3,490
1984		3,686	3,655
1985		3,708	3,670

A = Actual figures
B = D.H.S.S. figures
C = Includes 300 Glasgow graduates due to curriculum change
D = U.G.C. figures
E = Allows for 106 Aberdeen entrants from 1973 on six year course.

would be 60,000 by 1971 and they also noted that the greater part of the
increase was expected to occur before 1965, by which time there would be
between 58,000 and 59,000 civilian doctors. This was consistent with
their recommendation that the growth rate in hospital medical staff would
decline after 1965. In fact, according to the estimates made by the Todd
Commission (1968) there were already 62,700 doctors in 1965. Willink
had thus underestimated the growth in numbers of doctors, even before the
phase of reduced expansion which they envisaged would have taken place.
The Todd Report estimated that the actual number of doctors available by
1975 would be approximately 68,100, but the number needed would be 78,100.
In practice, by 1975 there were approximately 66,250 doctors working in
the National Health Service, so that the Todd estimate for the actual
total active stock* was low, but the real increase had only been achieved
as a consequence of increased dependence on overseas doctors. According
to the Todd appraisal of the situation, therefore, there remained a
'deficit' of several thousand doctors in 1975.

HOSPITAL MEDICAL STAFF

Growth in both the junior and senior hospital grades has consistently
been more rapid than was anticipated by any of the reports on manpower.
For example, the Todd Commission estimated that over the 10 year period
1965-1975 an additional 8,300 hospital doctors would be needed, thus
implying a 1975 hospital total of 33,034. In fact, Department of Health
figures for 1975 show that the total number of senior and junior hospital
staff in England, Scotland and Wales, including those holding locum appointments, was 36,594 - 3,500 more than anticipated by Todd. Willink
quoted the number of consultants and S.H.M.O.s in Great Britain in 1955 as
9,881, and the number of hospital medical staff below the rank of specialist as 9,900, giving an approximate hospital staff total of 19,781. The
estimated increase required over the 10 years 1955-65 was at the rate of
160 a year each for both junior and senior staff, a total increase of
3,200 over the 10 year period, which would lead to a 1965 hospital staff
total of 22,981. The actual total for hospital staff in 1965 was 25,465,
showing a discrepancy of nearly 2,500. Consultant and S.H.M.O. numbers
had risen during the 10 year period by about 1,600, while junior staff had
risen by over 4,000.

GENERAL PRACTITIONERS

In contrast to the hospital service, numbers of doctors in general
practice remained almost static for a long period of time, so that the
expansion in this sector of the service, envisaged by Willink, did not
occur. The number of doctors engaged in general practice in Great
Britain was 24,216 in 1955, 24,260 in 1965 and 24,458 in 1970. The lowest
number recorded was in 1966 (24,010). After 1971, with the improvement
of terms and conditions of service in general practice, numbers began to
rise and the 1975 total was 26,135. The Todd Report had suggested that
restoration of the doctor-population ratio to what it had been in 1961
would require 26,500 general practitioners in 1975, but that to achieve
the proper relationship between numbers of assistants and trainees and
numbers of principals, without detriment to list sizes, would require an
additional 5,000 general practitioners by 1975, making a total of 29,260.
Taking the hospital service and general practice together, the

* i.e. including non-N.H.S. doctors.

Willink projections can be compared with the actual situation 10 years later as follows:

Actual number of G.P.s and hospital doctors
in Great Britain in 1965   49,725

Number of G.P.s and hospital doctors in
1965 according to Willink estimates of
growth and make-up of deficiency   47,935

Difference   1,790

        Thus in the two major sectors of the N.H.S. the numbers of doctors
in post in 1965 exceeded the number allowed for in the Willink estimates
of required numbers of graduates by almost 1,800. The growth had been
made possible by the very large flows into and out of the N.H.S. of overseas doctors which had no more been anticipated by Willink than had the
loss of British doctors to the New World.

UNIVERSITY AND RESEARCH STAFF

        The Willink Committee was informed that in 1954-55 there were about
1,600 whole-time staff in the medical faculties in British Universities,
of whom all except a few were medically qualified. It was estimated
(paragraph 58 of the Report) that 400 of these whole-time teaching staff
had honorary contracts with the hospital authorities. The implication
was that the remaining 1,150 or so doctors in the Universities were not
engaged in any form of clinical work, but this very probably represented
an imprecise breakdown. The Willink estimates for future requirements
included the University staff with hospital contracts as part of the
total for all grades of hospital staff. For the medically qualified
whole-time University teaching and research staff who were understood to
have no contracts with hospital authorities an increase of 1% a year was
recommended, following advice from the Committee of Vice-Chancellors and
Principals. This implied a need for an additional 12 doctors a year.
        The subsequent increase in financial support to Universities, and
the position regarding full-time and part-time clinical teachers was
chronicled by Christie (1969) in a Harveian oration several years ago.
More recent trends are revealed by the fact that in 1974, in England and
Wales, there were 6,322 medical staff in Universities, of whom 2,476 were
whole-time. The number of medically qualified University staff holding
identifiable N.H.S. appointments in various grades was 4,037, representing a whole-time equivalent of 3,208. 1,132 of these appointments were
honorary and 1,278 were full-time N.H.S. appointments. The figures imply
that the number of medically qualified whole-time staff in Universities
increased between 1955 and 1974 from about 1,500 to over 2,500 (including
Scotland), and that the number of medically qualified whole-time University staff with no clinical contracts, whatever the true figure may have
been in 1955, was about 1,500 in 1974. The number of whole-time teaching
staff with honorary N.H.S. contracts would on the face of things appear
to have increased from 400 to over 1,200 - an increase of over 40 a year
or about a quarter of the total annual increase in all grades of hospital
medical staff envisaged by Willink for the years after 1965.
        The Todd Report did not make specific estimates for the medical
manpower requirements of University teaching and of research. On the
advice of the Ministry of Health and the Scottish Home and Health Depart-

ment they estimated a total need of 210 a year for doctors in local authorities, the Medical Research Council, Universities, the Armed Forces,
prisons, industries and administration. In view of developments in
community medicine (see below) this estimate of 210 a year, to include
both replacement and expansion, seems to have been considerably too low.

Further unforeseen developments have taken place, for example the
development of the Medical Research Council's Clinical Research Centre at
Northwick Park. But the whole position of teaching and research in
relation to medical manpower illustrates the extreme complexity of the
inter-relationships. As with the provision of doctors for the Armed
Forces (whose long-term needs were on the whole quite accurately predicted by Willink) the exercise is one of substitution: patients who are
cared for by 'University' doctors, 'research' doctors or 'service' doctors
would otherwise have to be cared for by N.H.S. doctors. There are only a
certain number of people in the population to be cared for altogether and
every practising physician, regardless of the nature of his employment,
requires access to an adequate amount of clinical work. There is a delicate exercise involved in achieving a closer definition of contractual
clinical commitments of academic staff, without intruding unduly upon the
legitimate desire for freedom of movement that is necessary for good
teaching and good research. The frequent and easy movement of doctors, at
various stages of their careers and in both directions, between the Universities and the National Health Service, is a precious asset much envied
by other Nations. That it presents a challenge to the compilers of manpower statistics is evident from the present unsatisfactory state of
affairs. It also requires careful planning consideration in relation to
the career structure, since many doctors in University appointments are
potential contenders for more senior N.H.S. posts. These considerations,
however, constitute arguments in favour of greater future flexibility and
co-operation between the authorities concerned, rather than the reverse.

COMMUNITY MEDICINE

The Willink Report (1957), in discussing local authority staff
including the school health service, quoted the British Medical Association as saying that 'the total number of local authority medical officers
was unlikely to be materially altered unless there were a complete reorganisation of public health services'. The B.M.A. suggested that the
total requirement for whole-time medical officers would be met by an increase of 75, over the existing total, of those 'whose predominant employment' lay with local authorities, of about 2,500. There was further
estimated to be an existing deficiency of about 125 whole-time doctors in
the service. The Willink Committee did not think it necessary to allow
for an additional 75 posts, however, over and above the filling of the 125
vacancies and the part-time contribution that would be made by increased
numbers of general practitioners.

The emergence of community medicine as a new portmanteau specialty
was fully envisaged by the Todd Report (1968). Its development has been
intimately involved with the administrative changes in the National Health
Service in 1974, when the 'complete reorganisation' mentioned by the
B.M.A. in 1957 became a reality. The Department of Health and Social
Security now publishes annual tables of staff for the community health
service. These show that in 1975 there were 671 Regional and Area Medical
Officers, District Community Physicians, specialists and trainees in
community medicine in England and Wales. Of these, 660 were whole-time.
Additionally, in the Community Health Service in England and Wales there

were altogether 6,285 doctors, of whom 1,358 were whole-time and the
great majority of the remainder were on a 'part-time sessional' basis
(2,699) or an 'occasional sessional' basis (1,727). The whole-time
equivalent for these staff was given as 2,087. Included in the Community
Health Service total was the School Health Service in England and Wales,
in which there were altogether 2,410 doctors, of whom 1,089 were whole-
time, the overall whole-time equivalent being given as 1,525. The exact
interpretation of these figures in relation to the total medical manpower situation is not easy; many of the half-time or 'occasional sessional' staff clearly engage in other forms of medical work. Some staff
included in the tables were 'engaged on administrative work only' while
others were partly or wholly engaged in clinical work, and there were
some doctors known to be holding more than one appointment within the
Community Health Service. Nevertheless, the 1975 figures do account for
2,752 whole-time equivalents of medical manpower in England and Wales
alone. The number of doctors in community medicine in Scotland rose from
317 in 1972 to 559 in 1975 (447 w.t.e.). Altogether the increase in
full-time medical staff seems to have been of the order of 1,000 since
the Willink assessment was made.

OCCUPATIONAL HEALTH

The Willink Committee gave figures for factory doctors as follows:

	1949	1955
Full-time	240	465
Part-time	2,840	4,000
Total whole-time equivalents	550	905

    The Report discussed the difficulty of assessing and forecasting
requirements but suggested that an additional 40 whole-time doctors a
year might be needed for five years, after which an additional 20 a year
might be sufficient. This would have led to a total of about 950 whole-
time doctors by 1975 (starting from 1955). The actual position
(Archibald, personal communication) was that in 1976 there were probably
about 800 full-time doctors in occupational medicine in Great Britain,
the part-time contribution being much harder to assess (see Chapter 4).

OVERSEAS DOCTORS

    The Overseas Doctors Association in the United Kingdom, in its
evidence to the Royal Commission (O.D.A., 1977) quoted Dr. David Owen as
stating that the number of overseas doctors in the United Kingdom rose
from 12,900 in 1965 to 20,500 in 1975. In 1960, in England and Wales,
1,256 of the 2,919 registrars (43%) and 1,185 of the 2,343 S.H.O.s (50.6%)
were born elsewhere than in Great Britain and Ireland. The corresponding
figures for 1975 were 2,942 of the 5,121 registrars (57.4%) and 4,626 of
the 7,709 S.H.O.s (60%). In general practice, among unrestricted principals in England Wales in 1965 there were 2,255 (11.3%) born elsewhere
than in Great Britain or Ireland, and in 1974 there were 3,732 (17.4%).
As far as total numbers are concerned, in 1975, in England and Wales,
doctors born elsewhere than in Great Britain and Ireland numbered 2,283
senior hospital staff (17.1%), 9,253 junior hospital staff (50.1%) and
3,920 in general practice (18.1%). In Scotland, dependence on overseas

doctors was less, the figure for all junior hospital staff, for example, being 862 (30.7%). Both the relative and the absolute dependence on overseas doctors had thus increased, to a greater extent in England and Wales than in Scotland, and most particularly in the junior ranks of the hospital service. Regional distribution showed considerable variation; for example, the number of overseas senior registrars, registrars and S.H.O.s in the Northern Region was 590 out of a total of 923 (63.9%) while in the South Western Region the number was 253 out of a total of 769 (32.9%). There was also uneven distribution between specialties, one example being the difference between general medicine and geriatrics; of senior registrars, registrars and S.H.O.s in general medicine in 1975, 617 of 1,720 (35.9%) were born outside Great Britain and Ireland, compared to 561 of 682 (82.3%) in geriatrics. The difference was particularly notable at senior registrar level, where 35 of 57 geriatricians (61.4%) were from overseas compared to only 26 of 203 physicians (12.8%).

So much, then, for the prognostications uttered over the last 25 years about the imminent diminution of numbers of overseas doctors in the Health Service, and so much for the British Medical Journal's comment of 1969 (Editorial, 1969) that by 1978 foreign graduates in the hospital service would have been reduced to 4,000.

WOMEN DOCTORS

Women now represent about 30% of British medical graduates, as compared to the Willink estimate of 20%. The B.M.A.'s draft evidence to the Royal Commission (B.M.A., 1977) estimated that women doctors now, and in the future, would contribute 60% of a full work schedule during their careers; it has been suggested (Kyle, 1977) that this may be an under-estimate. Women still constitute a relatively small proportion of the total pool of medical manpower, and although they are now entering the profession at a faster rate than previously it will be a number of years before the overall percentage of women begins to rise appreciably. The impact will first of all be on the junior hospital grades and will only at a later stage be more widely diffused across the full range of career appointments.

According to the 1960 Census carried out for the Joint Working Party on Medical Staffing Structure in the Hospital Service (Platt Report, 1961) the total of 7,531 hospital doctors in the grade of registrar and below in Great Britain included 2,012 women (26.7%). Interestingly, the available figures for 1975 suggest that of the total of 17,803 doctors in the corresponding hospital grades in Great Britain (excluding locums) 3,710 were women (20.8%). The proportion of women among doctors born in Great Britain for the same grades in 1975 was 24.8%. The pattern of sex distribution among senior hospital staff can be illustrated by the con-sultant figures for England and Wales; in 1965 548 (6.5%) of the 8,477 consultants were women, and 10 years later, in 1975, 1,000 (8.7%) of the 11,482 consultants were women. The trend in general practice shows a somewhat brisk rise; among unrestricted principals in Great Britain, in 1968, 2,188 (9.7%) of a total of 22,529 were women, and in 1975 3,181 (13%) of 24,464 were women. Evidence that the movement of women towards general practice continues is provided by the fact that of 1,136 assist-ants and trainees in England and Wales in 1975, 423 (37.2%) were women.

RETIREMENT

It is difficult to derive accurate statistical information about

42

trends in retirement, although much hearsay evidence suggests that the tendency to retire early has become more prominent in the last few years. In fact, among unrestricted principals in general practice in Great Britain, 13.5% of the total number were age 60 or over in 1973, and 14.1% in 1975. In the hospital service, the percentages of the total stock in individual age groups are less meaningful, since the sizes of the grades change from year to year much more than in general practice, mainly due to the influx of younger people. Some data for recent years are shown in the following table:

YEAR	(a) Number of Consultants aged 65 or more	(b) (a) as % of total number for year	(c) Number of Consultants aged 60 and above	(d) Number of Consultants aged 50-59 10 years previously	(e) (c) as % of (d)
1973	147	1.36	1,420	2,454	57.9
1974	155	1.39	1,525	2,600	58.6
1975	176	1.53	1,642	2,850	57.6

It will be seen that the proportion of consultants who remained working at age 65 or above had certainly not fallen during the last three years. Since the number of people who join the consultant grade for the first time above the age of 50 is relatively small, it may be assumed that the great majority of consultants over the age of 60 in 1975 were 'survivors' of the cohort who were in the age group 50-59 in 1965. The table shows that the percentage of these 'survivors' who continued to practise had remained constant during the last three years. Such indications are only crude guides to the real state of affairs as, indeed, is the average length of tenure in the grade. For example, if half of all consultants elected to retire at age 60, the average length of tenure in the grade would only change by about 2½ years. Of the 413 permanent-paid consultants in England and Wales who left the grade in the year ending 30 September, 1975, 155 were age 60-64. Death and retirement accounted for 278 of the 413 losses, and 221 of these (79.5%) were 60 years old or more. It is probable that most of the retirements in the 60-64 age group are close to the 'normal' retirement age.

EMIGRATION AND IMMIGRATION

Doubts had already been cast upon the Willink assumptions by Seale (1961) and with considerably more accuracy by Abel-Smith and Gales (1964). Between 1962 and 1964 the average net outflow of British doctors was about 270 a year, but the net loss rose to almost 500 in 1964-65. Further figures were given by Mrs. Barbara Castle in 1975 in response to a Parliamentary question from Mr. Tom Litterick (Hansard, 1975) showing that between 1968 and 1971 the annual net loss of British doctors had been about 300. In 1976 Dr. David Owen, in response to a question from Mr. Ifor Davies (Hansard, 1976) supplied information up to 1973, showing that the net loss of British doctors had remained about the same. He indicated that provisional figures suggested that in 1974-75 there may, however, have been an increase to about 450. Mr. Roland Moyle gave further information in a written reply to a Parliamentary question on 22 November, 1977, indicating that the net outflow of British and Irish doctors in 1974 was in fact 350 and that provisional figures suggested a rise in net outflow during 1974-75 with a return to the 1973-74 level in 1975-76, (Moyle, 1977).

Figures for inflow and outflow of overseas doctors have always been more difficult to obtain with any degree of accuracy. This is because the C.M.R.C. Index, which is a valuable source of information (see Chapter 4), has up to now not included temporarily registered doctors. There is no doubt that there has been a continuous net gain of overseas doctors for a considerable number of years; figures for the period 1965-70 show that between 1,500 and 2,000 fully registered overseas doctors were entering the country each year, and it is estimated that this represented about half of the total. During the same period an average of rather more than 1,000 fully registered overseas doctors were leaving the country each year. According to Dr. David Owen in 1976 (Hansard, 1976) the number of fully (or provisionally) registered overseas doctors entering the country in 1972-73 was 1,760, while the outflow was 1,060. Dr. Owen stated that provisional figures indicated that the pattern and order of size of movement for 1972-73 had continued in 1974 and 1975. Allowing for temporarily registered doctors, this would have suggested a net gain of at least 1,500 doctors a year.

Changes in recognition of overseas medical schools for full registration with the G.M.C., and introduction of the TRAB test in June, 1975, have influenced the inflow position. There were considerable numbers of doctors still entitled to full registration, or exempt from TRAB for various reasons (e.g. W.H.O. or British Council sponsorship) and in 1976 the D.H.S.S. estimated that there were about 200 overseas doctors wishing to find posts in the N.H.S. each month who were not required to take the TRAB test. Some indication of the position at the end of 1976 can be derived from the General Medical Council's own figures. The numbers of overseas doctors granted full registration and temporary registration for the first time during the calendar years 1973-76 are shown below:

	1973	1974	1975	1976
Full Registration	1,972	1,930	2,741	3,134
Temporary Registration for first time	2,236	2,390	1,934	1,021
Total	4,208	4,321	4,675	4,155

The General Medical Council's Annual Report for 1975 draws attention to the fact that the total figure for temporary registrations granted during 1975 was made up to 1,380 between January and May, and only 554 after the TRAB tests began in June of that year. Of these 554, 168 had passed the test and 320 had been exempted. It is clear from the above table that the number of temporary registrations granted for the first time during 1976 was less than half of the annual number before TRAB was introduced and recognition was withdrawn from qualifications granted after 22 May, 1975 to graduates of 55 medical colleges in India which had previously been recognised for full registration.

There are also indications that the geographical distribution of incoming doctors is changing. During 1976 full registration was granted to doctors from 13 countries; 1,750 of these doctors were from India (56%) and Australia and South Africa each contributed approximately 10% of the total. Temporary registration was granted for the first time to doctors from 69 countries; India accounted for 17% of these, and the U.S.A., Egypt and Iraq each contributed 10%. It is also perhaps noteworthy that the highest number of applications to sit the TRAB examination in 1976 came from Egyptian doctors, followed by those from India.

DISTRIBUTION BETWEEN GRADES

The Chief Medical Officer of the Department of Health, in his Annual Report for 1971, referred to the agreement between the Joint Consultants Committee and the Health Departments on identification of national staffing targets and added, 'it is therefore lamentable to have to record that the increase in the number of consultants was only 2.7%, a lower figure than that achieved in 1970 and considerably less than the hoped-for 4%. Lamentable too that barely one consultant in 40 is under the age of 35, and that the average age of appointment to the grade is still over 37 years. Almost half the senior registrars are aged 35 or more. Even among registrars, two-thirds are over 30. Hospital authorities, and the profession alike must face up to the need to redress a system which is wasting too many of the most productive years of many young doctors' lives in frustrating pursuit of established careers and which denies them the opportunity to undertake responsibilities of which they are fully capable' (D.H.S.S., 1972).

This quotation illustrates a number of points. Firstly, the fact that agreeing upon a target by no means necessarily implies that it will be met. Secondly, that one of the major difficulties in the system is diversification of responsibility, exemplified by the fact that the D.H.S.S.'s Chief Medical Officer considers himself in a position to lay blame equally upon the 'hospital authorities' and 'the profession' for the evident failure to implement recommendations which had been made, at a different level altogether, by the Joint Consultants Committee and the Health Departments.

The actual expansion of the consultant grade between 1966 and 1975 was almost always below 3% a year and only once (1973) exceeded 4%. Meanwhile, growth of the junior grades continued apace. From 1965 to 1975 the number of consultants in Great Britain rose from 10,110 to 13,190 (an increase of 30.5%). Taking all senior staff - consultants, S.H.M.O.s and medical assistants, the increase was from 11,519 to 14,752 (28.1%). During the same ten years the total junior hospital staff (including J.H.M.O.s and house officers) rose from 13,946 to 20,548 (an increase of 47.3%). On this basis, the ratio of total junior staff to total senior staff over Great Britain as a whole changed from 1.21 to 1 in 1965 to 1.39 to 1 in 1975. Much of the increase in junior staff was due to expansion of the S.H.O. grade, particularly during the 'embargo' on increases in the registrar establishment during the early 1970s. Again, however, it should be noted that figures for successive years show that increases in the number of registrars did occur during this period, and the rise was most notable between 1974 and 1975. Part of the reason for this, as now accepted by the Health Departments, was that there was some under-counting of medical staff in 1974 but although this may mollify some anxieties about the extent to which the system was running out of control, it does not inspire confidence in the statistics on which such conclusions must be based.

In May, 1973, the Department of Health 'decided to take action on a recommendation of the Central Manpower Committee aimed at improving the geographical distribution of training grade posts for hospital medical

45

staff'. Although this was largely an exercise in regional redistribution, it did make reference to the existing national ratio, of registrars and senior registrars to consultants, as being 71 to 100, and set a target ratio of 90 to 100. The practical results of this initiative were negligible, largely due to the difficulties of reaching agreement on an appropriate course of action at local level and of effectively monitoring the progress of events centrally. The actual figures for England and Wales in 1975 showed a total of 7,438 registrars and senior registrars and 11,482 consultants - a ratio of 65 to 100. The number of senior house officers in 1975 exceeded the number of senior registrars and registrars combined.

The medical assistant grade proposed by the Platt Report (1961) began to be implemented in 1966. The numbers of appointments since that date are shown graphically by Forsythe (1976). The total number of medical assistants in England and Wales rose from a little over 400 in 1966 to 1,072 in 1975. There was a dip in 1973, which coincided in time with a move to appoint consultants in accident and emergency departments, some of whom were drawn from the medical assistant grade. There continues to be controversy about the proper place of this grade in the hospital service, and indeed about its whole future. Appointments are made only on a personal basis, taking account of the individual circumstances of each case. There has certainly been no enthusiasm on the part of the Central Manpower Committee to permit a large scale expansion of the grade; some requests for medical assistant grading have been greeted with the response that if a specialist diploma is not held the applicant is not sufficiently qualified, while if the diploma has been obtained the applicant should be seeking a senior registrarship with a view to becoming a consultant. Medical assistants are unevenly distributed between specialties, and Forsythe (1976) has drawn attention to the relatively high dependence of psychiatry, anaesthetics, geriatrics and ophthalmology on this grade of staff.

Negotiations concerning the hospital practitioner grade have been drawn out over a very long period of time, and it was only during 1976 that the first appointments began to be made. This was, even then, with caution and considerable misgiving on the part of many people.

It was reported in Parliament in October 1977 (Moyle, 1977a) that 227 appointments to the grade of hospital practitioner had been made in England and Wales by 30 September, 1977 (1,490 posts occupied by general practitioners in hospitals had been recommended for hospital practitioner grading). The D.H.S.S. was at that time discussing the report of a working party set up to examine the difficulties affecting implementation of the grade. The whole basis of the grade remained open for discussion, particularly in regard to the wide variety of degrees of responsibility that might be encompassed, and the question of whether or not appointments should be restricted to principals in general practice.

In Scotland there has for some time existed the category of 'limited specialist' to enable specialist services to be provided in remote areas where it would be unrealistic to expect adequate recruitment or job satisfaction at consultant level. Although the Willink Report (1957) said virtaully nothing about the role of the general practitioner in the hospital, the Platt Report (1961) envisaged the possibility of general practitioners, with suitable qualifications and experience, being appointed to part-time hospital consultant posts. The Godber Report (1969) also felt that 'it should be open to doctors in this grade to apply for part-time training posts directed to vocational registration in a hospital specialty'. It seems likely that the true role of the general practitioner and the 'limited specialist' will not finally be resolved until definitive policy decisions have been made about the future of the medical assistant grade and the possible establishment of different levels of specialisation.

DISTRIBUTION BETWEEN SPECIALTIES

Although it has been generally recognised for many years that different branches of the medical profession vary considerably in the rewards and satisfactions that they are able to offer, with consequent disparity between competition for posts and the needs of the service, very little constructive action, either positive or negative, has been taken to redress the balance. Indeed, it has remained true since the beginning of the Health Service that consultants in teaching hospitals and in 'popular' specialties are the most likely to obtain distinction awards and it is usually the case that they, and those who choose to practice in salubrious districts, will command the largest private practice.

Almost the only example of a positive influence on the career choice of doctors is provided by the 'Family Doctors' Charter' (B.M.A., 1965) which greatly improved the remuneration and conditions of service for general practitioners. There is no doubt that since the late 1960s this has turned the attention of an increasing number of British graduates, including many of the brightest and best, towards general practice rather than the hospital service. A reflection of this is the decline in numbers of applicants for hospital posts, even in previously well-subscribed specialties such as general medicine and general surgery. The trend has no doubt recently been accentuated by concern over working conditions in hospitals, and perhaps in some cases about the future of private practice.

Within the hospital service, specialties vary considerably in the amount of work that they demand from their consultants, particularly at night and at weekends, and also in the opportunities that they provide for supplementing an N.H.S. salary in various ways. Thus, in some cases there would be arguments, purely from the point of view of encouraging recruitment, in favour of N.H.S. compensation in salary terms for relative absence of outside earnings, while in other cases there would be arguments in favour of extra duty payments. The form of consultant contract proposed by Mrs. Barbara Castle in 1975, which proved unacceptable to the profession, went some way towards improving the lot of the consultant who elected to work full time or to practise in a specialty (or for that matter a region) where private practice did not flourish. The subsequently negotiated junior hospital doctors' contract has far-reaching implications; if a similar principle were to be adopted at consultant level it seems probable that some 'shortage' specialties such as anaesthetics might benefit while others, such as radiology and pathology, would have difficulty in surviving at all.

GEOGRAPHICAL DISTRIBUTION

Many factors apply equally to both specialty distribution and geographical distribution. It is in general practice, again, that the most positive means have been adopted to secure evenness of geographical distribution, through the introduction of designated areas. The initial negative control, of restricting the setting up of new practices in wellfavoured areas, was later supplemented by financial incentives to practitioners going to under-doctored areas. It has several times been pointed out, however, that the effectiveness of this mechanism is debatable, since in marginal cases the recruitment of additional practitioners may result in loss of designated status. However, it remains true that no large-scale parallel to this system has ever existed in the hospital service.

The attempt of 1973 to redistribute registrar and senior registrar posts more equitably between regions has already been referred to, and likewise its lack of result. Attempts have been made through the agency of the Central Manpower Committee to correct the gross imbalances that have for many years existed in hospital staffing levels of different regions. Some measure of success with this exercise has been achieved, and more recently the allocation of manpower has been linked with the general question of resource allocation as reviewed in the D.H.S.S. document 'Sharing Resources for Health in England' (D.H.S.S., 1976). An important feature of these Resources Allocation Working Party proposals was the importance attached to the additional N.H.S. service costs arising from the clinical teaching of medical and dental students, and the consequent need for a special increment for teaching (SIFT) when financial allocations are considered.

The full effects of the efforts that have been made to provide a more equitable distribution of medical manpower between regions remains to be seen. It has not so far proceeded with dramatic speed. Comparison of individual regional staffing levels with those of previous years is made difficult by the reorganisation of the Health Service in 1974, with the consequent re-definition of regional boundaries. The Working Party on the Responsibilities of the Consultant Grade (Godber Report, 1969) gave a figure (Appendix C) showing the whole-time equivalent numbers of hospital medical staff in various grades for each existing Region at the time; the Sheffield Region was at that stage the most poorly staffed, with approximately 16.4 w.t.e. of senior staff (consultants, S.H.M.O.s and medical assistants) per 100,000 population. The highest figures for senior staff were in the North West Metropolitan and South West Metropolitan Regions, each showing approximately 23 w.t.e. per 100,000. Taking crude population figures for mid-1975, for the newly defined Regional Health Authorities, the range of senior medical staff figures, in whole-time equivalents, was approximately 16.4 - 27.2 per 100,000 population. The Trent Region (formerly the Sheffield Region) remained the lowest and the North West Thames Region remained at the top. Some understaffed Regions had clearly improved their position quite considerably, for example Manchester, Birmingham and Leeds. These are no more than very imprecise indications that while numbers of hospital medical staff in relation to population have risen throughout the country and a number of the relatively understaffed Regions have managed to improve their position, the range remains very considerable and inequalities clearly continue to exist.

REFERENCES

Abel-Smith, B. & Gales, K. (1964) *British Doctors at Home and Abroad*. London: Bell.
B.M.A. (1977) Submission of evidence to the Royal Commission on the National Health Service. *British Medical Journal*, 1, 299-334.
B.M.A. (1965) A Charter for the Family Doctor Service. *British Medical Journal (Supplement)*, 1, 89.
Christie, R.V. (1969) Medical education and the State. *British Medical Journal*, 4, 385-390.

Davies, Ifor (1976) PQ 2070/1975/6. *Hansard,* Vol. 907, Col. 629. 12 March,
1976. Written answer 6 November, 1975.

D.H.S.S. (1972) On the state of public health. *Health Trends,* 4, November
1972.

D.H.S.S. (1976) Report of the Resource Allocation Working Party. *Sharing
Resources for Health in England.* London: H.M.S.O.

Editorial (1969) Progress report on hospital staffing. *British Medical
Journal,* 4, 573-574.

Forsythe, M. (1976) Medical manpower and some of the effects. *British
Medical Journal,* 1, 174-176.

Godber Report (1969) *The Responsibilities of the Consultant Grade.* London:
H.M.S.O.

Goodenough Report (1944) *Report of the Inter-Departmental Committee on
Medical Schools.* London: H.M.S.O.

Kyle, J. (1977) *British Medical Journal,* 1, 855.

Litterick, T. (1975) PQ 4445/1974/5. *Hansard,* Vol. 988, Col. 253-254. 30
October, 1975. Written answer 6 November, 1975.

Moyle, R. (1977) Migration of doctors. *British Medical Journal,* 2, 1487.

Moyle, R. (1977a) Hospital practitioner grade. *British Medical Journal,*
2, 1427.

Overseas Doctors Association (1977) *ODA News.* Journal of the Overseas
Doctors' Association in the U.K. January - February, 1977, p.5.

Owen, David (1976) PQ 2070/1975/6. *Hansard,* Vol. 907, Col. 629. 12 March,
1976. Written answer 6 November, 1975.

Platt Report (1961) *Medical Staffing Structure in the Hospital Service.*
London: H.M.S.O.

Seale, J.R. (1961) Supply of doctors. *British Medical Journal,* 2, 1554-
1555.

Todd Report (1968) *Royal Commission on Medical Education.* Cmnd. 3569.
London: H.M.S.O.

Willink Report (1957) *Report of the Committee to Consider the Future
Numbers of Medical Practitioners and the appropriate intake of
Medical Students.* London: H.M.S.O.

4. The Present Position

Factual information on medical manpower is always to some extent out of date by the time it is assembled. The preparation of National Health Service medical manpower information has been considerably accelerated (particularly in the case of more specialised information, such as that concerning university medical staff). Data relating to the position at 30 September in any year is publicly available by the Spring of the following year. In 1977, the most up to date comprehensive 'stock' tables available related to 1971, but further tables were in preparation.

For the great majority of N.H.S. medical staff the 'present' manpower position may be taken as that at 30 September of the previous year. In fact, the information referred to in this book relates to 30 September, 1975.

Confusion often arises when figures relating to medical manpower are quoted. This is for two main reasons. Firstly, because there is sometimes failure to appreciate the distinction between stocks and flows. This distinction will be further developed in Chapter 8, but for the time being it should be remembered that the numbers of doctors entering or leaving the Health Service, or any part of it, do not necessarily bear any relationship to the numbers of doctors actually occupying posts within the service or the relevant part of it. Secondly, confusion can arise because of a failure to appreciate the different classifications of doctors that are used; the 'total number of doctors', for example may be falsely identified with the total number of 'active' doctors, or of 'civilian' doctors; figures relating to the National Health Service may be interpreted as relating to the British medical profession as a whole; numbers of doctors may be confused with whole-time equivalents, and it is sometimes not at all difficult to miss the point that while one set of figures refers to England and Wales an apparently comparable set, perhaps for a different year, relates to Great Britain.

The following simple diagram may serve as a useful reminder of the way in which the British medical profession is commonly divided for numerative purposes. Much of the ensuing description is based on this classification, although it must be appreciated that the information collected by individual agencies, or in specific ways, crosses the boundaries, for instance, between N.H.S. and non-N.H.S. doctors. For the sake of clarity and convenience, the discussion is confined to England, Wales and Scotland.

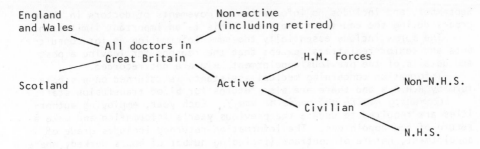

England
and Wales

Scotland

All doctors in
Great Britain

Non-active
(including retired)

Active

H.M. Forces

Civilian

Non-N.H.S.

N.H.S.

SOURCES OF DATA

The Department of Health and Social Security (England and Wales)

A great deal of information is collected every year by the D.H.S.S., in the form of various types of manpower returns. Although detail may be tedious, it is perhaps of some interest to know the kind of information obtained (in 1977) about various classes of medical staff.

Consultants and senior registrars. For these grades of staff employing authorities are either Regional Health Authorities, Area Health Authorities (Teaching), the Welsh Authorities or Boards of Governors in specialised hospitals in London. In all cases the employing authority notifies the D.H.S.S. of staff changes.

A separate form is completed for each change of appointment affecting each doctor. Forms are returned to the D.H.S.S. at the end of each month. Each form shows the nature of the change in appointment (new appointment to the employing authority, change of appointment within the authority, change of nature of work without change of appointment, or termination of appointment). The date of change is also shown. Details of the doctor include registered name, maiden name, national insurance number, date of birth, sex, place of birth (classified as Great Britain, Norhtern Ireland or Irish Republic, or elsewhere), nature of G.M.C. registration, any other employing authority with which the doctor is in contract, grade of appointment at time of change, field of practice (hospital, blood transfusion service, etc.), specialty, nature of contract (classified as whole-time, part-time or honorary), and number of notional half days or units of medical time. In the case of honorary appointments the nature of other appointments, for example with a university or the Medical Research Council, is shown. For senior registrars the form indicates whether the doctor is in the course of completing a recognised higher professional training programme. For appointments being terminated, the form shows the type of post that is being vacated and the reason for leaving; if the doctor is going abroad, the country to which he is going is shown.

Every year, each employing authority receives from the D.H.S.S. a composite print-out of the above information up to the end of June, and updates it to give the position at 30 September. The corrected information is returned to the D.H.S.S. by about the end of November.

Other hospital medical staff: (including consultant and senior registrar locums). Returns are made by Area Health Authorities, who may first obtain the necessary information from individual Districts. Information concerning all doctors is entered on a single form, and the return is made once yearly. It portrays the manpower position on 30

September, and includes no information on movements of doctors in these grades during the course of the year. This is an important limitation.

The forms include essentially the same information as for consultants and senior registrars, except that the reasons for leaving a post and details of the previous appointment held are not recorded.

Information concerning medical assistants is returned on a single form by R.H.A.s and there are also returns for blood transfusion staff.

Community health and medicine staff. Each year, employing authorities are required to update the previous year's information and make a return of new appointees. The information returned includes grade of appointment, nature of contract (including number of hours worked, where relevant, e.g. in the School Health Service), place of birth (classified as Great Britain, Northern Ireland or Irish Republic, and elsewhere), sex, date of birth and detailed specialisation of specialists in community medicine (capital building, information services and research, personnel and postgraduate medical education, health care planning, child health, social services, environmental health, or other).

General practitioners. Central indexes are maintained by the D.H.S.S. of principals, assistants and trainees.

For principals, the index shows name, unique identity number, national insurance number, sex, date of birth, country of birth (enabling a much more detailed analysis to be made than in the case of hospital medical staff), country of registration, year of registration, 'responsible F.P.C.' (i.e. the Family Practitioner Committee covering the bulk of the practice), and medical services provided.

Family Practitioner Committees make a quarterly notification to the D.H.S.S. of admissions and withdrawals, which enables the index to be updated at the beginning of January, April, July and October of each year. In most cases the quarterly returns give details of the previous posts of those entering a practice, or the reasons for withdrawal. Once yearly, at the beginning of October, F.P.C.s provide, among other information, details of the numbers of principals and assistants in each practice.

For assistants and trainees, quarterly returns are provided by F.P.C.s. These include details of name, unique identity number, national insurance number, sex, date of birth, country of birth, country of registration, year of registration and 'responsible F.P.C.' of the principal.

Information is supplied at 1 October by F.P.C.s concerning locums filling vacant principal posts or acting on behalf of principals who are temporarily absent due to illness or other causes. The return shows the locum's name, sex, date of birth and national insurance number, together with information about the absent principal.

Ophthalmic medical practitioners. Information is returned by Family Practitioner Committees on 31 December of each year, showing name, date of birth, unique identity number and whether the practitioner also provides general medical services to the F.P.C.

Other returns. Annual returns are made of vacant consultant and senior registrar posts (showing specialty, length of vacancy and position regarding advertisement) and of community medicine vacancies in the grades of regional and area medical officer, district community physician, specialist in community medicine and senior registrar.

With regard to potential emigration, additional quarterly returns are made of hospital doctors and general practitioners leaving N.H.S. posts with the intention of leaving Great Britain. These show grade, place of birth, sex, age and nature of G.M.C. registration.

On the basis of the information received, the D.H.S.S. carries out an annual exercise known as the 'N.H.S. Index'', which consists of comparing the records of N.H.S. doctors in England and Wales for the latest two years for which information is available. This provides some information about doctors who were working in the N.H.S. in one year, but not the other (i.e. about joiners and leavers) and also about movements between grades of appointment. At the moment, however, the information is of limited value since it is not sufficiently finely broken down. For example, the simple fact that a doctor has left the N.H.S. does not indicate whether he has retired, emigrated, moved to non-N.H.S. employment or is merely in the process of seeking a new N.H.S. post. For consultants and senior registrars, the D.H.S.S. has quarterly and annual analyses of numbers in post, and of joiners and leavers, showing the nature of previous employment or the reasons for leaving.

Non-N.H.S. doctors. The D.H.S.S. collects information annually concerning all doctors working in universities. The returns show the nature of the university appointment and the university subject. They are matched with appropriate N.H.S. returns in order to identify university medical staff also holding N.H.S. appointments, honorary or otherwise. In the case of university staff holding N.H.S. posts, it is possible to cross-relate the university post (professor, senior lecturer, etc.) with the N.H.S. grade (consultant, senior registrar, etc.) and to classify staff according to 'hospital specialty' as well as 'university subject'.

Lists are also held of doctors in the civil service, special hospitals, the Public Health Laboratory Service and industrial medicine.

Scottish Home and Health Department

On behalf of the Scottish Home and Health Department, the Common Services Agency of Scottish Health Services collects information in a form broadly similar to that obtained by the D.H.S.S. Tabulation and publication of the resulting information, however, is in a different form and the precise classification of specialties and sub-specialties is not identical. For the purpose of the C.M.R.C. Index (see below) information from Scotland is included, and in this respect Scotland as a whole is treated in much the same way as the individual English Regions.

General Medical Council

a) The General Medical Council annually publishes the Medical Register, which contains a list of those fully and provisionally registered doctors whose names appeared in the principal list of the Register maintained by the Council on 1 January of the year in question (but not those whose names appeared in the overseas list of the Register). In addition to this volume, the G.M.C. publishes fortnightly lists. Each edition of the fortnightly list shows doctors granted provisional registration and full registration (including those previously having provisional registration), doctors whose names have been altered and doctors whose names have been restored to the principal list (either on transfer from the overseas list, or after erasure from the register or at the end of a period during which registration has been suspended). The fortnightly lists give name, sex, date of registration, registrable qualifications with date and awarding body (e.g. university but not specific medical school). These lists do not include temporarily registered doctors.

b) Temporarily registered doctors are listed in the G.M.C.'s Register of 'temporarily registered medical practitioners'. This list is amended day by day and totals for new registrations are produced every month.

Doctors are granted temporary registration for the purpose of taking up a specified N.H.S. appointment. They are not entitled to engage in any other form of medical practice, and must re-apply for temporary registration in respect of each new appointment. Thus, the total number of temporary registrations granted during any one year is far in excess of the number of individual temporarily registered doctors in the country. The G.M.C.'s register does, however, show the date on which each relevant N.H.S. appointment begins and ends, and also what the appointment is.

C.M.R.C. Index

An index of doctors was compiled during the first world war, for defence purposes, and the present Central Medical Recruitment Committee Index dates from the second world war. The Index is now maintained by the British Medical Association on behalf of the D.H.S.S.

At present, the C.M.R.C. Index includes all provisionally and fully registered doctors. Its usefulness is greatly restricted by the fact that it has not up to now included temporarily registered doctors. At the end of 1975, however, the General Medical Council supplied the D.H.S.S. with current information relating to the approximately 7,000 temporarily registered doctors who were in the country so that this could be added to the C.M.R.C. file. Thereafter, information relating to temporarily registered doctors has been supplied on a continuing basis so that henceforth the Index will be comprehensive. The C.M.R.C. Index relates to Great Britain (i.e. it includes all doctors in England, Scotland and Wales) but is confined to civilian doctors. There are about 1,400 doctors in the armed forces who are not included.

Much work is currently being done on the C.M.R.C. Index by the D.H.S.S., and it is hoped that as time goes by it will become an increasingly valuable source of manpower information. The volume of work involved, however, in bringing the Index up to date and incorporating temporarily registered doctors is considerable. The information held on the Index for the period 1962-1972 includes D.H.S.S. reference number, name, date of birth, sex, country of first registrable qualification, year of registration, date of entry and type of entry to medical practice in Great Britain (e.g. from medical school, from armed forces, returning emigrant, immigrant, restoration to medical register etc.). The country from which immigrants arrived in Great Britain is shown. For those leaving, the reasons are shown (e.g. death, emigration or erasure from the medical register). Again, the country to which emigrants were going is shown. Wherever possible the occupation of each doctor is shown in the Index, according to broad general classifications (e.g. N.H.S. hospital senior staff, general practice etc.). In fact, ascertainment of an occupation is often difficult and time-consuming, and it is also often difficult to find out whether or not a doctor is still in Great Britain. It is intended to include more detailed occupational data in future, wherever possible, so that in due time the Index will provide a career record of each doctor. This will not, however, be available retrospectively beyond 30 September, 1973, and on a more limited scale from 1972. It will therefore be a considerable number of years before the Index could become valuable in this respect. In the meantime, however, it should provide better information about stocks and movements, and about doctors with more than one occupation.

At present, tabulations are available from the C.M.R.C. Index of migration information from 1962, and some stock tables are available from

1965 to 1971.

Other Sources

The National Census provides information which may sometimes be of value in relation to medical practice, for example numbers of hours worked (by sex) for different occupational groups.

Some information about specific groups of doctors is available from the relevant societies and organisations, for example in the case of occupational health and the pharmaceutical industry. The armed forces maintain records of their medical personnel. Many of the Royal Colleges and specialist Societies and Associations hold up-to-date lists of Fellows and Members, and it is often possible to obtain information about specialised groups of practitioners from these sources. The Medical Women's Federation has from time to time carried out surveys of women doctors, and other independent studies have been instituted, for example those of Brook (1976), on consultant psychiatrists, the Scottish Council for Postgraduate Medical Education (1974, 1976) on selected cohorts of graduates from Scottish medical schools, and Flynn and Gardner (1969) and Lawson and Simons (1976) on female and male graduates of the Royal Free Hospital. It is also possible, at least to some extent, to follow the progress of British graduates starting at the pre-registration stage through enquiries concerning career preferences (Parkhouse and McLaughlin, 1976).

The main disadvantage of all information of this kind is its tendency to be incomplete, due to the voluntary nature of the returns and the fact that it is usually collected for a specific purpose, at a given point in time, and not on a continuing basis. The Colleges hold very little information centrally about trainees, and gains and losses from individual specialties at this stage are poorly documented.

The Medical Directory is a useful source of reference, for tracing individual doctors and some other purposes. Inclusion in the Directory is, of course, voluntary and dependent upon individual doctors making the necessary returns. For this reason the information, as a statistical source of knowledge about medical manpower, is neither comprehensive nor consistently accurate.

VIRTUES AND PROBLEMS

One of the main purposes of a critical review must be to discuss the weakness and disadvantages of the existing system, since this form of analysis may indicate the directions in which improvement could take place. However, before discussing some of the current problems with medical manpower data, it should be emphasised that the amount of information available about doctors in this country is far in excess of what can be found elsewhere in the world. This is, of course, largely due to the existence of the National Health Service and tribute should be paid to the efforts that have been made over the last 30 years to improve the collection and presentation of data. For a number of important grades of staff remarkably comprehensive information is collected, and it will be clear from the above descriptions that further improvements in the system are envisaged.

For convenience, the problems may be summarised under a number of headings.

The most up-to-date information is at least six months old by the time it becomes available, and the delay in acquiring other forms of information may be considerably longer. Furthermore, much of the information which is published by the D.H.S.S., the General Medical Council and other organisations is not sufficiently detailed for research enquiries concerned with specific problems. For example, detailed examination of the age structure of the consultant population, in relation to sex and racial origin, would require far more information than is provided by the D.H.S.S. national tables for hospital medical staff. More detailed information can only be obtained through direct request to the body which holds the data, and this may well involve a considerable quantity of extra work. The staffs of the Department of Health and the General Medical Council are heavily committed in providing sufficient data for their own needs, and in formulating the basic information that should be made available to the public. Although it is often theoretically possible to satisfy specific enquiries for detailed analyses and breakdowns such requests may, in practice, have to wait many months or be declined because of more urgent priorities.

There is also, of course, the rather separate point that the bodies concerned, as sole proprietors of the data in question, can exert some discretionary control over what information is released, and how soon, in response to outside requests. This raises the two related questions of public accountability on the one hand and mischievous or time-wasting enquiry on the other. The Department of Health is itself, perhaps, in a particularly vulnerable situation in this regard, since the suspicion may arise of deliberate prevarication over the disclosure of uncomfortable or politically 'sensitive' information when, in truth, the problem is one of organisation and manpower. Some further remarks are made in relation to organisational difficulties (see below), but there is a general question concerning confidentiality. The D.H.S.S., although not an employing authority, receives information about doctors from the various employing authorities throughout the country. There is clearly a delicate question as to how much of this information the D.H.S.S. should release to enquirers without obtaining the permission of the employers. The employing authorities, in turn, may wish to obtain consent from the doctors themselves in some cases; it is certainly the case that the various employing authorities at present react differently to requests for information. The whole question of the confidentiality of data, both in relation to computer storage and otherwise, is at present under scrutiny and it might be that future recommendations or legislation will result in a clearer and more uniform viewpoint on this difficult matter.

Some types of information, about which up-to-date information would be of the greatest value, are particularly liable to be out of date. This applies to immigration and emigration statistics. There is always a good deal of hearsay evidence and 'soft' information relating to the number of doctors who have expressed the intention of emigrating, who have made enquiries from overseas High Commissions and other authorities, or taken the E.C.F.M.G. examination. In terms of hard fact, however, it may be very difficult under present arrangements to establish whether or not a doctor is still in the country and there is no good system of centrally-held information about temporary international movement of doctors. Actual available figures, therefore, tend to relate to the position two or three years previously and it is well known that the situation can change rapidly. It must also be emphasised that a great deal of temporary movement of

doctors takes place, both into and out of the country. At the time a
doctor leaves Britain it is by no means certain that he has gone for good;
the same is transparently obvious, in reverse, in relation to overseas
doctors coming in. Rapidly compiled 'emigration' data, based on the crude
numbers of doctors leaving the country, would therefore be grossly misleading. In order to obtain a true net figure, which is in any case
difficult, delay is inevitable.

In view of the importance of the whole question of doctor migration,
particularly bearing in mind the changes that are likely to occur in the
near future in the pattern of immigration from outside Europe, or emigration to the developing countries and our growing relationship with the
E.E.C., it would seem to be of great value to establish some system for
monitoring the movement of doctors into and out of the country, through
the agency of immigration officers. No such system at present exists; its
potential advantages might be outweighed by the time and effort involved,
the resentment that could be engendered, and the unreliability of the
resulting data. Nevertheless, the idea is perhaps worth consideration,
even if only on a trial basis.

One of the principal difficulties inherent in obtaining information
about particular groups of doctors, by means of surveys or research projects, is the time required to collect and analyse data. Even with the
best intentions it usually takes about three years to formulate and carry
through an enquiry of any size, and to prepare the results for publication.
When the resulting information relates to emigration intentions, career
choice, attitude to remuneration and conditions of service or other matters which are liable to sudden change the inherent limitations of the
method are obvious.

Inadequacy

Although the N.H.S. arrangements for collection of information on
senior medical staff are admirably comprehensive, the monitoring of the
other grades of staff in the hospital service leaves much to be desired.
The entry of all names onto a single sheet, to be returned to the
D.H.S.S. once a year, is well known to invite inaccuracy. For example, if
a newly graduated doctor were to move in February from Manchester to
Sheffield to occupy a pre-registration post, returning to Manchester in
August to take up an S.H.O. appointment he would be returned to the
D.H.S.S. in each of the two years in question as being in Manchester; the
fact that he had spent six months in Sheffield would pass completely without record. When information has to be obtained by Areas from Districts,
and particularly with the very rapid turnover of junior hospital staff
that occurs in some cases, it is no surprise that faults creep in. Even
within a single Region, as Postgraduate Deans have sometimes discovered,
it is a matter of considerable difficulty to maintain accurate, up-to-
date information about which junior doctors are occupying which posts at
any given time. It will also be apparent that the D.H.S.S. tables give
merely a snapshot impression of the staffing position at one moment in
time - 30 September of each year. They provide no indication of the
fluctuations in job occupancy that may be expected in any unit, hospital,
or district during the seasons and during periods of glut or famine.

The collection of adequate information about locums and vacant posts
presents similar difficulties. There are always a considerable number of
doctors in the process of changing from one job to another and, by the
same token, there are always a considerable number of unfilled posts
awaiting a new occupant. The number of doctors who technically appear to

be 'unemployed' at any one time is considerable, since they may be on leave, or in the process of moving from one part of the country to another, actively seeking a new appointment or deliberately making time to study for an examination; such details are often unknown and the true level of involuntary unemployment is thus difficult to ascertain.

The categorisation of 'vacant' posts raises difficult problems of definition. At senior registrar and consultant level the maximum number of posts that employing authorities are authorised to fill in any year is known, and also the number of posts occupied; precise information concerning vacancies is harder to specify.

Changes in the methods of presentation of data over the years, and differences between the D.H.S.S. and the S.H.H.D., also lead to difficulties in manpower estimation. For many good reasons the Department of Health is continually seeking better ways of tabulating manpower information, but the result is that it is often difficult to achieve a true comparison between the figures for different years. The fact that the precise breakdown of specialties and sub-specialties is different in England and Wales and in Scotland has already been referred to. In addition, there are possible difficulties over the precise categorisation of posts and those who occupy them. For example, a senior registrar in psychiatry may, at 30 September of a particular year, be occupying a post in mental sub-normality as part of a rotational training scheme; likewise, a registrar in general medicine may be temporarily occupying a post in cardiology. The question arises as to whether the person concerned should be returned as a senior registrar in psychiatry or mental sub-normality, as a registrar in medicine or cardiology. In practice, employing authorities classify occupants of posts, for the purposes of their returns, according to the training programme in which the post is established. This would clearly create difficulties in enumerating the number of trainees in a specialty such as obstetrics and gynaecology, where one year at registrar level is an elective year, which may be spent in posts belonging to any training programme other than obstetrics and gynaecology.

The precise nature of employment is a major inadequacy with much of the available date. This applies particularly to doctors holding more than one appointment, and doctors working outside the National Health Service, so that it is often impossible to assign a specific occupation, in detail, to a given doctor. The C.M.R.C. Index will only alleviate this problem insofar as it is possible to obtain the necessary information in the first place, and it appears that the machinery for doing this may still be lacking. It must also be remembered, in relation to the C.M.R.C. Index generally, that only after a considerable number of years will career information about individual doctors be recorded in any depth, and even then the amount of such information which is published or made readily available will presumably be decided by the D.H.S.S.

There is little doubt that the outstanding deficiency in existing data is the lack of coherent information about the progress of individual doctors within the system. The Departments of Health and the Employing Authorities are concerned with many things, including the numbers of doctors occupying posts at any one time - the numbers of 'pairs of hands' available to do the necessary work, and the numbers of doctors whose training must be provided for. From the point of view of doing a given amount of clinical work, whether the occupant of a specific post is the same person as in the previous year and, if not, what has become of last year's occupant, may be largely irrelevant. To assume that the Health Departments and Employing Authorities have no interest beyond this would, however, be unjust, and data about individual doctors are assembled. But it is true that much of the system of data collection and presentation has evolved to fulfil the primary function of showing the numbers of doctors working in specific places at specific times. The bulk of all our available information about medical manpower is collected from the N.H.S., by the N.H.S. and for the N.H.S. As is usually the case, when an attempt is made by an outside person to use the data for a different purpose to that for which it was originally designed, difficulties become all too apparent.

Incompleteness

Very little statistical information is available about certain groups of doctors particularly among those working outside the N.H.S. and, as already mentioned, those with more than one occupation. Because of the nature of medical practice in Britain over the last 30 years, in which the overwhelming bulk of the medical services to the community have been provided through the National Health Service, methods of measuring and comparing work contributions in the private sector have not evolved as in some other countries. In any event the precise details of an individual specialist's private practice (which can often best be assessed on financial grounds) is a sensitive subject and one concerning which it is generally felt that a good deal of personal privacy should be accorded. From the point of view of medical manpower in terms of organisation and dynamics - 'whole time equivalents' of work, travelling time, use of trained ancillary staff etc. - very little is known in an organised way about the private practice sector.

Some other groups have relatively little manpower information. In the field of occupational medicine, for instance, the estimate referred to in Chapter 3 was compiled from a knowledge of the main employers - for example the nationalised industries and the chemical industry which probably employ altogether about 220 doctors. It was acknowledged to be difficult to assess the part-time contribution of other doctors to occupational medicine, largely because there are many whose contribution is not more than 5 - 10 hours a week and often less. Many of these part-time doctors, but not all, are also general practitioners. The number of women doctors employed full-time in occupational medicine was thought to be very small - probably not more than 20 - 30. For this and some other branches of the medical profession there appears to be no systematic method of collecting manpower data.

Two other problems should be referred to again. Firstly, the incompleteness of knowledge about movement of doctors. This applies particularly to those occupying locum posts, those temporarily unemployed for various reasons and those changing at frequent intervals from one post to another. The current system of D.H.S.S. returns leaves large gaps in our knowledge about this situation. Some of the gaps can be filled at local or regional level as a result of painstaking enquiry but it is exceedingly difficult to be confident of the accuracy of any statement concerning movement, or to follow the detailed progress of an individual doctor. It would, of course, require a vast investment in time and labour to compile and maintain the necessary information and it is arguable whether or not it would be worthwhile. From the point of view of providing an effective health service it is important to know as precisely as possible what contribution is made by relatively 'casual labour' in terms of locum and short-term appointees, and what the quality of this service is. From the point of view of career guidance and future policy decisions relating to the career structure in general, it is equally important to be able to trace the paths of individual doctors through all their ramifications in order to understand the effects that these may have had, for good or bad, on career development and ultimate choice of specialisation. The best possible compromise needs to be found between the laborious collection of great quantities of statistical data which are never adequately analysed or put to good use, and the passive acceptance of a state of affairs in which too little is known and even less is done towards strengthening the system.

Secondly, there is the problem of incomplete responses to enquiries. It is relevant to refer to this again in the present context since, potentially, the survey or specific research project is a means whereby very detailed knowledge about movements of doctors and short-term fluctuations in manpower supply can be obtained. It is fairly unusual to obtain response rates of over 80% to questionnaires sent to doctors, even with vigorous attempts to follow up non-responders. Although such response rates enable a great many useful conclusions to be drawn, they can never be a substitute for complete information when statistical detail is needed. For example, exact information about the number of doctors who have emigrated, or who have changed their career choice from one specialty to another, or of the proportion of women whose careers have been influenced by marriage and childbearing, and many other important questions can never be resolved when there remain an appreciable number of the people concerned about whom no information is available. Much lower response rates have resulted from some enquiries, and when response rates are in the region of only 50% the resulting information is only of very limited value and can be positively misleading. Some of the doctors about whom it would be particularly valuable to have information are difficult to follow up or tend to respond poorly, for example, married women (who may be registered under their maiden or married name), overseas doctors and those who have emigrated.

Lack of Organisation

The D.H.S.S. holds no central record of the names and addresses of doctors in various grades and types of N.H.S. employment. This state of affairs arises from the nature of the Health Service itself, in which it is the individual Regional and other Health Authorities (and Boards of Governors), and not the D.H.S.S., who are employers. There may be arguments for or against the holding of central records of all doctors, and both the propriety and the value of the exercise would depend very much on the use to which such records were to be put. But from the point of view of medical manpower studies or enquiries the present state of affairs creates large problems. The problems are compounded by the fact that the employing authorities themselves are heavily burdened with administrative work and often ill-prepared to respond to requests for additional information. They may also have anxieties about disclosing such information to enquirers whose status, and the nature of whose work and sponsorship may be unclear. Each employing authority has the right to make its own decisions about how to respond to such enquiries and in practice the reactions differ considerably. If, for example, it were desired for perfectly respectable reasons to send a questionnaire to all registrars in general surgery, it would be necessary to write to each Area Health Authority, Area Health Authority (Teaching) and Board of Governors in the country explaining the purpose of the enquiry and asking them to supply the appropriate names and addresses. Experience suggests that some employing authorities would respond promptly, and others much more slowly;

some would refer the enquiry to an ethical or other committee before agreeing to disclose the information, and a few might refuse outright; some would need to be written to several times and at the end of the day there would remain some from whom adequate returns had not been obtained. Meanwhile, the time interval between receiving the first list and making the decision that no further useful information was likely to be forthcoming would be at least four months and, in our personal experience, more likely six. During this time perhaps one third of the registrars in question would have changed their jobs so that much of the information would be unusable by the time it had been assembled. Some more general comments about the reservations that may exist in relation to confidentiality, in supplying such information, have already been made.

This problem is illustrated in some detail since it seems to bring into focus many of the difficulties arising from a system which is centrally organised but peripherally administered. It may be that for statistical purposes it is sufficient for the Department of Health to know about the numbers of doctors in post and the movements that have taken place, without being able to identify individuals. But if that line of reasoning is to be followed then it might be said that the peripherally placed employing authorities, in many cases, appear to know remarkably little about their employees and are ill-equipped to supply the sort of information about them which one would normally expect a good employer to have at his fingertips. In any case, the argument breaks down when one considers the frequency with which the 'employees' of the system move from one 'employer' to another, so that it would always be a hopeless task to try and trace the progress of the individual through the good offices of any one employing authority. The undergraduate medical student, while at the university, has a Dean and a corporate body of staff in the medical school to safeguard his interests and monitor his progress with care. Arrangements in this regard are notably less satisfactory once the preregistration year is entered. Thereafter, in his new-found status of N.H.S. 'employee', pure and simple, the doctor floats in an administrative limbo between individual employing authorities who take note of his existence for a time, and a central bureaucracy that does not even know his name except retrospectively as an entry in an Index. Despite the appointment of Postgraduate Deans and the establishment of Regional Postgraduate Committees the universities have nothing like the same responsibility for the postgraduate student as for the undergraduate, nor the same control over his progress and movement. The Colleges and their Faculties, despite their guiding influence over training requirements and quality of individual posts, are again ignorant of even the names of many trainees in their specialties. All this, apart from its potential disadvantages to the trainee and to the system as a whole, creates major problems in the assembly and interpretation of manpower data during a stage - the stage of postgraduate training - at which it is particularly needed.

MANPOWER DECISION MAKING

There are overall economic considerations which determine the allocation of funds to the health departments and then there are decisions to be made about how much of the money is spent on manpower, including doctors. Political pressure, with or without a weight of public opinion behind it, may influence N.H.S. policy quite suddenly in particular directions, for example towards better care of the mentally handicapped or of children, or towards more emphasis upon primary care rather than hospital treatment. Such policy decisions or 'priorities' clearly have substantial medical manpower implications, so that there is immediately a conflict between the needs of the moment, or perhaps more precisely the perceived requirements of the immediate future, and the length of time needed to produce more doctors and train new specialists. It would be paradoxical in one and the same breath to plead for a greater influence over the selection of medical undergraduates with a propensity to engage in the types of medical work that fit the 'needs' of the community, and to reserve the right to alter these 'needs' at a moment's notice.

Employing authorities, and particularly the Regional Health Authorities are required to formulate their own manpower plans for the adequate provision of medical services within their own areas of responsibility. These are based largely on local assessment of the needs of the Region concerned, in relation to the comparative position of other regions and of the country as a whole. There are, of course, regular meetings between regions, for example of Regional Medical Officers with representatives of the Health Departments, and these serve as a means of exchange of views on medical manpower.

The local assessment of medical manpower needs, as far as the hospital service is concerned, is done at district level. This leads to the formulation of requests for additional staff and these are often put in order of priority after discussion at the Medical Executive Committee (approval is not required for reductions in medical staffing, but these must be notified to the D.H.S.S.). Area Health Authorities co-ordinate requests from their Districts, and requests from all Areas are considered at Regional level.

Each region has a Regional Manpower Committee, which is a professional committee of doctors and not a statutory committee of the Regional Health Authority. Its function is to advise the R.H.A. on matters relating to medical manpower but the ultimate responsibility for decision making rests with the employing authority, which is not in any sense obliged to accept the Regional Manpower Committee's recommendations. As far as junior hospital posts are concerned, there is the important question of recognition from the appropriate College or Faculty. The Regional Postgraduate Committee of each region has a series of sub-committees or Specialist Training Committees for the individual specialties; it should be the function of these committees to review the numbers and disposition of training posts in their special fields throughout the Region and to advise both the Regional Manpower Committee and the employing authority about requests for additional posts, both in relation to the likelihood of receiving college recognition and to the interests of regional training as a whole. At S.H.O. and registrar level the Colleges and Faculties recognise individual posts as being suitable for training (sometimes for limited periods of time, for example, for one year's training). In the case of senior registrars the emphasis is on recognition of training programmes, or rotational schemes, which normally incorporate all senior registrar posts in the specialty within the Region concerned. When additional posts at this level are under consideration outline manpower approval may be obtained from the Central Manpower Committee before the appropriate College is asked to give recognition for Higher Specialist Training.

The Central Manpower Committee was set up in 1972 to replace the former Advisory Committee for Consultant Establishments and its sub-committees. The composition of the Central Manpower Committee was later expanded to include representatives of undergraduate and postgraduate medical education as observers. Standing sub-committees were set up to deal with the problems of special grades of staff and particular aspects

of manpower. The Regional Manpower Committees and the Central Manpower
Committee function at different levels, and stand in somewhat different
relationships to the Regional Health Authority and the D.H.S.S. respectively. There was never a direct channel of communication between the
Regional Manpower Committees and the Central Manpower Committee. Membership of the Central Manpower Committee was not arranged deliberately on
a regional basis, so that it was inevitably the case that some Regional
Manpower Committees were far better informed of the activities of the
Central Manpower Committee than others. Likewise, in individual Regions
the amount of attention paid to the views of the Regional Manpower Committee by the employing authority has doubtless varied. In 1976 it was
agreed that the composition and functions of the Central Manpower Committee should be comprehensively reviewed (B.M.A. Annual Report, 1977). As
a result of this reconstitution, a number of the previous difficulties
should be resolved, including those of regional representation and communication.

Consultant, registrar and senior registrar appointments must all receive central approval, and all applications for personal grading as
medical assistant must also come before the Central Manpower Committee.
In the grades of senior house officer, and for clinical assistants, employing authorities have complete freedom to make appointments providing
that money is available.

The traditional policy with regard to consultant appointments was
that each individual application was considered centrally in relation to
all others from throughout the country. If the application was successful the employing authority was informed that it had authorisation to
advertise and fill the specific appointment in question and no flexibility
was possible. It became increasingly apparent that, particularly in the
'shortage' specialties, there was a gap between the number of posts considered desirable and approved, and the number for which suitable applicants could be found. At the end of each year employing authorities often
had a considerable number of unfilled posts on their books and there seemed to be little point in striving for further consultant expansion and
approving yet more new posts in this situation. The arrangements now are
that, although the number of additional posts in each specialty is determined centrally, Regional Authorities do not have to argue the case in
detail for individual posts but have freedom to decide on the allocation
of posts within the Region, according to local needs and opportunities.
If it is not possible to fill a post in a particular District an attempt
may be made to fill the post next in order of priority in that specialty
elsewhere in the Region. It is probably too soon to assess the effects
of this policy change. Additional senior registrar and registrar posts
are approved, where appropriate, providing educational approval has been
obtained.

The Central Manpower Committee takes a general view of the policies
which should, in its opinion, govern the numbers and distribution of new
posts in the various specialties. For an individual specialty the assessment tends to be based firstly on the numbers of appointments likely to be
needed to maintain the existing stock, based on probable retirements in
the immediate future. This is then related to the existing senior registrar establishment and the extent to which senior registrarships are
filled, with particular regard to the numbers of people approaching the
completion of their training and therefore eligible for consultant status.
In the light of this information, an estimate is made of the extent to
which the senior registrar 'market' would support the establishment of
additional consultant appointments over and above those needed for stock

replacement. Thus, the creation of additional posts in a specialty is determined to a large extent by the probability of such posts attracting suitable applicants and being filled. This analysis of the 'supply' situation is presumably matched against some analysis of the 'demand', since for various reasons it may appear that from time to time a greater degree of expansion is required in some specialties than others, always providing that it could be achieved. Having come to an overall decision about the number of new posts to be approved in a specialty, the distribution between regions is recommended according to their position in relation to the national average for staffing in the specialty concerned and other considerations including, no doubt, the numbers of requests actually received from each region. The general way in which the C.M.C. proceeds with these deliberations is known to the regional authorities, who are often fairly well aware of the order of magnitude of the numbers of new posts that are likely to be approved in a given year.

PROBLEMS WITH THE DECISION MAKING PROCESS

At different levels, there are more-or-less loosely defined criteria by which the demand for additional medical staff is measured. Firstly, at hospital or district level, there is a local assessment of 'need'. This is the estimate most directly related to knowledge of the amount and type of work that actually has to be done, and the ways in which it is hoped to improve and develop the service in relation to the prevailing local circumstances. It is for the local medical staff to advise the Area Health Authority, through the available network of channels of communication, about specific priorities, for example whether it is more urgent to have an improved geriatric service or an additional radiologist. It would make a fascinating study to analyse the ways on which these priorities are finally decided, and the extent to which the professional opinion of the medical staff takes precedence over the more general view of the non-medical members of the committees through which recommendations pass, or vice versa. The outcome, in any event, is no more than a provisional decision since for all staff above the level of S.H.O. it then becomes subject to scrutiny at regional and central levels. There is next a regional concept of the staffing 'norms' or levels that should apply to the region as a whole and the individual specialties within it, in relation to the population to be served and the national average. There is something to be said for this concept as a means of working towards more even distribution of staff and other resources; its application may reveal striking differences, between hospitals or Districts, which have grown up over the years. But there is the danger of inhibiting local initiative and of appearing to take insufficient account of local circumstances. Criteria may be difficult to establish; the use of population figures to set a 'norm' for child health services may not be an unreasonable starting point, but it is almost meaningless in relation to anaesthetics. Thirdly, at national level, 'targets' were set for the development of medical manpower in the National Health Service at the time of the setting up of the Central Manpower Committee: 4% growth a year in the number of consultants and $2\frac{1}{2}$% a year in junior staff, for the hospital service. These 'targets', however, were based not on a preconceived vision of the total numbers of doctors needed, but on a laudable intention to change the ratio between senior and junior staff. As far as total numbers are concerned, the system is essentially 'demand driven' at central level, since it is recognised that the exact need for doctors cannot at present be defined.

The interplay of these different criteria gives scope for lengthy discussion of all aspects of a request for additional manpower, some of which might well be overlooked if authority were to be vested in a single, all-powerful decision-making body against which there were no appeal. But there is little doubt that the present process is too cumbersome and insufficiently clear in its objectives. A more fundamental objection, perhaps, is the difficulty of making the existing arrangements work according to plan. There is undoubtedly need for much better and more rapid feed-back of information about the progress of events - about the extent to which 'targets' are departed from and the reasons why. A general view of medical manpower prospects for the N.H.S. as a whole must clearly emanate from the centre, on the basis of the overall economic position. Allocation between specialties should take far more account of the operational viability of the medical team as a whole, with particular emphasis on the need for adequate supporting services. It is probable that the Regions themselves should have a far closer involvement with the allocation of manpower on a regional basis; once these decisions are made the detail is best worked out at local level, with as little further interference as possible.

Even more fundamental is the criticism that all the present criteria, for needs, norms and targets, are essentially based on adding something to the existing state of affairs, without really looking at how the existing state of affairs came about and what relationship it bears to the true 'need'. There is, in fact, considerable difficulty in arriving at any proper figure for the 'establishment' of medical posts in the N.H.S., as opposed to the number of posts currently occupied. There are a number of easily recognisable difficulties about determining the exact establishment. Although a post may exist on paper, it may not have been filled for some years and no attempt may be being made to fill it; an additional post may be authorised but not yet filled, and will not be funded until a suitable applicant has indicated his willingness to accept the appointment; a case may have been made and accepted for an additional post but despite 'manpower approval' funds may not be available; changes that have occurred, for various reasons, may be known locally but not yet recorded centrally and may be interpreted differently by different authorities; other sources of information, maintained for specific purposes, may not accord with D.H.S.S. data. For example, the number of 'training' posts in a specialty, according to the Postgraduate Dean's office or according to the College's list of recognised posts may not correspond with the Regional establishment of S.H.O.s and registrars. But the fact that the precise 'establishment' of posts is difficult to define is no justification for abandoning the attempt. Merely to look at the existing number of doctors in various grades, and make an assessment of the likely availability of money and good candidates from year to year is no basis for proper manpower planning. It is living from hand to mouth in a way which demands complex administrative arrangements to prevent the situation running completely out of control; and success in this, even then, is by no means assured. It is understandably regarded as important to know how many doctors are available to do the work, and in this sense figures for numbers of staff in post are of more practical value than 'establishment' figures. But job occupancy can vary so much that as a basis for planning these figures would be meaningless. An example is provided by senior registrarships in anaesthetics; about two years ago, during a period of generalised recruitment difficulty, it is known that in one Region thirteen of the eighteen senior registrar posts were filled. Two years later the number of posts had been increased to twenty one and all were occupied.

In any rigorous analysis of the medical manpower situation there must be three stages in looking at the question of 'need' or 'demand'. Firstly, it is necessary to know the number of people actually available from time to time to do the work that has to be done. This is essentially a determining factor in planning the range of services that can be offered, or the need to invoke alternative forms of manpower, on a short-term basis. Secondly, it is necessary to know what the current establishment of posts is, so that the percentage occupancy can be determined, the reasons for shortfall can be analysed and future recruitment prospects can be assessed. Thirdly, there is a need to determine what the established number of posts should be in order to provide a determined range of services in a way which best combines effectiveness with job satisfaction. This is a different matter from merely setting a 'target' of 4% growth over the existing number of consultants; it is a matter of looking in detail at the work of the team and the pattern of care, in health and sickness, that it would like to be able to provide. It is only on some basis such as this that 'needs' can properly be assessed and manpower 'targets' can be set.

The first stage of this analysis involves a great deal more understanding than we currently have of the elasticity of the system. In a single specialty, in an individual hospital or District, there is a certain amount of work to be done and there are perhaps one or two consultants to do it. To a large extent the local people set their own standards in terms of improvements that they can bring about and the additional volume of work that they are prepared to bring upon themselves. There comes a point at which it is clear that an additional consultant is needed. The work has become too much for one or two people; to begin with it may be rather light for two or three, but the slack will be taken up in various ways and both a better service to the patient and a more rewarding career for the consultants will result. It is important to realise that to speak in terms of a 4% growth in the consultant establishment is utterly meaningless in relation to the men and women who actually provide patient care. There will come a point when they will ask for a 50% increase or a 100% increase in their particular consultant establishment; nothing less is possible. At the second stage, that of relating the numbers of people in post to the 'establishment' it may be said that the Central Manpower Committee makes considerable efforts, but the problem is complicated by lack of sufficiently accurate knowledge about what the establishment is, or what it actually should be.

Some of the problems of communication within the existing system can be inferred from the structure already outlined. A request for a junior hospital post will be looked at by the Regional Manpower Committee and also by the Specialist Training Sub-Committee of the Regional Postgraduate Committee. The views of the College will be sought and a visit of inspection, for educational purposes, may be arranged. The Regional Health Authority will take account of the views of both the Regional Manpower Committee and the Specialist Training Sub-Committee but will in all probability turn also to the Joint Advisory Committee on Senior Registrars. If and when these hurdles have been cleared, the request for an additional post will be submitted, if the R.H.A. so decide, to the Central Manpower Committee and the D.H.S.S. This is by no means automatic; Regional Health Authorities are under no obligation to transmit to the Health Departments requests that they have received from Areas. This has been particularly true in the case of registrar posts, where requests have been so severely discouraged that in many cases they got no further than Regional level, although it is apparent that other requests which were sent forward to the

66

Department of Health were in some cases approved. The same situation can arise at consultant level, where, despite the large numbers of requests for additional posts received from Areas and Districts, the requests made to the D.H.S.S. may be tempered by some knowledge of the likely allocation. It is also pertinent to mention that employing authorities are expected to be able to fund the posts that they ask for, so that there would be little point in requesting 20 additional posts in a specialty if the money could only be found for five.

It is apparent that there may be communication difficulties between the Regional Manpower Committee and the Specialist Training Committees; that the Postgraduate Dean's assessment of a training post may not coincide with the views of the College; that communication between Regional Manpower Committees and the Central Manpower Committee has heretofore been non-existent; and that unless the D.H.S.S. and the Central Manpower Committee are adequately informed by employing authorities about local assessment of requirements they cannot be expected to have any real concept of the demand in various parts of the country. To trace the progress of a number of requests for additional posts, over the last few years, and to assess the relative importance of opinions expressed by different bodies at different levels in reaching a final decision (together with a follow-up of whether or not the post was successfully filled) would be an interesting and revealing study.

Some long-standing difficulties can be directly related to a lack of clear policy at national level. Perhaps the outstanding example is that of the junior hospital grades. The differences of opinion as to whether S.H.O.s and registrars should properly be regarded as 'trainees' or as 'pairs of hands' was brought into focus by the Platt Report (1961) but has been discussed extensively both before and since. Conflict of interest inevitably arises between those responsible for training - the Colleges, the Postgraduate Deans and the Specialist Training Committees - and those responsible for providing a service to the community - the employing authorities and in many cases the consultants themselves who feel that the viability of their units depends on an adequate supply of supporting medical staff. From the training point of view there are arguments both for and against the deployment of junior staff in non-teaching hospitals, at various stages. There are also strong differences of view among trainees themselves about the relative merits of well-planned and highly organised postgraduate training programmes extending over all the relevant years together, and a free-enterprise, open competition arrangement in which each man carves his own path by applying for jobs of his choosing and by using his industry and initiative to gain the 'edge' over his contemporaries, not forgetting the art of being in the right person's favour at the right time. A detailed discussion of postgraduate medical education in Britain would form the subject of a book in itself, but it is obvious that there will never be satisfactory arrangements for manpower planning or design of the career structure until the philosophy of the junior hospital grades has finally been argued out and agreed.

The next most obvious lack of clearly defined policy relates to the future of the career grades. Although the declared policy of the medical profession and the Departments of Health at present is that there should be no permanent sub-consultant grade, the future of the medical assistant grade, or any alternative grade, remains in doubt. In the case of the hospital practitioner grade, there have been differences of viewpoint between general practitioners and hospital specialists. The range of work that may be undertaken by a hospital practitioner and the extent to which he is supervised are so loosely defined and subject to such wide variation

67

that absence of clearly formulated policy is again evident. As with the junior hospital grade, no satisfactory manpower plan can be expected to emerge until the whole future of the career grades in the hospital service has been determined.

As a final comment on problems of policy, the current attitude to the allocation of additional posts will serve as an example. As indicated above, the policy is pragmatic. The number of additional posts approved for a given specialty depends largely on the numbers of applicants likely to be available from the senior registrar grade. In practice, all requests for additional consultant posts are approved if the supply is adequate, and the reservations concerning supply relate (in 1977) to specialties such as geriatrics, radiology, anaesthetics, mental handicap and some branches of pathology. The assumption underlying this view is that the number of 'eligible' senior registrars is related to the anticipated number of consultant vacancies. First of all it should be noted that, in principle, the argument is a circular one, since it should theoretically require only two or three years to build up a larger cadre of eligible senior registrars or to reduce the number if this were thought desirable. In practice, the constraint is often upon recruitment to the posts available. Secondly, the argument assumes that the number of senior registrars in post corresponds with the senior registrar establishment; it is known that there are sometimes wide differences and that the situation may vary considerably from time to time. Thirdly, the argument assumes that virtually all consultant appointments are made from among senior registrars of three or more years' standing - that is, those who have completed the Colleges' and Faculties' requirements for training. This, again, is known not to be the case in practice. An appreciable number of consultant appointments are made from outside the senior registrar grade and the available figures suggest that the number of 'eligible' senior registrars would not support some of the expansions that have already taken place. For example, between 1 October, 1974 and 30 September, 1975 the number of paid N.H.S. consultants appointed in general medicine was 47, while the number of senior registrars with three or more years' tenure during the same period was 21. Admittedly, there were an appreciable number of holders of academic appointments in general medicine with senior registrar status. But in anaesthetics the number of paid consultants appointed was 90 and the number of senior registrars with three or more years in the grade was 26, with only a small number of 'eligible' 'honorary' senior registrars in academic posts. Even if all senior registrars with two or more years in the grade are counted, the total was only 62. The comparable figures for the year ended 30 September, 1973 were 86 paid consultant appointments, 24 senior registrars with three or more years in the grade and 63 with two or more years. Fourthly, the argument implies that the senior registrar establishment will continually be adjusted according to the availability of career outlets, and this represents a return to the circular argument, since there appears to be no means of assessing the availability of career outlets independently of the supply of senior registrars. Despite recent economic problems, and concerns for the hospital manpower programme, the 1976 figure for England and Wales showed a rise of 5.6% over 1975 in the total number of senior registrars. The number of consultant posts also continued to rise (by 3.5%), and the new appointments made during the year 1975/76 were not appreciably less than in previous years. It should be added that specialties differ considerably, so that overall statements of this kind can be misleading, but nevertheless a purely demand-driven arrangement of this type must ultimately have limitations.

The mechanical basis for the current manpower expansion plan is thus open to question, but so also is the underlying philosophy. The specialties in which there is likely to be no difficulty in filling additional consultant posts are the over-subscribed specialties where senior registrarships are constantly filled. The specialties with recruitment difficulties are those depended upon to provide support for additional consultants in the well-provided specialties such as medicine and surgery. It has for many years been recognised at local level that uncontrolled expansion in the numbers of surgeons and physicians will lead to intolerable loss of morale and, indeed, to breakdown of services, unless the supporting specialties such as pathology, radiology and anaesthetics can be appropriately strengthened. Many individual hospital staff committees have for some time adopted the policy of referring all requests for additional posts in the primary specialties for consideration by the supporting Divisions before recommending approval. The importance of these considerations, and the vital need to consider the delivery of health care as an activity of the hospital team as a whole, are not lost upon the Central Manpower Committee in principle; yet the philosophy of limiting the number of additional posts in specialties where recruitment may be difficult - notably the support specialties - while allowing growth in other specialties is entirely contrary to this spirit. It is at least conceivable that in the extreme there could be a danger, if political and other pressures were brought heavily to bear, that jobs might be created for certain groups of doctors, such as obstetricians or married women, simply because they had been trained and could not find career outlets, rather than because there was a demonstrable need for their services and a demonstrable ability to provide them with the resources or the manpower support that they would require.

POST SCRIPT

At a recent meeting a speaker reporting on a survey remarked that he had been unable to follow up some of his cases, a fact which might perhaps give new hope to those who feared that we now lived in a society which threatened such complete lack of privacy and independence that nobody could possibly get lost. The whole question of staff records is beset with problems concerning confidentiality and the right to demand personal information. In a free country we do well to acknowledge the fact that some people simply do not want to provide data about themselves, just as all good families have members who do not wish to keep in touch however enthusiastically their genealogically-minded relatives pursue them. This has to be reconciled with the evident advantages of knowing about how doctors are distributed and employed, and the factors that influence their career paths. This chapter has been much concerned with these advantages, insofar as they relate to manpower planning. Whether the manpower planning and forecasting that might be facilitated by such data would itself have significant advantages is perhaps a different question. The obvious concern of individuals at present about numbers of doctors and about possible unemployment, and the public concern about uneven distribution of medical manpower suggest that we are, on balance, moving towards a desire for better information about ourselves. This progress, if such it be, must go hand in hand, as in so many cases, with a true understanding of when and when not to use the new power that we create. It might be worth suggesting that at this stage a full study of what use information about doctors really is, or might be, in various ways, would be of no small value.

REFERENCES

B.M.A. (1977) Annual Report of Council 1976-77. *British Medical Journal,*
1, 1096.

Brook, P. (1976) Where do Psychiatrists come from? *British Journal of
Psychiatry,* 128, 313-317.

Flynn, C.A. & Gardner, F. (1969) The careers of women graduates from the
Royal Free Hospital School of Medicine, London. *British Journal of
Medical Education,* 3, 28-42.

Lawson, A. & Simons, H.A.B. (1976) The careers of men graduates from the
Royal Free Hospital School of Medicine, London. *Medical Education,*
10, 348-358.

Parkhouse, J. & McLaughlin, C. (1976) Career preferences of doctors graduating in 1974. *British Medical Journal,* 2, 630-632.

Platt Report (1961) *Medical Staffing Structure in the Hospital Service.*
London: H.M.S.O.

Scottish Council for Postgraduate Medical Education (1974) *Survey of Career Experience of Scottish Medical Graduates (Year 1962).* SC(74)3.

Scottish Council for Postgraduate Medical Education (1976) *Outline of a
Report on surveys of the career experience and training of the 1965
and 1970 graduates of the Scottish University Medical Schools.*
SC(76)27.

5. Women Doctors

Prior to the Second World War medically qualified women were few and, although they had an advantage over female teachers in that they were not compelled to retire on marriage, most women interested in medical work were confined to the 'caring' profession of nursing. So it is only during the past twenty-five years that the species 'woman doctor' has become a lively subject for discussion. Yet it is interesting to observe that, despite the great quantity of literature produced during the last two decades, there has never been any systematic monitoring of numbers, choice of career or of career patterns, emigration (or indeed, immigration of women overseas graduates), and ways of coping with what Celia Oakley (1976b) calls 'the same pressures as men plus some obvious additional ones'. One sentiment is constantly reiterated: 'There must be really effective monitoring of the career progress, both of women as a whole and of each individual part-time trainee, and this needs to be centrally organised in collaboration with the regions' (Arie, 1976); and again 'serial longitudinal studies of the careers of women doctors, in which goals achieved are compared with initial aspirations and expectations, are necessary' (Forster, 1975).

Lack of clear thinking about medical manpower, and a medical career structure which makes a mockery of many attempts at career planning, make for great difficulties in assessing the 'need' for women doctors and their likely place in the health service of the future. Meanwhile, it is interesting to trace, through the literature available, the considerable changes that have taken place in the fortunes of women doctors, since the speed and scope of these are not always appreciated.

In 1962, Kahan and Mac Faul reported that while 100% of unmarried women doctors were working whole-time, only 60% of those married and 16% of those with children were working whole-time; yet in 1976 Celia Oakley said 'today 93% of women under 30 are still practising medicine (compared with only 75% who are over 30), and yet because women are marrying younger this is probably the age when they are having their families, and when formerly they would have given up work' (Oakley, 1976). It is indeed relevant to ask (Forster, 1975), 'are the academic achievements of women medical students and doctors relative to men obtained from a study in the mid-1960s relevant to the intake and revised curricula of the middle and later 1970s?'

To begin at the beginning, in schools, there is evidence of what a study of women students at King's College Hospital Medical School (Clack et al, 1976) called self-selection. This may result from conformity to

71

social expectations, pre-selection by headmistresses who advise only
'high fliers' to apply to medical schools, and from the traditionally
inferior science teaching and laboratory facilities in girls schools.
The Goodenough Report (1944) recommended that one-fifth of the medical
school intake should consist of women, and suggested that 'the medical
schools may at their discretion exceed their quota for women students to
the extent by which their quota for men is not filled' (as happened during
the Second World War). The Report advised in general that, 'the proportion of women may well vary from school to school and from time to time
according to the quality of the students of both sexes applying for admission and to the public need for doctors. We propose it should be left
to the U.G.C. to decide on questions relating to compliance with this
condition, including the reasonableness at any given time of the proportion of men and women students in any school'. Despite this early broad-
mindedness, it is undoubtedly true that only a very few years ago it was
often necessary for girls to obtain higher school-leaving grades than
boys, in Advanced Level G.C.E. subjects, to gain admission to medical
schools. In 1974 the Committee of Vice-Chancellors and Principals in the
United Kingdom advised, 'that any remaining measure to limit the number
of women medical students to a fixed proportion of the whole or to require
higher grade school leaving qualifications is prejudicial and inappropriate
to modern conditions and should be discontinued'. Together with the Sex
Discrimination Act of 1976, and a note from the D.H.S.S. (1976), this
should ensure that all applicants for medical courses now have an equal
chance regardless of sex. Add to this the fact that school science facilities have improved beyond all recognition, and that girls are becoming
generally more career-orientated and aware of their opportunities (perhaps
because of the sex-mix and competition in comprehensive schools) and it is
no surprise to find it widely predicted that by the end of this decade 50%
of the medical school intake will be women.

Because of recent concern about manpower shortages, however, and the
feeling that 'woman means waste', (although the figures here seem to be
changing rapidly), there has been a somewhat punitive reaction coupled
with a reminder that each medical graduate now costs anything up to
£40,000 to produce. Instead of the former plea that a university education benefited a woman and her family whether she worked or not, and the
general view of only a few years ago that all young children need their
mother at home, we find Jefferys and Elliott (1966) expressing the view of
women students that, 'in accepting one of the limited opportunities for
training for a profession whose skills are greatly in demand they incur an
obligation to the community which they must do their utmost to discharge',
and Ulyatt and Ulyatt (1973) saying, 'women are divided into positive and
negative types' - the negative ones, naturally, being those who give home
commitments priority. The Ulyatts conclude their study by saying that
when girls are interviewed for selection to medical school the only concern
is with academic achievement and intellectual ability to complete the
course; but this is not enough, 'potential wastage' must be identified at
this time and 'it would be possible to accept girls who are discovered to
have no fear of neglecting and so harming their families rather than girls
who regard constant personal maternal care as the only safeguard against
abnormality and delinquency in their children'.

There is perhaps more commonsense in the B.M.J.'s comment (Editorial,
1974) that women doctors 'can have the best of both worlds if they wish to
strive for them as so many have done and are doing. But let the element
of choice remain, so that not even moral coercion is applied to those who
do not wish to conform. Women must be allowed to judge for themselves,

according to their own needs and instincts, the priorities and timing of the parts of their lives they give to their families and to the community. Perhaps the most potent factor of all will be their own need for self-fulfilment'. In 'Women in Medicine', Carol Lopate (1968) writes 'What may make the prospect of becoming a physician worthwhile for the young woman is not necessarily the financial gain or guaranteed security - although these may be pleasant dividends. It is the enrichment of her life, the full use of her gifts, the sense of self-expression which cannot be dismissed easily, even after she considers the obstacles it may bring. Perhaps this enrichment is the line of attack which those seeking more women in medicine should take'.

If the number of women graduates does rise by the end of the decade to 50% of the total, this very rapid change will obviously have to be taken into account by any future manpower Commission or Institute. There is, however, the contrary view, expressed by the Regional Medical Officers (1976) in their evidence to the Royal Commission, that 'if there are no restrictions other than high quality "A" level passes in physics, chemistry and biology, then both in number and quality achieved the balance of advantages lies overwhelmingly with the men'. It may be that in free and open competition, where the 'average' as well as the 'high fliers' of both sexes apply, the percentage of successful boys will rise in the absence of a quota system.

England is actually among the world leaders in terms of percentages of women medical graduates. Highest on the list comes the U.S.S.R., where Kissick (1964) found in 1964 that 60% of doctors were women. According to W.H.O. statistics (1974) this figure rose to 72% in 1973, a trend followed by satellite communist countries. In India, Carol Lopate (1968) noted: 'Since World War II, and especially since independence, the figure for women entering medicine has soared. Because of the emphasis that Mahatma Gandhi placed on equal opportunity for women, as well as the easy availability of domestic help, the economic advantage of having two income-producing persons in the family, and the better academic record of women, 35% of all physicians in India are now women'. The social implications of this in India would make an interesting study, as would the problems and career patterns of Indian women doctors in Britian. In 1962 Judek (1964) found that only 5.6% of Canadian medical school graduates were women, although it is interesting to note that 20.7% of doctors immigrating into Canada were women. By 1968, Nelson-Jones and Fish (1970) found that women constituted 15.2% of applicants in Canada and 16.4% of admissions, and Fruen, Rothman and Steiner (1974) reported that in Toronto the proportion of women applicants accepted (28.8%) was higher than the proportion of men accepted (20.8%). The numbers of women have also risen in the United States; Dube (1973) reported that while in 1967 women formed 10.4% of applicants and 9.8% of admissions, in 1972 they formed 16% of applicants and the same percentage of admissions. It is equally true in Britain that the girls who apply, albeit 'pre-selected', have a good chance of success. The Universities Central Council for Admissions (1976) reported that in 1975, while 32% of the candidates were women, they gained 35% of the places. A recent study at Kings' College Hospital Medical School endorsed this: in 1967, 20% of the medical student intake was female, rising to 38% in 1975. The proportion of women applicants was only 17% in 1967 rising to 29% in 1975, and in 1975 one in fifteen female applicants as against one in twenty-two male applicants was admitted (Clack et al, 1976). The authors compared these findings to those of Jefferys, Gauvain and Gulesen (1965), where men had a slightly better chance of admittance, and of Aird and Silver (1971) who found that the same proportion of women

73

were admitted as applied.

Not only do the 'high flier' girls have better 'A' levels than 'average' boys (Aird and Silver, 1971) but their medical school final examination results are better (Stanley and Last, 1968). The Kings' study gave additional evidence of this, showing that women students tended to have higher 'A' levels in zoology and biology, higher scores for effort at the end of the clinical year and higher marks in medical and surgical final examinations. The authors pointed out that perhaps men take their school examinations and undergraduate years more lightly and that better academic achievement does not necessarily mean better doctors.

What happens after graduation? There is no doubt that performance does not live up to promise, either in the quantity of work done or in the quality, if that is to be judged by postgraduate qualifications obtained. It is currently thought that the average woman doctor's professional con- tribution is only half to three-quarters of that of a male counterpart, with the consequent loss of 'available doctor time', although a recent report (Regional Medical Officers' evidence to the Royal Commission, 1976) commented, 'As in all "battles of the sexes" the exchanges have been notable for their warmth of opinion rather than factual evidence'. Stanley and Last (1968) noted that, 'only 30% of women compared with 42% of men acquired additional qualifications' after graduation.

First, the problems of women doctors have to be identified and then constructive remedies proposed; there has been no lack of studies on both subjects. These have included studies in individual hospitals (Kahan and Mac Faul, 1962; Aird and Silver, 1971; Flynn and Gardner, 1969; Clack et al, 1976); in university centres (Robb-Smith, 1962; Timbury and Ratzer, 1969; Whitfield, 1969; Eskin, 1976); and by Region (Eskin in Lincolnshire, 1972; and in the Sheffield Region, 1974). There have been reports of schemes to encourage women doctors to return to work, in the South West Metropolitan Region, (Essex-Lopresti, 1970), in the North West Thames Region (Clark, 1976) and in Oxford (Rue, 1967). There have been studies by husband and wife teams (Kenneth and Frances Ulyatt, 1971; Thomas and Beulah Bewley, 1975); and many studies by women about women (Flynn and Gardner, 1969; Eskin, 1972, 1974, 1976; Henryk-Gutt and Silverstone, 1976; Timbury and Ratzer, 1969; Kahan and Mac Faul, 1962; Lawrie and Newhouse, 1965; Shore, 1974; Lawrie, Newhouse and Elliott, 1966). Nor has Britain alone been concerned; Macdonald and Webb (1966), and Nelson-Jones and Fish (1970) have reported on Canada; Kissick (1964) on Russia, and Bhatt, Soni and Patel (1976) on India, where the fact that 39% of the female graduates of one medical college had emigrated served to make our British problems look insignificant. Very many medical writers, sociologists and psychologists in the United States (e.g. Steppacher and Mausner, 1974) seeking causes for the 'excess' suicide rate in American female professionals, including physicians, have suggested that, 'women are insufficiently integrated into a predominantly masculine profession and consequently have a need to prove themselves worthy of acceptance; additionally, they have a role conflict between home-making and a professional career, as well as an ambivalent attitute to success'.

The career problems of women are not confined to medicine. Frada Eskin (1976), comparing the employment status of women medical graduates and women science graduates in the University of Sheffield 1960-65, con- cluded that, 'the employment prospects of women in medicine are not as gloomy as might be imagined'. Women science graduates fared much more badly: 'the underemployment of women graduates is common to all profess- ions but political and financial considerations have created the recent upsurge of interest in medical graduates because of the chronic manpower shortage'.

Be this as it may, the changing social and career expectation of girls themselves must be the most important and durable factors in the present developing situation. Between the wars there was a generation of women in the professions whose men had been killed in the trenches; girls' schools - and there were very few coeducational schools - were staffed entirely by spinsters. The dying out of that generation and the new social outlook have completely altered the pattern of school staffing and the career pattern of women teachers. If the same sense of historical perspective is applied, we can appreciate the immense development in numbers and of opportunities to practise for women medical graduates. Many women do have a clearer comprehension of values in their own lives, and in their contribution to the community, than they are credited with by male enthusiasts and statistical jugglers. Some do not wish to become what Celia Oakley (1976b) calls 'type A, totally committed doctors. There are still a few men and more women who would never have chosen to pursue a career which demands total commitment for many years' and, 'many regard school clinics and family planning work as being nearer to real medicine than psychiatry or community health, now set on pinnacles'.

It is useful to try to identify some of the problems common to all women professionals who want to combine the duties and pleasures of maternal and marital commitments with the self-fulfilment and obligations to the community that their independent work entails. The reasons for minimal performance may be a combination of many factors: a natural urge to care for children; the still mainly inflexible career structure of the N.H.S., with insistence on full-time or resident experience for specialist examination eligibility; and the disapproval of husbands. A W.H.O. Conference (1968) on Methods of Estimating Health Manpower stressed, 'the necessity to evaluate social value systems which differ even across West European countries' and noted that, 'the Commissie Opvoering Productiviteit found in the Netherlands that the majority of men were opposed to the full-time employment of married women'.

There are also financial considerations. During the B.M.A. Conference on Medical Manpower Celia Oakley observed that, 'punitive general taxation and the recent introduction of separate tax assessment for married women have already partly solved the problem' (Oakley, 1976). Indeed, most women nowadays have to work to contribute to the family budget and, since the improvement of remuneration for junior doctors, women practitioners have found it feasible to make a profit rather than just breaking even, or showing a loss, after domestic help, car and other expenses have been paid.

Arie (1976) said, 'We are all part-timers now - gone is the 24 hours a day, seven days a week personal service of the G.P., and gone is the full-time commitment of the hospital doctor'. This should make easier the arrangement of part-time posts for married women, but some specialties do not lend themselves readily to less than full-time commitment. Oakley (1976b) advocated that G.P. principalships should be available to part-timers whose training merited them, but felt that, 'Part-time specialist medicine is quite another story. Talk of part-time training programmes is very topical but quite unrealistic for most disciplines. This seems obvious. How would the surgeon become skilled? Could the physician keep abreast let alone learn as fast as the subject is expanding? Responsibility in medicine means more than lack of irresponsibility in patient care. It means having a conscience to keep abreast with progress and a conscience to advance the subject'. She observed that even 'successful' women do not feature on committees - of 560 members of Royal Colleges' Committees, central policy committees and the G.M.C. only 3% were women. Likewise, Sir

Stanley Clayton (1975) said at the Sunningdale Conference, 'part-time posts in surgery and obstetrics, in which manual skills have to be developed, are impracticable. Some psychiatrists have spoken highly of this - but while several people may explore the psyche of one patient, only one can explore the abdomen'. It is apparent, therefore, that some specialties are more demanding in this respect than others, and the less than ruthlessly determined woman will probably opt for one of the 'shortage' specialties. For example women manage so well in anaesthetics, taking on increasing workloads as their domestic responsibilities permit, that there is talk of it becoming a 'female' specialty.

Hence, the discussion naturally leads to consideration of the career structure, to the provision of supernumerary posts in the training grades and to the establishment of a two-tier career-grade system of 'specialists' and 'senior-specialists' or 'consultants'. In a letter to the B.M.J., Helen Sutton (1976) said, 'clinical assistant posts bypass the cumbersome machinery of established training posts but these doctors do senior registrar or consultant work', and 'the present clinical assistant posts carry neither status nor independent clinical responsibility'. Celia Oakley further commented, 'The less than fully committed man or woman doctor would be professionally fulfilled and have the pressures removed by a structure which allowed for part-time or full-time appointments outside the rat race' and therefore 'some posts need to be less demanding than others in terms of hours on call, the academic standard which is required to be attained and maintained, and the competition for vacant posts' (Oakley, 1976b). George Dick's view was that the establishment of a specialist grade would allow for greater flexibility, bring us in line with E.E.C. requirements and 'dispense with the need for clinical assistant, medical assistant and the proposed hospital practitioner grades - this would solve the problems of many doctors, including those with domestic ties, who have undergone retraining, and by whom consultant posts are often difficult to obtain' (Dick, 1977). Hastings (1977) supported the case for an altered career structure with a two-tier specialist and consultant system: "Why do we believe that consultants should be a minority elite, supported by a hierarchy of junior staff? What is wrong with the European concept of a health service staffed by specialists and G.P.s, with everyone else in training? But 'specialist' is just a new name for a sub-consultant grade, it will be argued; and the answer is yes, it will be a grade below consultant, but one with status and clinical responsibility. Moreover, I envisage many (if not most) of the career specialist posts being occupied by women doctors who acquired their specialist training part-time while having children, and many of them will work part-time for the whole of their careers'. Brocklehurst (1976) questioned 'whether hospital doctors really need to be supported by junior staff - in many American hospitals for instance there are no juniors'. Many women are comparatively immobile because of the geographical commitment of their husbands to places of work; they could contribute to the work of hospitals staffed essentially by specialists and consultants, without dependence on a constant, obligatory flow of junior doctors as 'trainees'.

Jean Lawrie (1976), as President of the Medical Women's Federation, wrote, 'Postgraduate medical training is only available through jobs in the N.H.S. There is therefore a special obligation on those who administer and finance the N.H.S. to make sure that those U.K. graduates who seek training can obtain it'. The D.H.S.S. issued a memorandum in July 1972 entitled 'Women Doctors Retainer Scheme' 'designed to help women doctors to maintain their professional training and skills during the years when they could not undertake a full-time or even an ordinary part-time post'.

A minimum commitment of seven 'education' sessions and 12 paid 'service' sessions was stipulated and a £75 grant given to cover the expenses of registration, membership of a medical defence organisation and subscription to a professional journal. The response was poor. Clark (1976) found in the North West Thames Region that only 11 out of 270 non-practising doctors had applied; Eskin (1974), in the Sheffield Region, found 'out of a total of 120 women doctors known to be unemployed only 8.3% made enquiries about the scheme'; and Henryk-Gutt and Silverstone (1976) reported that there were only 208 women doctors in the scheme altogether.

The D.H.S.S. 'Retainer Scheme' was meant to complement the 1969 Retraining Scheme: 'the Secretary of State considers that all reasonable steps should be taken to reduce this waste of medical manpower' (having found in 1965 that 28% of women doctors compared with 3% of men doctors under 65 were not working). The Retraining Scheme authorised the creation of supernumerary and part-time posts, but again its success has not been marked. The delays in processing applications, which were sometimes up to a year, became notorious, and if the doctor had to move for domestic reasons the application had to be negotiated entirely afresh. To add insult to injury the end result of the prolonged negotiations, in some cases, was a discovery that funds were not available to implement the post. Arie (1976) reported that between 1969-75 only 185 part-time registrar and 128 senior registrar posts were established. Henryk-Gutt and Silverstone (1976) commented that the splitting of existing posts was a little-used option as these were difficult to fill; and, 'the supernumerary doctors did not feel they were part of a team, their contribution did not seem important, and they were excluded from certain aspects of work. Also male colleagues felt women had an unfair advantage as they did not have to compete for posts'. In its Evidence to the Royal Commission, the Association of Anaesthetists echoed this comment: 'making exceptions for women is not a satisfactory solution; it introduces the need for 'definitions' of family responsibilities: with the implications for private practice opportunities under the existing contract arrangements it creates resentment in men who would also like a part-time contract'. They called for 'greater flexibility in contracts, as whole or maximum part-time are impracticable for most married women'. A further paper published by the Central Manpower Committee (1975) concluded that, 'a national review of training facilities would be needed', that 'lady doctors may have to accept that only the less popular hospital specialties will be open to them', and that, 'most lady doctors will enter fields which do not require long periods of training, e.g. general practice and some areas of consultant medicine, e.g. family planning, school doctors'. These facts of life women doctors had already discovered for themselves.

The next D.H.S.S. initiative was a Conference at Sunningdale in July 1975 entitled 'Women in Medicine', 'to take a fresh look at the position of women in the profession', since as Mrs. Barbara Castle said, 'the sensible use of the talents of women doctors is an economic necessity'. This Conference was followed by a Draft Circular (D.H.S.S., 1976) which asked again for encouragement of all doctors to complete pre-registration training, use of the Doctor Retainer Scheme, re-entry courses, training on a part-time basis, establishment of part-time career posts, planning of needs and opportunities in general practice, and continued career counselling and guidance. The accelerated establishment of Regional Counsellors was advised - one of whom, Dr. Mary Duguid from the Mersey Regional Health Authority said at Sunningdale: 'The D.H.S.S. and the Colleges who are so anxious about future staffing should try to look upon women doctors as their equivalent of the North Sea Oil - the foreign oil is beginning to dry up. The home produce is a little more expensive and difficult to get into use at first, but investment will finally pay off in a more satis-factory solution of manpower problems'.

Several regional schemes have been independently launched in recent years - of which perhaps the best known is Dr. Rosemary Rue's in Oxford, where, in 1975, 122 women were in part-time training (Rue, 1975). Dr. Rue identified the groups of unemployed women doctors as those who married and had a child immediately after qualifying, part-timers unsuitably em-ployed, and those who had been out of work for a long period. She comm-ented that the value of retraining schemes was that 'once involved then the appetite is whetted for further work'. Yet in a report of the results of the training scheme from 1973 to 1975 we find that while 15 women had attained clinical assistant posts only one had become a consultant, and it is difficult to avoid the thought that this may have happened in the natural course of events. Peter Clark (1976), Consultant Pathologist at Barnet General Hospital, ran a very successful one year clinical intro-ductory course in the North West Thames Region and found 'need for a pro-per register of married women doctors' if contact was to be maintained. Essex-Lopresti, in 1970, also reported success in a scheme for recruiting women doctors in the South West Metropolitan Region.

Individual schemes must be regarded as helpful, and the D.H.S.S. has provided a framework intended to help recruitment in this field, yet the results cannot be judged satisfactory. This is, no doubt, partly because eager planners want instantaneous results, and lose a sense of perspective; they should rather acknowledge the scale and pace of the changes which have occurred over the past quarter of a century. It is also partly be-cause women do not wish to be cajoled or bludgeoned into returning to work; as Sir Stanley Clayton (1975) said at Sunningdale, 'one is tempted to ask if women are really so frustrated. The doctors who have chosen domesticity talk least about the problem and I doubt whether you will tempt more than a proportion of them back'. And their instincts may well prove right. Once panic about a manpower crisis has subsided the cry for women doctors to return to work may become a little more subdued. Even while the panic lasts there will be cynics who see the entry of more women into the medical schools as a convenient future means of 'losing' surplus doctors and shielding the male practitioners from unemployment.

A comparison might again be drawn with the history of the teaching profession, in that the employment of women doctors will no doubt in part be sensitive to the law of demand. In 1957 Willink wrote, 'it is clearly important to ensure that the number of new recruits entering medicine is sufficient but not in excess of requirements at a time when expanding de-mands upon the limited pool of suitable young men and women are being made by other professions especially teaching, science and engineering'. In the fifties a shortage of teachers, to deal with the 'post-war bulge' and the rising birth-rate, was anticipated by the D.E.S., so training grants were given to students who promised to teach for at least five years; married women were enticed back with favourable part-time teaching arrange-ments and equal pay. Now, with the discovery that 'the Department has got its figures wrong again', recently established and expanded teacher train-ing colleges are being closed, and there are said to be 10,000 surplus newly-qualified teachers unemployed. It goes without saying that part-time and married women teachers can be dispensed with; their claims to employment are conveniently placed below those of men with a family to maintain and a career to establish, and of young newly-qualified teachers who would otherwise swell the Government numbers of unemployed. Perhaps all is a question of timing: the Regional Medical Officers, in evidence to

the Royal Commission, made the point, 'if an increase in the percentage
of women medical students led to a reduction in "doctor availability" the
effect would be limited to the junior grades initially since it would be
a long time before any significant influence was felt on career grades in
a predominantly male work-force of 70,000'. And, by then, who knows? We
may have a logical and satisfying career structure, a rationally reorganised system of training and of regional hospital staffing, a common-sense
administrative framework, and an independent institute of manpower planning producing accurate and up-to-date information.

REFERENCES

Aird, L.A. & Silver, P.H.S. (1971) Women doctors from the Middlesex Hos-
    pital Medical School 1947-67. *British Journal of Medical Education,*
    5, 232-241.
Arie, T. (1976) A new deal for half our doctors? *Lancet,* 2, 1073-1075.
Bewley, B.R. & Bewley, T.H. (1975) Hospital doctors' career structure and
    misuse of medical womanpower. *Lancet,* 2, 270-272.
Bhatt, R.V., Soni, J.M. & Patel, N.F. (1976) Performance of women medical
    graduates from Medical College, Baroda, 1949-74. *Medical Education,*
    10, 293-296.
Brocklehurst, J.C. (1976) Expansion of the medical schools. *British Medi-
    cal Journal,* 2, 1390-1391.
Central Manpower Committee (1975) *Women Doctors.* Paper by the D.H.S.S.
    CMC/1/75/1.
Clack, G.B., Pettingale, K.W., Ryan, K.C. & Tomlinson, R.W.S. (1976) A
    study of women students at King's College Hospital Medical School.
    Medical Education, 10, 450-455.
Clark, P.A. (1976) Medical Manpower II - Women in medicine. *British Medi-
    cal Journal,* 1, 78-82.
Clayton, S. (1975) The problem of part-time training. In *Women in Medi-
    cine.* Conference organised by the D.H.S.S., 4-5 July.
D.H.S.S. (1972) *Women Doctors' Retainer Scheme.* H.M.(72)42.
D.H.S.S. (1976) *Women in Medicine: Improving opportunities for doctors
    with domestic commitments to practise in the N.H.S.* London: D.H.S.S.
Dick, G. (1977) A 'specialist' grade. *British Medical Journal,* 1, 53.
Dube, W.F. (1973) Women students in U.S. medical schools; past and present
    trends. *Journal of Medical Education,* 48, 186-189.
Editorial (1974) Women in medicine. *British Medical Journal,* 3, 590-591.
Eskin, F. (1972) A survey of medical women in Lincolnshire 1971. *British
    Journal of Medical Education,* 6, 196-200.
Eskin, F. (1974) Review of the women doctors' retainer scheme in the
    Sheffield Region 1972-73. *British Journal of Medical Education,* 8,
    141-144.
Eskin, F. (1976) Comparison of employment status of women medical gradu-
    ates and women science graduates, University of Sheffield 1960-65.
    Medical Education, 10, 456-462.
Essex-Lopresti, M. (1970) Recruitment of women doctors for hospital ser-
    vice. *Lancet,* 2, 204-206.
Flynn, C.A. & Gardner, F. (1969) The careers of women graduates from the
    Royal Free Hospital School of Medicine, London. *British Journal of
    Medical Education,* 3, 28-42.
Forster, D.P. (1975) Misuse of medical womanpower. *Lancet,* 2, 818.

Fruen, M.A., Rothman, A.I. & Steiner, J.W. (1974) Comparison of character-
     istics of male and female medical school applicants. *Journal of Medi-
     cal Education*, 49, 137-145.
Goodenough Report (1944) *Report of the Inter-Departmental Committee on
     Medical Schools*. London: H.M.S.O.
Hastings, C. (1977) Open letter to the Chairman of the B.M.A. Council.
     British Medical Journal, 1, 181.
Henryk-Gutt, R. & Silverstone, R. (1976) Career problems of women doctors.
     British Medical Journal, 2, 574-577.
Jefferys, M. & Elliott, P.M. (1966) *Women in Medicine*. London: Office of
     Health Economics.
Jefferys, M., Gauvain, S. & Gulesen, O. (1965) Comparison of men and wom-
     en in medical training. *Lancet*, 1, 1381-1383.
Judek, S. (1964) *Medical Manpower in Canada*. Ottawa: The Queen's Printer.
Kahan, J. & Mac Faul, N. (1962) Middlesex women graduates, 1947-61.
     Middlesex Hospital Journal, 62, 192-194.
Kissick, W.L. (1964) Current status of medical education in the U.S.S.R.
     Journal of Medical Education, 39, 1069-1077.
Lawrie, J.E. (1976) A new deal for half our doctors? *Lancet*, 2, 1356.
Lawrie, J.E. & Newhouse, M.L. (1965) Working women doctors. *British Medi-
     cal Journal*, 1, 524.
Lawrie, J.E., Newhouse, M.L. & Elliott, P.M. (1966) Working capacity of
     women doctors. *British Medical Journal*, 1, 409-412.
Lopate, C. (1968) *Women in Medicine*. Baltimore: The John Hopkins Press.
Macdonald, E.M. & Webb, E.M. (1966) A survey of women physicians in
     Canada, 1883-1964. *Canadian Medical Association Journal*, 94, 1223-
     1227.
Nelson-Jones, R. & Fish, D.G. (1970) Women students in Canadian medical
     schools. *British Journal of Medical Education*, 4, 97-108.
Oakley, C. (1976) Medical Manpower II - Women in medicine. *British Medi-
     cal Journal*, 1, 78-82.
Oakley, C. (1976b) Pressures of work on doctors and family. *British Medi-
     cal Journal*, 2, 541-542.
Regional Medical Officers' Evidence to the Royal Commission (1976) *Medi-
     cal Manpower in the N.H.S.* Memo of evidence from the R.M.O.s of the
     Regional Health Authorities, England.
Robb-Smith, A.H.T. (1962) The fate of Oxford medical women. *Lancet*, 2,
     1158-1161.
Rue, R. (1967) Employment of married women doctors in hospitals in the
     Oxford Region. *Lancet*, 1, 1267-1268.
Rue, R. (1975) Organization and service problems. In *Women in Medicine*.
     Conference organised by the D.H.S.S., 4-5 July.
Shore, E. (1974) Medical manpower planning. *Health Trends*, 6, 32-35.
Stanley, G.R. & Last, J.M. (1968) Careers of young medical women. *British
     Journal of Medical Education*, 2, 204-209.
Steppacher, R.C. & Mausner, J.S. (1974) Suicide in male and female physi-
     cians. *Journal of the American Medical Association*, 228, 323-328.
Sutton, H. (1976) A new deal for half our doctors? *Lancet*, 2, 1201-1202.
Timbury, M.C. & Ratzer, M.A. (1969) Glasgow medical women 1951-54: their
     contribution and attitude to medical work. *British Medical Journal*,
     2, 372-374.
U.C.C.A. (1976) *Thirteenth Report, 1974-75*. Cheltenham: Universities Cen-
     tral Council on Admissions.
Ulyatt, K. & Ulyatt, F.M. (1971) Some attitudes of a group of women doc-
     tors related to their field performance. *British Journal of Medical
     Education*, 5, 242-245.

Ulyatt, K. & Ulyatt, F.M. (1973) Attitudes of women medical students compared with those of women doctors. *British Journal of Medical Education*, 7, 152-154.

Whitfield, A.G.W. (1969) Women medical graduates of the University of Birmingham 1959-63. *British Medical Journal*, 3, 44-46.

W.H.O. (1968) *Methods of Estimating Health Manpower*. Report on a Symposium held in Budapest, 15-19 October. Geneva: World Health Organization.

W.H.O. (1974) *Health Statistics Annual Report 1973*. Vol. iii. Copenhagen: World Health Organization.

Willink Report (1957) *Report of the Committee to consider the future numbers of medical practitioners and the appropriate intake of medical students*. London: H.M.S.O.

6. Career Choice

'if to do were as easy as to know what were good to do' wrote Shakespeare, 'chapels had been churches, and poor men's cottages princes' palaces'. The same difficulty faces the young doctor when deciding his choice of career, and the problem is compounded by his lack of knowledge concerning the bewildering number of possibilities open to him. As Martin and Boddy (1962) said 'Medicine is probably unique among the professions in the range of opportunities that it offers to its graduates. The qualified medical practitioner may pursue his career in the hospital ward, in the laboratory, or in the community. He may assume the variegated responsibilities of the general practitioner, or elect specialist training in fields which range from anaesthetics to psychiatry, from thoracic surgery to pathology. He may devote himself wholly to clinical practice or give varying parts of his time to teaching and research'. Faced with such a complex variety of choices (about some of which he will know very little) it is not surprising that the medical school applicant who could state confidently 'I have always wanted to become a doctor', a few years later when asking himself what <u>sort</u> of doctor he wants to become, is often irresolute and baffled. Martin and Boddy go on: 'The processes that lead to a final career decision, in which personal preference (itself a product of a number of influences), estimates of one's own abilities in relation to the supposed difficulty or competitiveness of particular specialties, and probably entirely fortuitous events, interact, are fairly complex'.

Career choice starts in school, where 'self' and 'pre' selection is fairly rigorously enforced by the necessity to achieve a high academic level in the relevant A Levels. As Roger Ellis of Marlborough College (1977) said, 'many more want to become doctors than there is room for in our medical schools', and this seems intuitively to be a good reason for expansion on the principle often expressed by politicians that higher education should be freely available to those who want it and can benefit from it; although Hirsch (1977) has said, 'People abroad were amazed at the naivety of the Robbins expansion, with its built-in failure to make a distinction between what is possible for the individual and possible for society at large'. A registrar from London, Dr. Olsen (*The Times*, 1976) observed, 'there is a spectre of mass medical unemployment .... some doctors might be forced into unacceptable occupations, even taking on the work of hospital porters'. This, were it to become a reality, would certainly obviate the necessity of 'career choice' for those concerned, although the author did not seem to have considered possible objections from the relevant Unions!

82

The real issue is the conflict between the philosophy that a university education, being by definition something much more than a vocational training, should be available to those whose academic record and potential may be said to merit it, and the more material view that numbers of professional trainees must be controlled. If we truely believe in 'The Idea of a University', then there must be a place somewhere for those who want to study medicine as an academic discipline in its own right, who may have no formed intention of a specific career in relation to this and who are willing to risk unemployment or 'diversification'. If the price we pay for state-aided medical training and near-monopoly government employment of its products is a loss of this Idea, then ultimately it may be a high price indeed. But we shall need to know where we stand on this point, to make manpower plans and to determine our attitude to 'early career choice'.

Of the selection of medical students, Sir Cyril Clarke (1977) said, 'I would plump for the parson's child - public spirited, well disciplined and accustomed to relative poverty'. Perhaps unfortunately, Deans have to be more realistic, and to quote 'Scrutator' (1977), 'Deans are unhappy at turning down enthusiastic idealistic school leavers simply on their A Levels, but with so many good applicants, they say, how else can they choose? We do know that A level scores correlate with pass rates in subsequent examinations. But are we so certain the academic training we provide will turn out the sort of doctors we may need in the 1980's'. There was a plea for 'far more variation in courses offered by different universities'; this is a valuable suggestion, and it is virtually certain that the pattern of subjects offered for study and the relative importance assigned to each in the medical school curriculum has a considerable influence on the many primary choices of career, at least. This is when the 'pecking order' of the medical hierarchy becomes first visible, although it is interesting to note how it can be manipulated - general practice, instead of being the fate of those who 'fell off the ladder', is now highly esteemed, and the proposed three year vocational training scheme will perhaps enhance its status further: less pressure of work, better conditions in Health Centres, higher remuneration plus extra payments, the possibility of hospital practitioner work, all combine to promote an attractive image.

The gaining of a place in medical school results from a combination of personal preference and high academic ability. Background factors, such as a medical tradition in the family, were undoubtedly of importance formerly, when personal contact with a particular medical school and an appreciation of the importance of rugby football formed pleasant links of continuity, and sons often followed fathers and grandfathers to the same teaching hospital and perhaps into the same specialty. Today the stern realities of A level grades, the availability of State maintenance grants and halls of residence, and the ambitions of career masters to search out prospective talent in their schools, mean that all would-be medical school entrants of both sexes tend to have an equal chance of success.

Entrants to medical school often hold preconceived ideas about specialties: surgeons may be regarded as autocratic, decisive and practical, physicians as intellectually broad-minded, paediatricians as kindly and approachable, psychiatrists as calm and detached (Becker et al, 1963; Zimny and Thale, 1970). There will also be developing ideas of the relative status and prosperity of different branches of medical practice; for instance, Martin, Mayo and McPherson (1967) found that first year medical students regarded general practitioners as being poorly paid and of low status. However, Dean (1972) and Martin and Boddy (1962) noted that interest shifted towards general practice during the undergraduate course.

Since that time other factors (see Chapter 2) have increased the attractiveness of general practice, and the British Hospital Doctors Federation (*The Guardian*, 1977) commented, 'doctors are turning their backs on a career in hospital medicine .... even surgery has ceased to attract British applicants .... young doctors can go into general practice and earn more money and have a life that gives more job staisfaction without constantly being under intolerable pressures'. An increasingly materialistic attitude to medical careers, with loss of early humanitarianism, has been noted during progress through the medical school (Eron, 1955; Becker et al, 1963), and Simpson (1972), who ably reviewed the psychological effects of the undergraduate course, referred ironically to the 'pre-cynical' and 'cynical' phases of the curriculum. It is perhaps not surprising that dreams of high idealism should be tarnished by contact with reality, but the 'cynicism' appears to be short-lived and to fade after graduation, particularly with some types of practice (Gray, Moody and Newman, 1965; Gray, Newman and Reinhardt, 1966).

Once the school leaver becomes a medical student, the factors influencing him, and his reactions to them during the next decade, will obviously determine the pattern of his life's work. The Honourable J.W. Fulbright (1975) in an Oxford address said, 'through the creative power of education we can expand the breadth and depth of human wisdom, sympathy and perception' and he quoted the Hazen Foundation Report (1977) 'Reconstituting the Human Community' - 'What each of us needs is a new moral vision capable of giving us at least some notion of where we may be going and some sense of the value of our place in the changing world in which we live'. Regrettably, these ideals may often seem irrelevant when the student is faced with the difficulties of absorbing a bewildering amount of factual knowledge and practical experience in a vast number of subjects; and those in which examinations have to be passed will of course, seem to be the most important. Yet those who plan the medical school curriculum must have a vision of the future and an awareness of the changing needs of society: 'the universities have a special responsibility. Medical men and women need education as well as training, and the universities need imagination and determination to meet a double challenge: to make and enlarge centres of excellence and exert their influence on continuing medical education which must show constant changes' (Vaughan, 1969). The responsibility lies with the educators to encourage and guide their students, pre and post-graduate since the division is artificial, so that they find professional fulfilment and satisfaction in their final choice of career.

An important pre-requisite in the medical school curriculum is the availability of factual knowledge about, and experience in, as wide a range of specialties as possible. Attention has been drawn to the lack of 'early exposure' of students to anaesthetics, radiology and pathology because of the low priority accorded in medical school curricula and examinations. It is sometimes difficult to interest or involve consultants in teaching students, especially in former non-teaching hospitals where there is a lack of tradition and frequently much overwork. Increased numbers of medical students require increased numbers of teachers, and if sufficient interested consultants cannot be found, and given enough time and support for their teaching activities, then compulsory attendance can only lead to further lack of interest in their specialties. The low level of patient contact in many less-popular specialties is worth noting; most future doctors want contact with patients as people, and preferably as people who can be cured. Patient management is often seen as 'positive' only if leading to cure; hence the relative unpopularity of geriatrics which is of necessity long-term and unproductive of any real 'cure', and psychiatry where 'cure' is often intermittent and unpredictable. These specialties suffer from the recruitment disadvantage of dealing with the old, the alcoholic, and the mentally and physically defective - the 'second-rate' or low-status members of the community.

Rosemary Hutt (1976), in a comprehensive review of career choice, wrote, 'the interest shown by researchers and policymakers has arisen in part from the problems of geographical and inter-specialty maldistribution which have persisted since the inception of the Health Service, and as plans for increasing the total numbers of British doctors are beginning to take effect, the attention of medical manpower planners may well be more sharply focused on ways of ensuring that this increased supply is used to the best possible advantage'. Those who work in the shortage specialties have sometimes offered their own remedies: 'the only solution to this intractable problem is to offer a cash incentive in the form of a higher differential salary scale for anyone concerned with geriatric medicine and to throw away the mythical distinction award and replace this with an automatic seniority award' (Datta, 1976). Mrs. Barbara Castle, as Secretary of State, by no means always rejected the idea of cash incentives to encourage doctors to work in shortage specialties or in unpopular locations. It must undoubtedly seem reasonable from the point of view of those responsible for staffing the N.H.S. that if undergraduate emphasis could be laid on unpopular specialties, and means found of 'directing' doctors to understaffed regions then many problems would be solved. It would also, at least partially, solve the emigration problem if all graduates had to undertake to work a specified number of years in this country as a return for their medical training, as might be feasible with a system of student loans rather than grants.

But the dangers are real: 'Already almost a monopoly employer of doctors in Britain, the State will be only too eager to become the monopoly educator also. Academic freedom in medicine is rather a nebulous term and in one country or another is being encroached on by the State - but there must be freedom to reward success so that areas of excellence will flourish and will expose mediocrity. State control carries many advantages to the community and the profession, provided decisions are based on knowledge and good judgement rather than on political expediency, and providing the incentives to personal efficiency are maintained, and the hazards of uniformity are avoided' (Christie, 1969). And commenting on the American scene, *The Times Higher Education Supplement* (1976) said, 'medical education in the United States is under public scrutiny as never before ..... attempts (by Congress) to reform the pattern of medical training to improve the uneven distribution of specialists and increase the number of general practitioners by setting quotas ran into strong opposition ..... from the medical schools (who) enlisted some of the weightiest figures in the academic world to protest against 'unwarranted interference with the academic decisions of the schools'''. The Mayo Foundation Annual Report (Mayo, 1976) provides an example of this reaction: 'Increasing governmental regulation of medical practice could seriously limit medical centers such as Mayo through geographical restrictions on service to patients, stipulations as to the numbers and kinds of specialists trained, and curtailment of the patient care activities of physicians who must devote time to implementing federally-mandated programs'.

Indirect influences are a different matter. The constant struggle to improve conditions in shortage specialties and unpopular regions and the voluntary enlistment of medical schools and their graduates in development and incentive-based schemes has surely much to offer. A strong pull is both more effective and more acceptable than a clumsy push. Just as high quality medicine as a whole cannot survive by strangling private practice in order to give monopoly to a State system which can be as bad as it likes, but only by creating a Health Service good enough eventually to compete with what the private sector is able to offer, so the future salvation of the 'shortage' specialties must come not through direction of labour but primarily through increased attractiveness.

The influences during medical school and early postgraduate training which determine the ultimate decision of career choice may be fortuitous. The influence of senior staff members was noted by Coker et al (1960), particularly in the case of bright students who tend to be given special attention (Last, Martin and Stanley, 1967). Undoubtedly, the help and interest of a senior member of staff has sometimes illuminated a particular specialty; the enthusiasm of a fellow-student has often proved contagious so that one particular year in one particular medical school has produced an outstanding number of trainees in one or another field; but of paramount importance is self-appraisal and the acknowledgement of a need for continuing self-education. This relates not only to initial career choice - the assessment of personal qualities and aptitudes against practicalities and prospects - but to the open-mindedness that is needed to respond to the changes in medical careers that time and progress will require: 'A doctor must learn throughout his working life, not simply to keep abreast of the growth of medical knowledge but also to cope with the gradual changes in the patterns of practice and in the expectations of patients ..... At present there is little likelihood that many doctors will review their own performances carefully and critically to determine their educational needs. Such action requires a change in attitude, which will not occur spontaneously and will not result from exhortations, whether from "super docs" or from the D.H.S.S. Attitudes of this kind need to be vigorously promoted and their seeds must be sown as early as possible. It is in our medical schools that the process must begin. Students must learn to recognise the limitations of their own knowledge and abilities, and to admit their areas of ignorance. The attitudes which they develop to independent learning must ensure continuing self-education so that they can adapt to the constant changes in medical practice. At present we do not promote these qualities in our students: this is the greatest indictment of our present system of medical education' (Editorial, 1976).

Of equal importance to medical school training is the availability of good postgraduate programmes and advice. The Christ Church Conference (Nuffield Provincial Hospitals Trust, 1962) gave a vital lead by recognising the importance of giving all doctors advice and training in their chosen specialties, not only in junior posts but as a continuing process throughout their careers. Since then much valuable work has been done to different degrees across the country by Postgraduate Deans and Postgraduate Councils, especially in Scotland and Ireland. But many problems remain, especially for women graduates and overseas doctors, and many opportunities for recruitment and stimulation of enthusiasm are lost. It might indeed be said of the Todd Report, as The Times Higher Education Supplement (Cullingford, 1977) said of the James Report, 'it is both sad and worrying to find that arguments for the improvement of the training of students buckle under falsely remembered principles and snap under the pressure of administrative convenience'.

Since the inception of the N.H.S. a number of studies on career choice have been carried out, on a general basis, in individual medical schools and by sending biennial questionnaires to graduates of British medical schools first contacted during their pre-registration year (Parkhouse, 1976, and further studies to be published). A survey of all senior registrars

in 1975 (Parkhouse et al, in preparation) should give a general picture
of preferences, causes of change and final decisions in career choice.
Other work is in progress (Hutt, 1976). The Association for the Study of
Medical Education carried out a survey of final year medical students for
the Todd Report (1968); they found that students from rural areas tended
to favour general practice, that women preferred (perhaps of necessity)
general practice and public health, married students showed a greater preference for medical science and research, children of medically qualified
parents more often chose anaesthetics and surgery. Other studies of career preferences at the undergraduate stage have been reported (e.g. Martin
and Boddy, 1962; the Ogstons, 1970 and 1971; Geertsma and Grinolis, 1972).
Oates and Feldman (1971) found that the career choices of students at the
State University of New York Upstate Medical Center had changed considerably between 1967/68 and 1972, family practice and internal medicine having
gained in popularity while interest in all other specialties had declined.
Most of these findings derived from medical students are of limited value;
this has been pointed out in relation to career preferences expressed at
the pre-registration stage (McLaughlin and Parkhouse, 1972, 1974; Parkhouse
and McLaughlin, 1975, 1976; Parkhouse and Palmer, 1977). These studies
showed that only about 30% of graduates had made a definite career choice
by the time they neared the end of the pre-registration year. There were
marked differences in the pattern of choices between medical schools, and
from one year to another even among the graduates of the same medical school.
Subsequent enquiry only two or three years later reveals a considerable
number of changes of career choice (Parkhouse, 1976, and further studies to
be published). Similarly, Last and Stanley (1968) noted an increased diffusion of career choices after graduation compared to those expressed at the
undergraduate stage, although preferences for general practice and surgery
appeared to be better sustained than others. Stanley and Last (1968) found
that 69% of single men, but only 46% of married men intended to work towards
a career in a hospital specialty. There is no doubt that in many cases marriage is the ultimate determining factor in career choice and particularly
so for women doctors.
      Sir Derrick Dunlop (1975) said in addressing the first Nottingham
medical graduates 'the catholic mantle of a medical qualification, provided
we don it right, can be made to fit all our tastes, talents and idiosyncras-
ies'. Doctors can specialise, 'journalise' or enter politics; 'if we love
the human race we can become family practitioners; if we hate it, morbid
anatomists'. Naturally enough, studies have been made of personality in relation to career choice, for example by Walton (1966, 1967, 1969) in Edinburgh
and others. Although attempts at prediction on the basis of vocational interest scales have been relatively unrewarding (Athelstan and Paul, 1971),
there is evidence of the kind of association between personality and preferred type of medical work that commonsense and general experience would
suggest (for references see Hutt, 1976).
      In a descriptive sense, the external factors influencing career choice
are fairly self-evident. Financial considerations apply in regard to the
improved position of general practice, and in the varying opportunities
for private practice and for obtaining distinction awards in different
hospital specialties. Although the distribution of distinction awards is
considerably more even than it was only a few years ago, there are still
many holders of these rewards, particularly at the higher level, in the
'prestige' specialties. There are differences in promotion prospects between specialties, and difficulty here may lead either to a change of
career intention, or simply to emigration. Surgery tends to be a particularly firm specialty choice, often decided upon at or even before the beginning of the undergraduate course and adhered to inspite of strong com-

petition for senior posts; hence, perhaps not surprisingly, Last (1967) found a high proportion of surgeons among emigrants. Conditions and location of work are important, and it is no surprise that psychiatric and geriatric units fare badly in comparison to teaching hospitals in close proximity to university departments and other academic facilities. There are also the intrinsic differences between 'people' orientated specialties and those concerned with laboratory or statistical work, between positive curing and amelioration, between preventive medicine and the treating of the already ill - although in many cases there is bound to be overlapping so that one choice will include many of these possibilities.

What is less clear is the extent to which these various factors operate, in different circumstances and among different groups of doctors. Although many studies have been made it is difficult to obtain a comprehensive picture which is sufficiently up-to-date to be of value. As with the analysis of supposed 'trends' in general (see Chapter 8) there is ample experience to show how quickly a change in a single factor - the price of housing and availability of mortgages, or improved remuneration in general practice - can alter the extent to which doctors are willing to move in pursuit of training or hang on to the hope of an eventual consultant appointment during many years of hospital training. Information about the factors determining choice of career, if it is to be genuinely useful, must be sufficiently rapidly produced and brought up to date often enough to be responsive to these effects. Lawson and Simons (1976), studying the careers of men graduates from the Royal Free Hospital, remarked, 'for the location of the work there was a marked aversion to large provincial communities, London, South and South West England being favoured'. This is a view among only one group of graduates, and the apparent enthusiasm for work in London would not be supported by other comments. It is also likely that the greatly expanded intake of many of the provincial medical schools, which brings in many young men and women with considerable pride in the surrounding communities from which they come, will do something to ameliorate the recruitment problems of these areas.

Perhaps there will always be a 'pecking order' in the status and remuneration of various specialties, and, within these specialties, of different localities. But the increasing output of British graduates, with its greater diffusion across the country, and the diminishing opportunities for emigration to some formerly attractive places, may well mean that the problems of the present 'shortage specialties' will diminish. Further efforts are still needed to look at the attractiveness and the working conditions of different specialties, and improve them where necessary, to reduce inequalities between and within regions, to disseminate accurate information about available career choices at an early stage and to provide a counselling service, where needed, at both pre- and postgraduate levels.

REFERENCES

Athelstan, G.T. & Paul, G.J. (1971) New approach to the prediction of medical specialization: student-based strong vocational interest blank scales. *Journal of Applied Psychology*, 55, 80-86.

Becker, H.S., Geer, B., Hughes, E.C. & Strauss, A.L. (1963) *Boys in White: Student Culture in Medical School*. Chicago: University of Chicago Press.

Christie, R. (1969) Medical education and the State. *British Medical Journal*, 2, 385-390.

Clarke, C.A. (1977) Wrong ways to choose right medics. *Times Higher Education Supplement*, 21 January.

Coker, R.E., Back, K.W., Donnelly, T.G. & Miller, N. (1960) Patterns of influence: medical school faculty members and the values and specialty interests of medical students. 35, 518-527.

Cullingford, C. (1977) Whatever happened to the James Report? *Times Higher Education Supplement*, 8 April.

Datta, S.B. (1976) Careers in geriatrics. *British Medical Journal*, 2, 883.

Dean, T.M. (1972) Attitudes of medical students towards general practice. *British Journal of Medical Education*, 6, 108-113.

Dunlop, Sir Derrick (1975) *University of Nottingham Gazette*, No. 86, September.

Editorial (1976) Getting postgraduate education right. *British Medical Journal*, 1, 116.

Ellis, R. (1977) Doctor manpower (correspondence). *The Times*, 23 March.

Eron, L.D. (1955) The effect of medical education on medical students' attitudes. *Journal of Medical Education*, 30, 559-566.

Fulbright, J.W. (1975) *Fifty Years On*. R.B. McCallum Memorial Lecture, Pembroke College, Oxford, 24 October.

Geertsma, R.H. & Grinols, D.R. (1972) Specialty choice in medicine. *Journal of Medical Education*, 47, 509-517.

Gray, R.M., Moody, P.M. & Newman, W.R.E. (1965) An analysis of physicians' attitudes of cynicism and humanitarianism before and after entering medical practice. *Journal of Medical Education*, 40, 760-766.

Gray, R.M., Newman, W.R.E. & Reinhardt, A.M. (1966) The effect of medical specialization on physicians' attitudes. *Journal of Health and Human Behaviour*, 7, 128-132.

The Guardian (1977) Doctors are shunning hospitals, 16 February.

Hazen Foundation Report (1977) *Reconstituting the Human Community*. Connecticut: Hazen Foundation of New Haven.

Hirsch, F. (1977) *The Social Limits to Growth*. London: Routledge & Kegan Paul.

Hutt, R. (1976) Doctors' career choice: previous research and its relevance for policy-making. *Medical Education*, 10, 463-473.

Last, J.M. (1967) Overseas movement of British doctors. *Social and Economic Administration*, 1, 4, 20-28.

Last, J.M., Martin, F.M. & Stanley, G.R. (1967) Academic record and subsequent career. *Proceedings of the Royal Society of Medicine*, 60, 813-816.

Last, J.M. & Stanley, G.R. (1968) Career preferences of young British doctors. *British Journal of Medical Education*, 2, 137-155.

Lawson, A. & Simons, H.A.B. (1976) The careers of men graduates from the Royal Free Hospital School of Medicine, London. *Medical Education*, 10, 348-358.

Martin, F.M. & Boddy, F.A. (1962) Career preferences of medical students. *Sociological Review Monograph*, 5, 21-32.

Martin, F.M., Mayo, P.R. & McPherson, F.M. (1967) Professional stereotypes of first-year medical students. *British Journal of Medical Education*, 1, 368-373.

Mayo (1976) Annual Report of the Mayo Foundation, Rochester, Minnesota, p.13.

McLaughlin, C. & Parkhouse, J. (1972) Career preferences of 1971 graduates of two British medical schools. *Lancet*, 2, 1018-1020.

McLaughlin, C. & Parkhouse, J. (1974) Career preferences. *Lancet*, 1, 870-871.

Nuffield Provincial Hospitals Trust (1962) Conference on postgraduate medical education. *British Medical Journal,* 1, 466-467.

Oates, R.P. & Feldman, H.A. (1971) Medical career patterns: choices among several classes of medical students. *New York State Journal of Medicine,* 71, 2437-2440.

Ogston, D. & Ogston, W.G. (1971) Honours graduates in medicine of the University of Aberdeen 1931-60. *British Journal of Medical Education,* 5, 30-33.

Ogston, D., Ogston, W.G. & Ogston, C.M. (1970) Origin and employment of the medical graduates of the University of Aberdeen 1931-69. *British Medical Journal,* 4, 360-361.

Parkhouse, J. (1976) A follow-up of career preferences. *Medical Education,* 10, 480-482.

Parkhouse, J. & McLaughlin, C. (1975) Career preferences of 1973 graduates. *Lancet,* 1, 1342.

Parkhouse, J. & McLaughlin, C. (1976) Career preferences of doctors graduating in 1974. *British Medical Journal,* 2, 630-632.

Parkhouse, J. & Palmer, M.K. (1977) Career preferences of doctors qualifying in 1975. *British Medical Journal,* 2, 25-27.

Scrutator (1977) The week. *British Medical Journal,* 2, 711.

Simpson, M.A. (1972) *Medical Education: A Critical Approach.* London: Butterworths, 62-66.

Stanley, G.R. & Last, J.M. (1968) Careers of young medical women. *British Journal of Medical Education,* 2, 204-209.

The Times (1976) Warning of jobs threat to doctors, 29 March.

Times Higher Education Supplement (1976) Medical schools: cutting out the dead wood, 3 December.

Todd Report (1968) *Royal Commission on Medical Education.* Cmnd. 3569. London: H.M.S.O.

Vaughan, J. (1969) The future of postgraduate medical education. *Lancet,* 2, 995-999.

Walton, H.J. (1966) Differences between physically-minded and psychologically-minded medical practitioners. *British Journal of Psychiatry,* 112, 1097-1102.

Walton, H.J. (1967) The measurement of medical students' attitudes. *British Journal of Medical Education,* 1, 330-340.

Walton, H.J. (1969) Personality correlates of a career interest in psychiatry. *British Journal of Psychiatry,* 115, 211-219.

Zimny, G.H. & Thale, T.R. (1970) Specialty choice and attitudes toward medical specialists. *Social Science and Medicine,* 4, 257-264.

7. Immigration and Emigration

There is a case to be made for an integrated study of world patterns and trends in the migration of doctors and the social, political, economic and religious factors which cause them, as an extension of the World Health Organisation 'Multinational Study of the International Migration of Physicians and Nurses' (1976). It would be valuable, for example, to maintain up to date information on the numbers of Filippino graduates in the United States and Canada, and the inward and outward flows; on the numbers of Ghanaian students trained in the U.S.S.R., for philanthropic or ideological reasons; to know what anxieties about overproduction or excessive costs of medical care have determined the imposition of restrictions on entry of overseas doctors to North America; to have information about the extent to which the work of the Medical Missionary Societies, the Grenfell Mission in Labrador and those working in Africa and Asia, has been replaced by V.S.O. and the establishment of medical schools in developing countries with the assistance of staff, either attracted by advertisement or seconded by Government, from the developed countries. There are innumerable factors influencing the international migration of doctors, and for our manpower planning purposes we need to know which of these are important to Britain.

THE IMMIGRATION PROBLEM

The vast entry of overseas doctors to Britain has largely taken the nation unawares since the Willink Report of 1957 (see Chapters 1 and 3). In 1969 Gish estimated that 'almost one fourth of all doctors then employed by the National Health Service were born, and mostly trained, outside the British Isles'. In 1977 there were estimated to be about 25,000 overseas doctors in Britain. There has been a great deal of acrimony about the employment of this large influx: on the one hand reports of communication difficulties and low standards of training, with hearsay evidence that the best Asian graduates go straight to the United States, and on the other hand complaints about lack of training and teaching, being used as 'pairs of hands' and poor career prospects. This question first became prominent in public debate in 1961 when, in a famous speech in the House of Lords, Lord Taylor of Harlow said 'they are here to provide pairs of hands in the rottenest, worst hospitals in the country because there is nobody else to do it' (*Hansard*, 1961). No doubt the well-established, older Asian doctors may themselves feel that the great increase in incoming numbers has implied some lowering of standards, and hence a threat to their own position in society. The Community Relations Commission (1976) said, 'the adverse publicity which has been aimed at overseas doctors in recent years, and the growing impression that they are given a second-class status can therefore bring difficulties into doctor/patient relationships, as well as damage to good community relations in general'.

The history of the registration of overseas doctors was reviewed in the General Medical Council's Annual Report for 1975 (G.M.C., 1976). The 1886 Medical Act first made statutory provision for the registration in this country, under reciprocal arrangements, of overseas qualified doctors. By 1970 reciprocal arrangements were established with 23 countries and recognition extended to the primary medical qualifications granted to students of over 90 overseas medical schools. Although originally the system had been mainly used to allow British doctors to practise overseas, it came to allow a large annual inflow of overseas doctors; and 'the recent multiplication of overseas medical schools, with diverse standards and objectives, has made the system less acceptable'.

As the scrutiny of standards became progressively more difficult the G.M.C., in 1971, initiated a review of all the qualifications it had recognised and this led to a progressive reduction of recognition; in 1972, as a result of political developments, recognition was withdrawn from six schools in Pakistan and Bangladesh; on January 1st, 1972 there followed withdrawal of recognition, for full registration in the U.K., of medical degrees granted in Sri Lanka. On May 22nd, 1975 recognition was withdrawn from 55 Indian Colleges as, after protracted correspondence, the G.M.C. (1976) 'was no longer able to effectively satisfy itself as to the standard of qualifications currently granted in India, although this did not reflect on the standards of earlier years'. It is interesting to note that the immediate reaction was a rapid rise in applications for full registration from Indian doctors who had qualified before this date and from doctors from other overseas countries. In 1973 full registration was granted to 1,972 doctors; in 1974 to 1,930 doctors; but in 1975 to 2,741, the main rise being after the TRAB tests began (see Chapter 3).

The actions of the G.M.C. were endorsed by the Merrison Committee (1975) which noted, 'Entry to the register for home educated doctors is controlled by controlling educational institutions. The problem in relation to doctors educated overseas is the extent to which the G.M.C. ought to accept the standards of educational institutions overseas. Our changing relationships with the Commonwealth and with the European Economic Community are obviously relevant in this connection .... It seems to us that the only possible posture for the G.M.C. to adopt for the registration of overseas graduates is that it must ensure that the overseas doctor has reached a standard of competence which is at least equivalent to that of the minimum standard required for the registration of a doctor trained in the U.K.'. The Merrison Committee pointed out that 'a range of competence' will be found as among all medical graduates. It was acknowledged that 'the present level of care offered would have collapsed long ago without the crucial contribution of overseas doctors', but the report went on to say, 'this is obviously a matter of concern to the public who may be treated by overseas doctors, to members of the medical profession whose successful practice will often depend on colleagues' competence, and to overseas practitioners themselves whose effectiveness as doctors may be reduced by doubts about the value of their qualifications'.

The Health Departments stated that in 1974 there were 13,300 overseas born doctors in the N.H.S. in Great Britain (the total number in the U.K. being considerably higher). Some were permanently established in career posts: 3,450 in general practice and 1,900 in hospital career grades, about

14% of each group; 8,000 were in hospital training grades (42% of the total), and some of these eventually settled in career posts (Merrison, 1975). The Todd Commission (1968), as noted in Chapter 1, had estimated that some net immigration would need to continue to ensure maintenance and development of the N.H.S.; although the Merrison Report was hopeful that reliance on overseas doctors would diminish as the output from our medical schools increased, the latest estimates suggest an immigration rate of 4,000 - 4,500 per annum with a continuing net gain.

The granting of 'full' and 'provisional' registration by the G.M.C. has exactly the same significance for overseas doctors as for practitioners qualifying in this country; quite separate is 'temporary' registration which allows a doctor to work only in a specified capacity and is limited to a particular appointment, although this can be at any level in the hospital hierarchy. When the doctor is from a medical school about whose standards some uncertainty exists the G.M.C., in deciding whether to grant registration, is able to seek reports and take account of his linguistic ability, relevant professional experience, character, mental health and clinical competence.

Although statutory provision for temporary registration of overseas doctors was established in 1947, it was only after 1960 that the numbers became substantial (G.M.C., 1976). Some years ago the D.H.S.S. instituted one month's clinical attachment for all overseas doctors before they could be employed by hospital authorities, so that reports are available to the G.M.C. in considering renewal of temporary registration. However, apart from the extra work involved for the consultants, there has been doubt about the effectiveness of this scheme.

The B.M.A. suggested limiting the entry of overseas doctors by imposing a test akin to a U.K. undergraduate examination; the Committee of Vice-Chancellors and Principals (Merrison, 1975) noted 'the widespread belief that present conditions of registration of foreign doctors are unsatisfactory'; the Royal College of Nursing referred to the 'dangers of misunderstanding and the differences in ethical principles and cultural background' and gave as an example a doctor from abroad who interpreted the use of colloquialisms in a psychiatric patient as a sign of confusion and disorientation. The Merrison Report concluded that 'an overseas doctor may be allowed to practise in this country with a knowledge of medicine less than the minimum that would be required of his counterpart educated in the British Isles .... and even when his professional knowledge and skill is sufficient he may lack understanding of patients and grasp of the language, attitudes, values and conventions of the community in which he practises'. The Report blamed the G.M.C. for allowing medical standards to be overridden by the manpower requirements of the N.H.S. during the preceding 20 years. The D.H.S.S. made its position very clear: 'The arrangements for the admission of overseas doctors must neither impede nor deter those whose medical education and ability are of an appropriate standard and character for work in the N.H.S.' (Merrison, 1975). Neither the training needs of the overseas graduates, whose experience here may be totally inappropriate to conditions in the underdeveloped countries, nor the requirements of a logically planned career structure were referred to in this comment.

The Merrison Report endorsed the G.M.C.'s proposals for granting full and provisional registration, and also the establishment of a Temporary Registration Assessment Board to test both professional and linguistic capacity before temporary registration was granted. This scheme was to be operated in conjunction with an improved Clinical Attachment Scheme as instituted by the D.H.S.S. The results of 'TRAB', as it has come to be called, have been illuminating; the proportion of failures has been very high, and this combined with the desire of the underdeveloped countries to retain their own graduates, by legislation if necessary, has already made a difference to the numbers involved. Of the 1,019 doctors who applied to take the TRAB tests from June 1975 to February 1976 inclusive, seven passed from Bangladesh (54 applicants), 42 from Pakistan (96 applicants), 100 from India (236 applicants); while from Iraq 49 passed (103 entered) and from Egypt 46 (out of 215) passed. As noted in Chapter 3, the G.M.C. figures for the calendar year 1976 show that Egypt headed the list with the largest number of applicants; this suggests that there may be a significant increase in the number of Middle Eastern doctors in the British Health Service in the immediate future.

The General Medical Council made proposals which were accepted by the Merrison Committee (1975) for modifications in the procedure for controlling entry of overseas doctors to Britain, and these recently became the subject of debate in relation to the Medical Bill which followed the Merrison Report (*Lancet*, 1977a). The recommended changes in registration of overseas-trained doctors have been accepted as an amendment to the original Bill (*B.M.J.*, 1978); when implemented, the revised regulations will make full registration available to doctors who have either obtained a foreign medical qualification from a school inspected and approved by the General Medical Council, or who have passed a British qualifying examination, for example, the M.R.C.S., L.R.C.P. Temporary registration will be replaced by limited registration, which will be granted for periods of time at the discretion of the General Medical Council and specifying the types of employment covered in the case of each applicant. It is envisaged that doctors granted limited registration will be eligible to apply at a later stage for full registration on the grounds that they have gained additional experience in Britain or in the meantime passed a British qualifying examination.

The position concerning doctors from other E.E.C. countries has been reviewed by Gawn (1978). An Order-in-Council of 1977 empowered the General Medical Council to grant full registration to 'properly qualified' doctors entering Britain from other E.E.C. countries. There is no sound legal basis for refusing such registration on the basis of linguistic incompetence, but the E.E.C. Medical Directives did place upon Member States the responsibility of ensuring that, 'the persons concerned acquire, in the interests of their patients, the linguistic knowledge necessary to the exercise of their profession in the host country'. Accordingly, the present arrangement in the United Kingdom is that, apart from exceptional cases, registration will be terminated after six months unless the doctor concerned has been able to satisfy the General Medical Council of his linguistic competence. No such requirement exists in the case of visiting Britain on a purely temporary basis. A further problem concerns 'Third Country Doctors'; that is, those who are nationals of an E.E.C. country but whose medical qualification was obtained outside the E.E.C. Such doctors are not at present automatically entitled to registration in any E.E.C. country, but are considered individually as was the case before the E.E.C. Directives were implemented. In Britain, the Overseas Doctors Association and the British Medical Association have strongly urged that the Government should press for a change in this ruling.

Bearing this historical perspective in mind, can we analyse what is happening to the overseas graduates in our hospitals, what contribution they make, what effect their presence has on the N.H.S. career structure system and what they themselves gain from the experience?

The first conclusion is that, although the G.M.C. has perhaps belatedly

endeavoured to upgrade standards of admission, there has been a complete
lack of systematic monitoring of the numbers involved, with a view to
establishing quotas. In 1961 Lord Platt said, 'in view of the extent to
which the Hospital Service is dependent upon young doctors from overseas
whose stay here is temporary, and the uncertainty whether this help will
continue to be available on the present scale, we consider it essential
that information about the number of those helpers from overseas should
be collected every year so that if and when the number falls this may be
detected without undue delay, and such steps as may be necessary taken to
make the loss good' (Platt Report, 1961). But estimates of the numbers
involved have fluctuated greatly so that we have no more precise knowledge of quantity than we have of quality.

The difference in achievement between British and overseas graduates
can be seen in the examination results of the Royal Colleges. The Merrison Report (1975) quoted the figures of the Royal College of Psychiatrists,
showing an 81% pass rate for British graduates as against 47% for overseas
doctors, and those of the Royal College of General Practitioners where,
from 1972 to 1974, the consolidated figures gave an 82% pass rate for U.K.
graduates and 21% for overseas graduates. Other specialist examiners
could echo these findings. The 1972 tables for the Foreign Medical Graduate examinations in America (Merrison, 1975) showed the same position:
94% of U.K. candidates passed, 41% of those from India and 25% of those
from Pakistan. What do these figures tell us?

That most of the overseas graduates work in the more unpopular specialties and in the less agreeable parts of the country is evident. The
great majority are in busy non-teaching hospitals, which now usually have
postgraduate medical centres and libraries, but where access to university
centres may be difficult. Also, as Dr. Nicholas Bosanquet (1975) has
pointed out, 'immigrant doctors certainly do man the unpopular specialties
but their other function is to provide a broad base to the narrow topped
pyramid of hospital medicine', a fact very relevant to the career structure
of the service (see also Chapter 2). Whether such training as they receive is relevant to their needs depends upon their ultimate career intentions, which are often undefined or subject to change in response to varying opportunities and circumstances. For those returning home, we need to
note that, 'Western medical education has in the past been orientated towards the individual. It is obvious that in order to provide motivation
for investigations into health problems of developing countries, education
must be more orientated to the community and include medical economics.
In many European countries the syllabus is still limited to the national
pattern of disease and social factors' (Farquhar et al, 1976). And, 'there
is a need for doctors to work in rural areas, to be efficient administrators
and to have had public health training, to be orientated towards community
health and preventive medicine and to work with para-medical teams' (Sebai
and Baker, 1976).

While the main preoccupation is staffing of the N.H.S., it does not
seem likely that we can adequately fulfil our obligations either to the
needs of overseas doctors themselves or to their countries of origin. In
June 1974 a report from the Consultants and Specialists Association (1974)
said 'It is an historical fact that many of the developing countries of
the world look to Britain as a developed country which is able to help
them in many ways. Most of these are countries which are members of the
Commonwealth, or which have in the past been members of the Commonwealth,
and of the erstwhile British Empire. One of the services which we in
Britain can offer to these less well developed countries is that of assis-
ting in the training of doctors who will ultimately return to their own

countries to practise. This is a duty which we owe both for historical reasons and also because it is our place as a developed country to assist those nations which are at the moment less fortunate'. The Report noted that these overseas doctors had supplied a very large part of the service requirements at junior level among the medical staff of our hospitals, but predicted that as world medical services developed, and as the result of altered political attitudes here and overseas, the numbers would decrease, probably to half over a period of ten years. The Report concluded by saying: 'In an ideal situation one would like to see appointments for overseas trainees controlled and monitored in the same sort of way as the pre-registration appointments are controlled at present. If this were to come to pass we could expect a further reduction in the service provided by these doctors and a further gap in the service needs of the hospital service would arise. We recommend that consideration should be given to the setting up in teaching and non-teaching hospitals of special training appointments for overseas doctors. These appointments would not form part of the establishment posts for the training of consultants to serve the Health Service although it should be possible for doctors to pass from one type of post to another'. Other proposals for ways in which residual training capacity in the junior hospital grades might logically be used to accommodate overseas doctors have subsequently been made (Parkhouse, 1976).

In the United States, the problems facing immigrant doctors were analysed in a paper by Lassers and Nordan (1975). The United States has, of course, in common with other developed countries, its own system of Board examinations which foreign medical graduates must pass before they are permitted to practise, and this is an arrangement which many members of the medical profession would like to see adopted in Great Britain. In an effort to understand difficulties and assist integration of doctors from totally different cultures the problems were listed by Lassers and Nordan as being, firstly a need for personal adjustment to changes in life style and separation from family and friends. Secondly, there are cultural differences, so that customs and traditions native to the overseas doctor may prevent him understanding, or even being aware of the problems his patients face. This is what Desai (1969) called 'cultural dissonance'. For example, the Lassers and Nordan paper reported that when a child on the unit was dying and there was a discussion on how the parents might be helped, an Indian resident asked 'What's the problem, why don't you just tell them to call in the mourners?' Similarly, differences in child rearing and the permissiveness allowed to teenagers often cause misunderstandings, and there is an unawareness of the cultures of the various sub-groups within the population. Thirdly, there is the language problem. Lassers and Nordan found that even when competence was fairly good there were misunderstandings of finer points. For example, there was a lack of expertise in library information-gathering and the use of relevant books; trainees would give a word-for-word recitation of an article which they did not really understand. There were difficulties when interviewing patients and poor contact was made: one wrote 'my background was poor and I was afraid to get involved. I knew about words that can be positive or negative in my language, but I did not know what these words would be in the English language. I was afraid to start talking with a patient and at a certain point did not know what to ask or what to say'. Fourthly, there is the student-instructor relationship: a lack of responsiveness and reluctance to tell senior colleagues and teachers that they were not being understood, because of the deference traditionally accorded to figures in authority: 'Only within strict limits can a question be asked; to do so a student must know neither too much nor too little - too much would challenge the teacher's knowledge of the subject, too little would demonstrate the student's own ignorance. As a result, it was often difficult for us to know who understood and who just nodded his head politely in ignorance' (Mittel, 1970). Fifthly, there was a lack of interest because the problems dealt with had little relevance for the overseas doctors in terms of their future work. The recommendations made by Lassers and Nordan were for one-to-one teaching, and a willingness to discuss problems with overseas trainees and 'not to process them as a kind of second-class citizen' (Char, 1971). It needed to be recognised that individual understanding often transcended language and cultural differences - as one patient said, 'I don't always know what he's saying, but I know that he cares about me, and that's the important thing'. Yet this was not always the case, as life may be held more cheaply in a land of dire poverty and a high rate of mortality might be accepted.

Much of the above analysis could be applied directly to the situation in Britain. In particular, it is necessary to appreciate that the possession of a basic level of linguistic competence, sufficient for most purposes of communication with patients and colleagues, does not necessarily imply that learning at a postgraduate level will be easy. Overseas trainees in the hospital specialties not infrequently admit, on questioning, that in attempting to prepare themselves for higher examinations they have made no real attempt to understand the subject matter; because of their traditional patterns of teaching and learning at home they have found it easier to try and memorise whole sections of the appropriate books.

There is naturally much concern in the developing countries over the emigration of their newly qualified graduates: 'more than 90% of each graduating class of the Palilavi Medical School in Shiraz, Iran, goes to the United States for residency training - the majority of these remain permanently in the United States' (Ronaghy et al, 1974). And Baham Joorabchi (1973) of the same medical school, says 'developing nations around the world invest extremely limited capital and manpower resources in schools of medicine and in subsidising the cream of their student body during the costliest of all educational endeavours. They naturally expect to benefit from the services of the product of such education. Yet these countries, suffering from a variety of illnesses and health hazards no longer seen in more developed parts of the world and with only one physician for 10,000 or more (of the population) lose their medical graduates at an alarming rate to the Western World'. In the United States alone Somers (1971) estimated that in January 1971 there were 48,000 foreign medical graduates, and they were entering at the rate of 8-10,000 per annum which was equivalent to the total output of the United States medical schools. Most of the entrants came for training but many remained and in 1969, 23% of all physicians licensed to practise in the United States were foreign medical graduates.

To combat this problem efforts are being made to establish postgraduate training centres in the less developed countries themselves. The Ibadan Medical School in Nigeria (which was established in 1948) began postgraduate training in 1962, drawing recruits from the six medical schools that had been set up in the country. But many graduates still go abroad for training and tend to stay, so that a survey in 1974 found that one-third of all the graduates from the Ibadan School were resident abroad. Osunkoya (1974) said in his report, 'the most important problem is the shortage of teachers. It is hoped that the developed countries such as Britain will be able to offer some assistance in this respect'.

97

As a result of this loss of manpower the authorities in developing countries are pressed into training more and more doctors in systems already strained by overproduction, or may be compelled to implement unwise legislation in an effort to curb the outflow. Peiliang Kuan (1970) noted that of the medical graduates of the National Taiwan University of 1965, 61.5% remained abroad in 1970 and commented 'the Chinese government does not propose to take steps to restrict young doctors going abroad, but it is looking for a possible way to attract the medical emigrants to return to Taiwan'. Mofidi (1970) said 'the physicians' migration has adverse effects on the recipient countries: aside from the dubious allegation of lower quality of care obtained from the F.M.G.s[*], these countries' shortage of health manpower is masked and goes uncorrected'. The newly qualified doctor goes first for postgraduate training unobtainable at home and because physicians trained abroad are in greater demand by universities, the government and especially the consumer; he then finds that in this new way of life he can earn more than he ever would even in some highly placed government post at home and has access to sophisticated facilities and skilled personnel trained in highly specialised fields. In his own country there may be few jobs available that he would wish to take; in Iran for example, 95% of the doctors practise in the urban centres while 70% of the population is in the rural areas: 'While altruism might sustain the returning physician for a short while it is, to say the least, unreasonable to expect him to ignore his years of training and to practise bush medicine with inadequate drugs or supplies; or to do without professional support and opportunity for continuing education and research. The near impossibility of supporting a family, and providing for their future on the meagre government salary - the only source of income in rural practise - is of course a basic issue (Joorabchi, 1973). Similarly in India, Rao (1974) found a reluctance among doctors to work in rural areas and little interest in teaching or research careers; 'most of them preferred setting up in private practice and using their training fruitfully', because of the high value they attached to status and prestige. Some caution is indeed necessary before accepting the facile view that by taking foreign doctors the affluent nations are inevitably depriving the great rural masses of India and Asia of much-needed medical care. As Reinhardt (1975) commented from the United States, 'Available data suggest at least tentatively that the migration of foreign-trained physicians into the United States effectively constitutes a transfer of medical manpower from reasonably well-to-do urbanities in the donor countries to well-to-do and sometimes not so well-to-do urbanities in the United States. That flow had admittedly served to fill certain gaps in the distribution of American physicians and has hence been welcomed by the formulators of health manpower policy in this country; but the flow also seems to represent the product of the push away from relatively over-doctored centres in countries that cannot fully absorb their own physicians to the latters' satisfaction, and of the pull towards the economic rewards and professional prestige associated with medical practice in the United States'.

It is arguable, nevertheless, that we do the underdeveloped countries a disservice when we train their graduates to our own pattern, ignoring the irrelevance of this to the health care needs of the trainees' country. This is emphasised in a recent report by Voluntary Service Overseas (*The Observer Review*, 1977) which criticises the export of 'medical colonialism' and the emphasis on curative rather than preventive medicine; the example is quoted of an African country sending three doctors to England at great

[*] Foreign Medical Graduates

98

expense to study advanced cardiology while 'grass root' medicine was starved of funds. Senewiratne (1976), from Sri Lanka, takes a different view: 'preventive and social medicine is taught by good teachers of general medicine - there is an over-emphasis which seems to be creeping into the new British curriculum. The poverty and disease of our country is more a reflection on the way the country is run than on the way the doctors are trained. Changing the medical curriculum cannot provide either protein or employment'.

As long ago as 1961 the Nuffield Conference on Postgraduate Medical Education (*Lancet*, 1962) stressed the importance of British postgraduate medical education not only to 'the people of this island' but to many other countries because 'the excellence of the education available to graduates at all levels in our hospitals will inevitably influence the present and future quality of the National Health Service; because we have an obligation to contribute generously to the training of graduates for Commonwealth countries; and because the good name of this country depends to some extent on how far we exert ourselves to ensure that the young doctors sent here from abroad are provided with a solid foundation for their professional work'. But it is not in the interests of the developing countries for us to import their graduates in wholesale numbers to provide a 'cushion' for our Health Service; it would be far more helpful for us to second doctors and administrators to assist them in establishing training centres of their own which would develop curricula relevant to local needs and upgrade the status of locally trained doctors. In 1963 the Working Party on Medical Aid to the Developing Countries under the Chairmanship of Sir Arthur Porritt (Report, 1963) said 'the best and most economical way of helping the developing countries to improve their medical services is to raise the standard of teaching at their own teaching centres and to train their own teachers, so that this central influence may permeate the whole of their medical systems'. And again, at the Second Commonwealth Medical Conference at Kampala in 1968, the British Government stated its preparedness to try to make such assistance available. A number of arrangements have, in fact, existed for some years whereby strong and useful affiliations and exchanges have been developed between British medical schools and centres abroad; a list of these was given in Appendix 17 of the Todd Report (1968). The current focus of interest in this respect is the Arab World.

But if overseas graduates are to remain in their own countries for postgraduate education and practice, or if they visit Britain only to obtain defined postgraduate training or experience relevant to conditions in their own country, then the career structure for our own graduates, greatly increasing in number as the years go by and perhaps half of them women, will need to be drastically revised. This, in turn, attaches new importance to choice of career and the factors that influence it.

EMIGRATION OF BRITISH DOCTORS

Reinhardt's reference to the 'push and pull' forces of migration has been mentioned. 'The "push" is the imbalance between the expectations engendered by medical education and the reality of the working and social environment of practice: the "pull" is the thirst for further postgraduate education and experience, for higher economic reward, and the opportunity to practise the highly technological medicine the student has been taught' (Fendall, 1975). So we find migration from India to East Africa, from Pakistan to the Arab countries and West Africa; Britain receives physicians from the less developed countries and donates them to North America and

Australia, accompanied by many of our own medical graduates; and there is also an outflow from Western society to the less developed countries through Government sponsorship, technical assistance, voluntary agencies and international organisations which attract out of the country a number of mature and experienced people. The difficulty is, of course, in disentangling all these skeins of cause and effect, and in tracing the changing pattern over the years so that we can estimate the numbers of our own doctors emigrating now and likely to do so in the future, and assess the changes here and abroad which could alter the present trends.

A publication of the Office of Health Economics (1966) noted, 'one factor tending to create a shortage of doctors in Britain is medical emigration on a scale not officially recognised until recently'. Reference had been made to the problem by the Willink Committee in 1957, which recognised that scant information was available about numbers but concluded 'there is no doubt that the opportunities for doctors from Great Britain to obtain employment overseas have been diminishing in the recent past and will continue to do so in the future'. The Council of the B.M.A. expressed a contrary view but had little evidence to support it, and the Pilkington Committee (1960) stated, 'it was suggested to us in evidence that British medicine was in danger of being seriously depleted by emigration but investigation proved the extent of emigration to have been much less than had been suggested, although completely satisfactory figures are difficult to obtain'. This is not surprising as the statistics used were derived from the Board of Trade and were based only on passengers by sea, excluding air travellers altogether; and the calculation was based on numbers emigrating to the British Colonies and Commonwealth, and ignored the United States and other developed countries.

Davison (1961) and Seale (1962) estimated that during the five years up to 1961 the equivalent of one-third of British medical school graduates had emigrated. Two years later, further studies confirmed a high rate of emigration, although not quite at the rate first conjectured when re-migration and 'double-counting' were allowed for. Abel-Smith and Gales (1964) said, 'In June 1962 the Minister of Health stated that about 6% or 7% of graduates of the 1950s were resident abroad. We found the percentage to be one-fifth. If the planning of medical school intake is based on the Ministry's figures, then a substantial increase is urgently required'. In 1964 Seale, and Abel-Smith and Gales estimated that 5,000 doctors born and trained in the British Isles (4,000 from Britain and 1,000 from Ireland) had emigrated over the previous ten years and not returned, 75% of these from the hospital service; this was equal to one quarter of the output of British-born graduates in British medical schools over that period. Davison (1962) wrote, 'If it were not for excessive emigration no shortage of doctors would exist; the manpower losses of nationalised medicine are to be written off in the same fashion as the financial deficits of our nationalised industries, by asking for more. If and when supplies of Asian doctors fail, Lord Taylor* suggests the advent of the Common Market will permit us to import Italian doctors to run our Health Service. Clearly, 14 years of socialism have made us completely shameless, for no one can believe these policies to be in the national interest'.

At that time the intense competition for consultant posts in Britain was undoubtedly a major factor. Many highly trained senior registrars in their thirties and forties, in the days when junior doctors were not so well paid as now, felt frustrated in their careers. The alternative was to 'drop off the ladder' into general practice. Many felt bitter at the

---

* Sunday Times, 31 December, 1961

100

financial sacrifice they had made on behalf of their families: we lost 'highly trained, experienced and competent men and women who had held several senior registrar appointments before finally leaving the hospital service. They had acquired new techniques and knowledge in advance of some older and longer established consultants but were themselves unable to obtain such a post. Further, the very specialised experience they had gained in their latter years in hospital had no application in general practice - many were unwilling to change to such work and often they were also unacceptable to established general practitioners' (Office of Health Economics, 1966). The Platt Report of 1961 (see Chapter 2) did much to relieve the bottleneck at senior registrar level, by focusing its attention on this grade, and since then the problems arising from the career structure have predominantly been in the lower training grades. It is ironic that in 1978 a senior registrar may face a drop in salary if he accepts a consultant post, and in a recent letter to The Times (Rickards, 1977) the President of the Hospital Consultants and Specialists' Association compared the applicants for a training post in general surgery at Wolverhampton in 1964, when 26 registrars all from British medical schools applied, to the response for the identical post recently advertised when the 21 applicants were all from overseas.

In 1967 a team from the Ministry of Health, headed by Dr. R.H. Barrett visited North America (*B.M.J.*, 1968a) in the hope of persuading medical emigrants to return to Britain. They found 'considerable dissatisfaction with the life of general practice' in Britain, and also 'with the prospects in a hospital career (*B.M.J.*, 1968b). Higher financial rewards and the availability, at that time, of academic posts with good research facilities, had attracted many emigrants. The commonest reasons for wishing to return to Britain were not, however, directly related to medical practice but rather to the benefits for children and the dislike of some features of life in North America (*B.M.J.*, 1968b).

It appeared from the Central Medical Recruitment Committee Index (Gish, 1970) that from September 1962 to September 1967 4,500 British and Irish born medical graduates left Britain and 2,900 returned, making a net loss of 1,600, the peak year being 1964-65 when 500 left permanently; the subsequent loss was about 400, or one-fifth of the total output of the British medical schools. Of these 75% went to developed countries - to North America, temporarily for experience or permanently to specialist posts, and to Australia, mostly to permanent posts in general practice. The other 25% went to developing countries - the younger ones involved in aid programmes or for adventure, and the older to sponsored jobs - and returned at the end of their tour of duty. Accurate statistics were even harder to come by in the early 1960s than now, when the World Health Organisation and the D.H.S.S. have done some valuable work. There is still, as Eysenck (1977) has said, a need for factual knowledge: 'A rational person would as far as possible construct his policies on the basis of ascertained fact, or at least on the basis of theories most strongly supported by facts. Unfortunately the sociology of knowledge is rather in the position of the Cretan who said that all Cretans are liars - a paradox which has puzzled philosophy students for many generations. If all theories are a reflection of the social scene, then the theory advanced by sociologists of knowledge also has no objective reality and therefore we need not take it seriously and can go on believing facts are facts, and theories can be more or less true to facts. Why this dislike of the objectivity of facts? The simple answer is that facts can be very bothersome'.

One of the most bothersome facts in our present economic position is the cost of educating medical graduates. Evans (1970) quoted a 1966 headline from 'Home News' - 'Brain Drain has saved the U.S. 357 million pounds sterling': the estimated cost of producing a doctor at that time was £28,000, and now it is quoted as at least £40,000. But money, both the cost of educating a doctor and, perhaps more important to him what he can earn, is only part of the problem. Lord Brain (1967) said 'the dark side of the N.H.S. is an ever growing unhappiness and dissatisfaction among consultants, junior hospital staff, and general practitioners, sometimes one group coming into prominence with its complaints and sometimes another; a dissatisfaction so great that we are losing a number equivalent to 33% of the annual output of our medical schools to countries overseas, and that those who go are often among the keenest and most ambitious of our young doctors'. Lord Brain observed that those who went were often among the most experienced and mature doctors, we lost thereby much valuable teaching potential to the detriment of doctors in training. He went on to condemn the neglect of data collecting: 'Whose task, then should it have been to have kept in review the progress of medicine .... this involves continuous research and collection of objective data .... the lack of which the Gillie Committee regretted. Such work is beyond the scope and power of branches of the medical profession. While it could perhaps have been done by other organisations, it was purely the responsibility of the Ministry of Health .... Something has been done by the Ministry in the way of collecting this kind of information during recent years. Valuable as this is, it came too late to prevent the crisis in which we are now involved'. Whether the necessary work is done independently, or by the D.H.S.S., the essential criteria are that the information should be accurate and up to date, and that it should be freely published; it may well be that the latter obligation would ultimately be the deciding factor in favour of an independent body.

Many independent studies have been done among groups of doctors. During a Survey Report on General Practitioners in the Reading Area, Crowe (1969) noted that of 231 local general practitioners, 96 (42%) had seriously considered emigrating, 20 had practised abroad and returned and 12 had trained abroad and settled in this country. The countries in which potential emigrants were interested were, in order of preference, Canada, New Zealand, Australia, Europe, the United States and South Africa. Last and Brodie (1970) found, in a survey of British doctors from 1961-69, that 12% had emigrated in the period 3 - 7 years after graduation and Canada was the most popular choice. Ogston, Ogston and Ogston (1970) stated that one-fifth of male Aberdeen graduates were working abroad, most as permanent emigrants, and concluded 'this level agrees with the estimates of emigration rates for all British medical schools made by Abel-Smith and Gales and by Seale; and also as in previous surveys (Seale, 1966; Ash and Mitchell, 1968; Whitfield, 1969) Canada and Australia were the most frequently chosen countries'. Drs. Marrigje J.A. Scobie - de Maar (unpublished report; see also Gish, 1970) found that during the period 1962-66, 2,759 British graduates had left and 1,484 had returned. Of these 1,828 had left for developed countries and 654 returned (36%); 931 had left for short-term appointments to developing countries and 830 had returned (89%). Canada had the lowest rate of returning emigrants, only 21%; the percentage from the United States was 52%, from South Africa 69%, and from Europe 80%. In Asia the numbers going and returning were equal and in Africa more returned than went (as at that time many African countries were in the process of achieving independence). As previously found, Canada, Australia and New Zealand tended to attract general practitioners while the United States attracted senior hospital and university doctors.

Whitfield (1969) in a Birmingham study, found that of doctors graduating between 1959 and 1963, 10% had emigrated with a sharp rise in the last three years. Two-fifths went to Canada, one quarter to Australia and one-seventh to the United States; their reasons were dissatisfaction with the N.H.S. and the long queue in England for consultant posts, the high income and hospital privileges abroad, the quickly achieved status in the New World without higher qualifications, the facilities for research and a conviction that Europe was irrevokably in decline. Whitfield stressed the difficulty of obtaining information; he reiterated Davison's (1961) suggestion that the British Medical Register 'should be reorganised so that each registrant pays an annual fee to remain on it and is required to give information of his type and place of practice', but concluded that many permanent emigrants had no interest in remaining on the British Register and that the task would therefore best be performed by medical schools for their own graduates, asking also what considerations prompted emigration and for what period the doctor intended to stay abroad.

In a letter from the Royal Free Hospital, Brumfitt, Hoffbrand and Wills (1976) remarked, 'unless radical changes are made there will soon be precious few true academics working in clinical academic posts in this country'. And in a survey during 1969 Gish and de Maar found increasing numbers of British and Irish medical school graduates taking state board examinations in America, especially Irish doctors tending to go to the United States instead of Great Britain; there were more from Scotland than England because the Scots had to move away to find employment and therefore found it easier to accept the idea of emigrating overseas; and more from London/Oxbridge than the provinces, possibly because the provincial schools drew students from different social or class backgrounds.

At a Macy Conference in 1970 (*Health Trends*, 1971) the representatives of 14 countries considered the migration of doctors. There was agreement that there should be no government or statutory restrictions, that there was a need for better comparable data, and that donor countries should supply information about currently available posts for emigrants.

The assessment of the numbers of doctors emigrating permanently has been rendered more difficult because many graduates, in common with other young people in search of experience and adventure, have travelled abroad without any firm personal decision having been made whether to stay, or return, or perhaps move on to another country. Indeed these decisions are impossible to make until the conditions have been experienced at first hand and the reactions of other members of the family - both elderly relatives left at home and the immediate family accompanying the emigrant - have been ascertained. Also the ruling in the United States that the holder of a temporary visa must return home at the end of his allotted stay and wait two years before being eligible to apply for permanent emigration, led many doctors to apply for permanent status as a safeguard in case they decided to stay. There has always been, among the best young people, a feeling of need for adventure throughout the world before settling down. The United States offered hospitality in short-term posts which provided contact with other medical ways of life, and there have also been overseas commitments of limited tenure to developing countries. Porritt (Report, 1963) said, 'Experience gained in overseas service, with the demands which it makes on the initiative and adaptability of the young doctor, often develops professional skill and personal character more quickly and more effectively than any equivalent period spent at home', and recommended that 'steps be taken to ensure that appointing bodies, as well as the men themselves, will be encouraged to regard overseas service in approved centres as an additional qualification for appointment to senior posts in this country'. The Report suggested that universities should be encouraged to introduce, gradually, a system of proleptic appointments. Fortunately this adventurous spirit still prevails, as shown by the excellent series of recent articles entitled 'Where Shall John Go' (*B.M.J.*, 1976, 1977a).

There have been more vested interests in promoting this sort of leave of absence; Mrs. Barbara Castle advocated the secondment of medical teachers to the new schools being established in the Middle East, and another Secretary of State has echoed the sentiment: 'Mr. Ennals has referred to one estimate suggesting that around 50,000 new hospital and health centre beds are being planned in the OPEC countries alone and that capital developments of around £3,000 million are planned for the next five years. The N.H.S., much admired overseas, could benefit from competing for this business. And, in some circumstances, it would be important to support exports by the release of staff for key assignments overseas or by arranging for training for overseas personnel .... Staff who take up an overseas post in these circumstances are likely to be given leave of absence without pay by their N.H.S. authority, and a few may be seconded by their authority, which will be reimbursed for all the expenses incurred .... The ability to release a British specialist may be crucial in determining the overall effectiveness of a British bid for a contract' (*Lancet*, 1977b). At the same time private and profitable arrangements are made by way of tempting advertisements in the national press.

Another factor which complicates the present pattern is membership of the E.E.C., with the elaborate negotiations and adjustments that have resulted. Although the period required for 'specialist' training varies between countries, all doctors of the member states are in theory freely interchangeable and medical skills command an international market. *The Times* (1976a) reported, 'There seems little doubt that freedom of movement of doctors, when it is working fully, will lead to a net loss to Britain. British doctors have a high reputation and there are shortages especially in anaesthetics, radiology and pathology in the community. The Government has authorised the G.M.C. to issue certificates of specialist training to British doctors wishing to move and during this first month there have been 200 enquiries'. In the same newspaper on the following day Mr. Walpole Lewin was reported as saying on E.E.C. movement: 'Are we to have a strong and vigorous medical profession that will monitor and improve our own standards and welcome our friends and colleagues in Europe who would wish to come here for postgraduate experience, or do we settle for a mediocre service which our own graduates will not find satisfying but which may well attract some of the surplus doctors from Europe who have failed to establish themselves in their own country' (*The Times*, 1976b). These countries are having their own problems in dealing with numbers, as Brearley (*The Times*, 1976b) noted: 'the output of medical schools in France and Italy could double the numbers of doctors in practice in these countries in the next decade'. Rowe (*The Times*, 1976b) reported that Denmark could not find enough places in its own system for training young doctors and while most European countries were cutting medical school intake only Britain was expanding. The Liberal Party evidence to the Royal Commission (*Lancet*, 1977c) said, 'Medical schools in Europe are so productive that many doctors may soon have difficulty in finding jobs and it is estimated that there will be a 40,000 surplus of E.E.C. doctors by 1981'. It proposed that 'a standing committee should be established to review manpower requirements as past predictions have been wrong too often'. In a recent comparative study of remuneration and health service financing, Klein (1977) quoted figures which 'confirm the position of Britain's doctors as the prolateriat of the international medical community, and so help to explain the current state of morale'.

A Special Representative Meeting of the B.M.A. (*B.M.J.*, 1977b came
to the conclusion that medical emigration into and out of Britain was
slowing down. Entry to the United States of America had been made much
more difficult with the new two-day visa qualifying examination introduced
in September 1977. *The Lancet* (1977d) reported, 'the setting up of bars
against the admission of foreign medical graduates in the U.S. provoked,
we are told, the chartering of a private plane to fly 75 medical men from
South Africa so that they could beat the deadline'. Australia, New Zealand and Canada also no longer have their doors wide open to British graduates. The *Toronto Star* (1974) reported a Federal Provincial Health
Conference during which the Health Minister, Marc Lalonde, spoke of restricting the immigration of foreign trained doctors - a measure necessary
if Canada was to avoid having a glut of doctors since, 'one in every three
doctors in Canada is an immigre. Great Britain provided in 1972 about a
third of immigrant doctors[*] .... priority must be given to Canadian graduates wishing to practise in Canada over foreign doctors'. Mr. Robert
Andras (1975) Canadian Minister of Manpower and Immigration said that
immigrants intending to come to the labour force must show evidence of
fulfilling a need in the community: 'in this respect the application of
immigrant regulations to doctors will be no more or less stringent than
the application to any other trade or profession'. And in June 1975, under
a headline 'No room in Canada for British G.P.'s' the Trudeau administration was reported as noting that Canada had accepted 300 or more doctors
annually from Britain for the last 10 years, seeking higher earnings,
better working conditions and enhanced professional satisfaction - a far
greater number than officially admitted by the D.H.S.S. - and that this
drain of expertise had 'represented an "invisible" loss totalling at least
£100 million' (*Daily Telegraph*, 1975). If the end of free medical migration is indeed in sight - and perhaps this remains to be seen - then some
of the uncertainties will disappear from the manpower equation. It ought
to be easier to calculate the output of medical graduates required and to
achieve a rational balance between career and training posts, and the
report of the Special Representative Meeting of the B.M.A. (*B.M.J.*, 1977b)
concludes, 'this should be top priority of the medicopolitical agenda'.

. . . .

The pattern that emerged during the 1950s and 1960s was of highly
trained junior staff, unable to advance to consultant status because of
the strength of competition, and unwilling to 'fall off the ladder' into
general practice in this country, emigrating to practise specialised medicine mostly in North America and to general practice in Australia and
New Zealand - a course of action reinforced by relative poverty at home
and Arabian Night tales of affluence abroad. This exodus was accompanied
by a flow of temporary emigrants seeking a year or two of experience and
adventure in centres where grants and opportunities were more readily
available than they are now. The strand of the pattern which ran via the
Colonial Service to the countries of the Empire had been replaced by that
via V.S.O. to developing countries and that flow, for example of volunteers
for missionary service and work in Vietnam, earthquake and disaster areas,
was practically all of a temporary nature without loss or gain in numbers
to the Health Service, and usually bringing in breadth of experience. Towards the end of the sixties, as recommended by the Platt Report (1961)

---

[*] this figure included those re-emigrating from a third country

the number of consultant posts increased and the senior registrar establishment was simultaneously reduced. The 'cushion' of overseas doctors in lower training grades did not provide as much competition; the number of British graduates had fallen because the 'post war bulge' had either been accommodated or had emigrated, and because of Willink's (1957) recommendations for reduced medical intake. Everything seemed to be set fair, except that the increasing dependence of the N.H.S. on overseas doctors, and its implications, was not widely appreciated.

More recently, poor morale and inadequate funding have led to increased emigration among senior staff; junior doctors, although well paid, see no glowing future in consultant jobs which mean only increased responsibility and overwork, and have anxieties that increased production of doctors without a better career structure will once again lead to chaotic and frustrating competiton. Outlets to developed countries are being blocked because of increased doctor production or economic recession elsewhere, and this applies equally to the New World countries and the European Economic Community. The flow of immigrants from underdeveloped countries seems at long last likely to dry up, because of restrictive tests here and a natural desire on the part of the producer countries to keep their own doctors.

We will no doubt continue to educate foreign medical students and train specialists, for financial reward as well as philanthropy, and likewise second doctors to help set up medical schools in the Middle East and other parts of the world. But is the home market to be flooded with British graduates competing for the popular specialties and localities, or can we achieve better distribution by specialty and geographically, to make proper use of our best medical manpower? Mr. David Ennals (1976) has referred to the problems which have 'exacerbated shortages in staff in geriatric medicine, psychiatry and the support specialties, most marked in anaesthetics, radiology and pathology in which demand is world high'. And is it really true that in these specialties 'there is nowhere for the next generation of doctors to emigrate' (Cundy, 1976)? Gish has written: 'Much still needs to be learned, however, about why certain categories of doctor emigrate - for example, by specialty, place of training, family background, etc. Also, why some return, why others go to particular parts of the world, and why the return rate differs from area to area. We also know virtually nothing about the value attached to a period of time spent abroad, either to the individual or to medical practice in Great Britain: this factor, combined with the work potential of women doctors, and the need to rationalise the hospital career structure are the most important elements in the science of medical manpower planning today. If emigration to developed countries is to be checked, it will be necessary to make it possible for doctors who have already developed a considerable level of expertise in a specialty to exercise that specialty. There is undoubtedly room for many more consultants, particularly in lieu of the many junior hospital doctors who are already doing work which is virtually indistinguishable from that of more senior men.... What is necessary is to allow qualified specialists, even if they are not consultants, to work at their specialties at least on a part-time basis, while carrying on a general practice (perhaps more specialised forms of general practice can be envisaged)' (Gish, 1970).

British doctors have always gone abroad in significant numbers and, particularly in the days of the Empire, medical services in large areas of the world were provided by the graduates of British medical schools. Likewise, foreign doctors have always wanted to come to Britain, temporarily or permanently, for many reasons. Some of the patterns and forces that govern these movements have been reviewed and some current reasons for disenchantment and confusion have been quoted. Sir George Pickering (1974) made the outspoken challenge: 'Would our highly trained doctors not be sensible to emigrate to Europe where they will be so much better than the others, and where they can earn large sums of money?' This surely makes the point that for the future, we need not only to have better information about the ebbs and flows of emigration and immigration, including all the professional, social and personal reasons that impel them, but to restructure, equip and finance the health services of this country in accordance with what we learn.

REFERENCES

Abel-Smith, B. & Gales, K. (1964) Emigration of doctors. *British Medical Journal,* 2, 53.

Andras, R. (1975) Letter from the Office of the Minister Manpower and Immigration, Canada, 16 January.

Ash, R. & Mitchell, H.D. (1968) Doctor migration 1962-64. *British Medical Journal,* 1, 569-572.

Bosanquet, N. (1975) Immigrants and the N.H.S. *New Society,* 33, 130-132.

Brain, Lord (1967) *Is there an Alternative?* B.M.J. Booklet. London: British Medical Association.

British Medical Journal (1968a) Emigration of British doctors to United States of America and Canada. 1, 45-48.

British Medical Journal (1968b) Return to Britain? 1, 1-2.

British Medical Journal (1976) Where Shall John Go? 2, 855-857; 1049-1051; 1185-1186; 1364-1366.

British Medical Journal (1977a) Where Shall John Go? 1, 94-96; 222-224; 629-631; 693-696; 963-965; 1074-1075; 1143-1145; 1206-1208. 2, 247-249; 1465-1466; 1530-1531.

British Medical Journal (1977b) A special representative meeting of the B.M.A. 1, 787-788.

British Medical Journal (1978) Most of Merrison. 1, 532.

Brumfitt, W., Hoffbrand, A.V. & Wills, M.R. (1976) A Professor emigrates. *Lancet,* 1, 1072-1073.

Char, F. (1971) The foreign resident: an ambivalently valued object. *Psychiatry,* 34, 234-238.

Community Relations Commission (1976) *Doctors from Overseas: A Case for Consultation,* London.

Consultants and Specialists Association (1974) *Hospital Medical Staffing.* Report from the Hospital Consultants and Specialists Association.

Crowe, M.G.F. (1969) *Your Views on the Future of General Practice: Survey Report of the Reading Area.* Wokingham: W.Harold Lee Ltd.

Cundy, J.M. (1976) Reduction of medical student intake. *British Medical Journal,* 2, 380-381.

Daily Telegraph (1975) No room in Canada for British G.P.s, 20 June.

Davison, R.H. (1961) Medical emigration: second thoughts on the Royal Commission. *Lancet,* 1, 1107-1108.

Davison, R.H. (1962) Medical emigration to North America. *British Medical Journal,* 1, 786-787.

Desai, A.S. (1969) *Attitudes and Learning Experiences of Foreign Students in American School and Social Work.* Dissertation submitted to the faculty of the School of Social Service Administration in candidacy for the degree of Doctor of Philosophy, University of Chicago, Chicago, Illinois.

Ennals, D. (1976) Emigration of doctors. *Lancet*, 2, 107.

Evans, J.P. (1970) Notes on the foreign medical graduate problem in North America. *British Journal of Medical Education*, 4, 249-251.

Eysenck, H.J. (1977) The facts of life. *Observer*, 6 March.

Farquhar, J.W., Hendrickse, R.G., Lindblad, B.S., Senecal, J. & Sterky, G. (1976) Teaching child health problems of developing countries to European medical students. *Medical Education*, 10, 122-124.

Fendall, R. (1975) Emigration of doctors. *British Medical Journal*, 1, 190.

Gawn, R.A. (1978) The E.E.C. Medical Directives: present state of implementation. *Health Trends*, 10, 1-3.

General Medical Council (1976) *Annual Report for 1975*, London.

Gish, O. (1969) Medical education and the brain drain. *British Journal of Medical Education*, 3, 11-14.

Gish, O. (1970) British doctor migration 1962-67. *British Journal of Medical Education*, 4, 279-288.

Gish, O. & de Maar, M.J.A. (1969) Graduates of British and Irish Medical Schools taking State Board examinations in America. *British Journal of Medical Education*, 3, 221-224.

Hansard (1961) Parliamentary Debates, 5th Series, vol. 235, col. 1131.

Health Trends (1971) Migration of doctors and medical manpower planning. 3, 35.

Joorabchi, B. (1973) Physician migration: brain drain or overflow? With special reference to the situation in Iran. *British Journal of Medical Education*, 7, 44-47.

Klein, R. (1977) Doctors and the economy. *The Times*, 24 March.

Kuan, P. (1970) Medical education in Taiwan. *British Journal of Medical Education*, 4, 164-167.

Lancet (1962) Postgraduate medical education. Conference convened by the Nuffield Provincial Hospitals Trust, 1, 367-368.

Lancet (1977a) The Medical Bill in the Lords, 2, 1370.

Lancet (1977b) Health reports, 1, 316.

Lancet (1977c) Liberal Party Evidence to the Royal Commission, 1, 377-378.

Lancet (1977d) Continuing controversy on foreign doctors, 1, 476.

Lassers, E. & Nordan, R. (1975) Difficulties in postgraduate training of foreign paediatric residents and interns in child psychiatry. *British Journal of Medical Education*, 9, 286-290.

Last, J.M. & Brodie, E. (1970) Further careers of young British doctors. *British Medical Journal*, 4, 735-738.

Merrison Committee (1975) *Report of the Committee of Inquiry into the Regulation of the Medical Profession*, London: H.M.S.O.

Mittel, N.S. (1970) Training psychiatrists from developing nations. *American Journal of Psychiatry*, 126, 1143-1149.

Mofidi, C.M.H. (1970) *Medical Manpower in Iran*. Public Health Papers No. 47, Geneva: World Health Organization.

Observer Review (1977) Third World Medicine: overseas opportunities, 13 February.

Office of Health Economics (1966) *Medical Manpower*, London, p.16.

Ogston, D., Ogston, W.D. & Ogston, C.M. (1970) Origin and employment of the medical graduates of the University of Aberdeen 1931-69. *British Medical Journal*, 4, 360-361.

Osunkoya, B.O. (1974) Postgraduate medical education in developing countries. *British Journal of Medical Education*, 8, 69-73.

Parkhouse, J. (1976) Do we need more doctors or not? *Proceedings of the Royal Society of Medicine*, 69, 815-821.

Pickering, Sir George (1974) Postgraduate medical education. In *The Way Ahead* Published for the Nuffield Provincial Hospitals Trust by the Oxford University Press, London, pp. 1-6.

Pilkington Report (1960) *Doctors and Dentists' Remuneration 1957-60.* Cmnd. 939, London: H.M.S.O.

Platt Report (1961) *Medical Staffing Structure in the Hospital Service.* London: H.M.S.O.

Rao, T.V. (1974) Work value patterns of Indian medical students. *British Journal of Medical Education, 8,* 224-229.

Reinhardt, U.E. (1975) *Physician Productivity and the Demand for Health Manpower.* Cambridge, Mass: Bollinger.

Report (1963) *Medical Aid to the Developing Countries.* Report by a Working Party, Chairman: Sir Arthur Porritt, London: H.M.S.O.

Rickards, J.F. (1977) No Britons apply for N.H.S. post (Correspondence). *The Times,* 1 March.

Ronaghy, H.A., Iqbal, A.A., Moradi, S.R. & Solter, S.L. (1974) Evaluation of student opinion regarding curriculum in an Iranian medical school. *British Journal of Medical Education, 8,* 127-130.

Seale, J.R. (1962) Medical emigration from Britain, 1930-61. *British Medical Journal, 1,* 782-786.

Seale, J. (1964) Medical emigration from Great Britain and Ireland. *British Medical Journal, 1,* 1173-1178.

Seale, J. (1966) Medical emigration from Great Britain and Ireland since 1962. *British Medical Journal, 2,* 576-578.

Sebai, Z.A. & Baker, T.D. (1976) Projected needs of health manpower in Saudi Arabia, 1974-90. *Medical Education, 10,* 359-361.

Senewiratne, B. (1976) Medical training in developing countries. *British Medical Journal, 1,* 43.

Somers, A.R. (1971) *Health Care in Transition. Directions for the Future.* Chicago: Hospital Research and Education Trust, p.7.

The Times (1976a) Disagreements delay free movement of doctors within EEC, 15 December.

The Times (1976b) NHS as attraction for surplus EEC doctors, 16 December.

Todd Report (1968) *Royal Commission on Medical Education,* Cmnd. 3569, London: H.M.S.O.

Toronto Star (1974) Ottawa to study quota on immigrant doctors, 15 February.

Whitfield, A.G.W. (1969) Emigration of Birmingham medical graduates 1959-1963. *Lancet, 1,* 667-669.

Willink Report (1957) *Report of the Committee to Consider the Future Numbers of Medical Practitioners and the appropriate intake of Medical Students.* London: H.M.S.O.

World Health Organization (1976) *Multinational Study of the International Migration of Physicians and Nurses.* HMD/76.4, Geneva.

8. The Future

'Planning can be defined as the process of deciding how the future should be better than the present'. (W.H.O., 1974b)

METHODS OF APPROACH

A great deal of work has now been done on manpower planning in medicine and the allied health professions, in a number of different countries. Hiestand (1966) commented that, 'the literature is already voluminous, but one is impressed more by what has not been learned than what has'. Regrettably, the same remains true a decade later. But progress has been made towards understanding the nature of the problems and appreciating the shortcomings and potentialities of each of the possible methods of approach. Much of the relevant work, with particular reference to European countries, is reviewed in a number of W.H.O. reports (1969, 1971, 1973, 1974a, 1974b).

Economists and social scientists tend on the whole to take a fundamentally different view of the planning situation from doctors and others who are professionally concerned with the inner workings of the system. In the extreme, one view is to decide how much money is likely to be available, or should be made available, for the health services and then to plan accordingly; the opposite view is to decide how many doctors and others are needed and then work out the costs. In practice, it is not profitable to pursue either policy in isolation, and compromise is needed. This point was well made by Klarman (1969), who reviewed the economic approach. Economists tend to be less restrained by traditional demarcations between professional groups, and have displayed very considerable interest in the possibilities of substitution of one form of manpower for another, in the hope of achieving the most efficient type of team at the minimum cost in relation to its effectiveness. As Klarman remarked, 'the primary difference between the economist's approach and that of others is that the former doubts the fixity of ratios between different types of health personnel and the ratio of such personnel to a population, and asserts the technical possibility of substitution among health occupations'. It is generally recognised, however, that there are limits to this substitution. A further very important comment was made by Klarman, 'another difference of approach is that the economist tends to favour a range of projections derived from the application of a given method of

110

estimation under alternative assumptions'. As mentioned in previous chapters of this book, it has become increasingly obvious that it is necessary to explore the consequences of a variety of different strategic approaches rather than merely trying to arrive at a single, categorical statement about how many doctors will be needed in a given future year.

A point that should be made at the outset is that there is a fundamental interrelationship between macro and micro-planning. Again, some form of compromise is necessary for almost all purposes. An extremely detailed manpower analysis of the internal ramifications of the system, in which every compartment and movement is assessed, usually presents enormous difficulties and becomes too unwieldy to be useful. But on the other hand, a very crude model which is concerned merely with the total population of doctors, and not at all with how they are distributed within the system, is almost invariably valueless. In practice, therefore, it is at least necessary to look at the major components of the system in order to understand what effects the development of a situation over a period of time is likely to have.

The first possible approach to manpower planning is on the basis of requisite professional standards. A classic study was that of Lee and Jones (1933). Starting from first principles, the process of planning on this basis may be summarised as follows (W.H.O., 1974b).

1. Objective setting, e.g. defining the diseases most in need of control and prevention within specific population groups.

2. Projecting problems and resources in the light of the probable future situation, e.g. changes in the population pattern.

3. Reviewing possible policy options in keeping with probable resources and constraints.

4. Deciding on policies.

5. Drawing up programmes.

6. Incorporating evaluation procedures to measure progress or lack of it.

7. Repeating the planning cycle.

A practical description of methods of manpower planning in the U.S.S.R., largely along these lines, is given by Popov (1971) and Bogatyrev (1969).

The total review of an existing health system in a developed society, for example in Great Britain, would be a massive undertaking and in practice the starting point for future manpower estimates tends to be more pragmatic. A piecemeal approach to the evaluation of existing services and means of delivery of health care is more feasible, and must be undertaken as a basis for future major policy decisions. To take but one example, studies of the possible organisation of the work of general practice such as those reported by Crombie (1972) and Bevan (1972) should be pursued.

Other, less basic approaches to future planning are based on such criteria as desirable doctor/population ratios, which may be broken into 'norms' for individual specialties and regions, overall economic estimates based on the proportion of the gross national product which should be devoted to health care, or simply the rate of growth in the numbers of doctors which is considered desirable or feasible on the basis of varying criteria. Each of these approaches is relatively crude, for reasons which have been partially discussed. As a comparative guide, for one region in relation to another or one nation in relation to others, doctor/population ratios have some merit as a macro-planning guide and have been used in a number of countries as well as Great Britain (e.g. Judek, 1964;

111

Surgeon General's Consultant Group, 1959).

Where a National Health Service does not exist, and the organisation of medical work is largely on an item of service basis, estimates of manpower requirement may be made on the basis of actual or desirable hours of work or caseloads for various types of doctors (U.S.A. Manpower Commission, 1974; Vandewater, 1975; Reinhold, 1976). This approach has its own difficulties. For example the public 'demand' for a particular type of service, such as general surgery, which is being met on a private practice basis by the specialists concerned may not reflect the 'need' of the community for this service as it might be assessed by an impartial observer. Bunker's (1970) study of surgical practice in the U.S.A. and Great Britain is pertinent to this. Anaesthetists would also comment that to measure their workload according to the number of cases anaesthetised in a year would be very misleading unless allowances were made for the different speed of surgery on the two sides of the Atlantic.

Whatever method of approach is employed, there are a number of weighting factors which must be taken into account. These include some already discussed in previous chapters, for example retirement age, the increase in proportion of women medical graduates, and the increasing tendency for doctors to work 'social hours'. Many other factors relate to the 'productivity' of doctors and possible future trends in this regard. The Australian Commission on Medical Manpower (1973) analysed many of the relevant trends in productivity under the following headings:

(a) Organisational Changes

    The use of paramedical personnel in community practice:
      Practice nurses
      Social workers
      Physiotherapists, etc.

    Paramedical personnel in hospitals and special centres

    Organisation of medical training:
      Undergraduate courses
      Internship
      Vocational training

    Domiciliary care

    Regionalisation in rural areas

(b) Advances in Medical Knowledge and Technology

    Multi-phasic screening
    Preventive medicine
    Therapeutics
    Medical records

(c) Conditions of Work

    Hours
    Earlier retirement
    Study leave

(d) Age and Sex Distribution of Doctors

An extended dsicussion of physician productivity in relation to the U.S.A. is provided by Reinhardt (1975).

Many of the factors listed above are equally relevant to the British condition, and each may have either a positive or negative effect on overall 'productivity'. On balance, the Australian conclusion was that there is no likelihood of a future net increase in productivity. In other words, it is wise to assume that for any given total number of patients to be treated, the necessary number of doctors will rise rather than fall.

Most of the above considerations are related more to the demand side of the medical manpower equation than the supply side.

The main factors governing supply are firstly, the manpower resources of the community - the numbers of school leavers with the intellectual and personal capacity to become doctors; secondly, the availability of money for medical school teachers, buildings and equipment; and thirdly, the feasible rate at which any desired expansion can be achieved. It is generally assumed that the first of these conditions presents no problems. Certainly, the demand for medical school places far exceeds the available number and the current increase in the medical school intake, far from endangering academic standards, has corresponded with an increased stringency of entry requirements. The second restraint is, in fact, vital in one sense but irrelevant in another. Although much has been made recently of the cost of training doctors, the amounts of money involved are insignificant compared to the cost of the subsequent employment of these doctors throughout their professional lives and the demands that they are likely to make for equipment and other resources (Maynard, 1977). The real need is to match the supply to the market demand for doctors; nobody would defend the expenditure of large sums of money on training doctors who are forced to emigrate through disillusionment with conditions of work in Britain or through sheer unemployment. But once the need for more doctors is established, the cost of training them should not be a major factor. The difficulty, as always, is to relate manpower predictions to the time-scale of medical training, which is uncomfortably long; this will be further discussed in relation to possible strategies of planning. The third constraint, the rate at which supply can be altered, is significant in relation to the expansion or contraction of existing medical schools and the creation of new ones, but other forms of control are potentially available in relation to the admission of doctors from overseas and the substitution, to a greater or lesser extent according to need, of alternative forms of health manpower. Politically, the control of supply through manipulation of international movement has always presented problems of which this country, as a free society, should perhaps be particularly proud. The consequent inconvenience, from the planning point of view, which has hitherto resulted from our association with the Empire and the Commonwealth may very well continue in future as a result of our membership of the European Economic Community. It is merely one more complicating factor in the overall prediction of supply and demand.

As a last general comment on methods of approach, the importance of further and more detailed micro-planning studies is emphasised by the reminder from the Hospital Junior Staffs Committee of the British Medical Association (H.J.S.C., 1977), 'there is, however, a paradoxical situation whereby there are areas throughout the country, both geographically and in certain specialties, where medical staffing is inadequate to meet service needs. This is a problem of maldistribution and not of total numbers. It is made worse by a chaotic and grossly imbalanced staffing structure so that there are too many doctors in the training grades to allow all who have completed adequate training schedules to get through to established career posts'.

MODEL ANALYSIS

All worthwhile future estimates and predictions depend upon the ability to visualise the system and its component parts in order to under-

stand the effect of various influences upon it. This implies the construction of a 'model' of the system, which may be carried in the mind or
set down in some form on paper. Most people who think about medical manpower have some kind of 'mental picture' of the system which doctors are
entering and leaving, and within which they distribute themselves and
obtain promotion. The great advantage of putting the picture on paper,
in as unambiguous a form as possible, is that others may apply similar
analysis and may compare their own 'mental pictures' with it.

Models may be simple or complex. They may be concerned with long-
term trends or short-term problems. They may deal with the whole system
or with parts of it. Since very different models, of differing degrees
of complexity, are appropriate for different purposes it is useful to
break down the components of the system in symbolic form so that any
suitable model can be put together from the relevant pieces.

In this context, 'the system' may be understood to mean the medical
profession of Great Britain as a whole or, depending on what information
is available and required, the medical staff of the National Health Service. As already indicated, a specific model may be concerned only with
a sub-system - e.g. psychiatrists or women doctors.

Analysis of the system

The system as a whole is made up of compartments, or cells, which
may be designated as rectangular boxes. Each cell contains classes of
doctors, which may conveniently be shown in capital letters. The cells
are related to each other, and possible movement in various directions
can be indicated by arrows between cells. From many cells movement is
also possible to the outside world - i.e. to locations external to the
system, which may be distinguished diagrammatically by being enclosed
within a curved boundary.

Thus, each cell will have an inflow and an outflow:

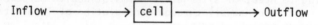

In practice, there will frequently be more than one possible inflow:

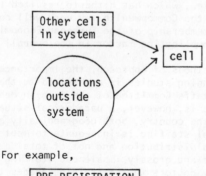

For example,

```
PRE-REGISTRATION
HOUSE OFFICERS  ─┐
                 ├→  S.H.O.
OVERSEAS DOCTORS ─┘
```

                    etc.

Likewise, each cell has one or more outflows:

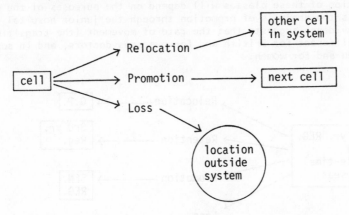

In this case, relocation and promotion have been shown as separate possibilities, since this is of importance in modelling the actual movements of doctors. Movement from the registrar 'cell' to the senior registrar 'cell' (promotion) is fundamentally different from movement to, for example, the general practice 'cell' (relocation).

e.g.

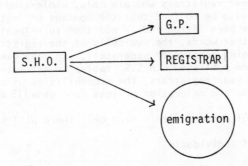

The actual designation of cells may depend on the purpose of the model. For example, within each grade of the hospital service there are potential sub-cells which for some purposes may need to be shown separately,

e.g.

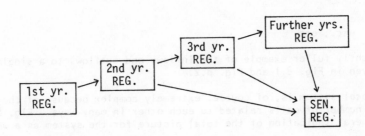

115

There may be one or more classes of doctor within each cell. Again, the designation of these classes will depend on the purposes of the model. An example is the analysis of promotion through the junior hospital grades, where evidence suggests that the rate of movement (the transition matrix) is different for British and for overseas doctors, and in some cases for men and for women.

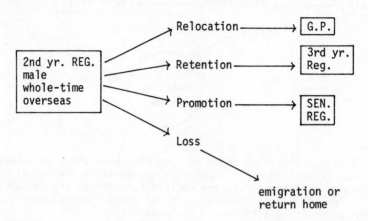

The above example depicts a very specific analysis of the possible movement of second year registrars who are male, whole-time and overseas graduates. It will also be noticed that the concept of 'retention' as a possible movement has been introduced in addition to relocation, promotion and loss. In other words, the sub-cells of the registrar grade, one for each year, are being considered separately. In many cases enough detail is available from published D.H.S.S. tables to estimate for a sub-cell, such as second year registrars, the probabilities of promotion, retention in the grade and relocation or loss (see page 119 and pages 120-21).

For each class of doctors within each cell there will be:

Number of individuals	n
Average tenure (years)	$\bar{t}$
Annual inflow (= sum of inflow sources)	ΣI
Annual outflow (= sum of outflows)	ΣO
∴ Annual fractional expansion	$\dfrac{\Sigma I - \Sigma O}{n}$

etc., etc.

A slightly fuller example of the inflows and outflows to a single cell is given in Fig. 8.1 and Fig. 8.2.

The total system is, of course, extremely complex because of the very large number of cells related to each other in many ways. Fig. 8.3 shows a general indication of the total picture for the system as a whole,

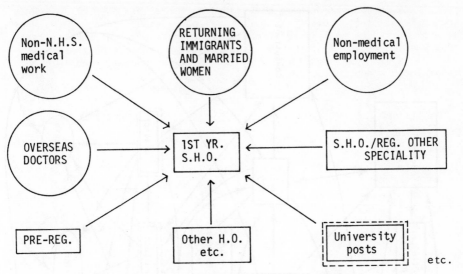

etc.

Fig. 8.1   1st year S.H.O. - inflow

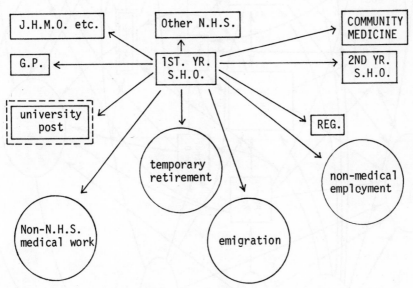

Fig. 8.2   1st year S.H.O. - outflow

but this should not be regarded as being necessarily either complete or accurate.

On the above basis, the system is capable of analysis from two points of view. Firstly, in terms of the stock of doctors in each individual cell or combination of cells. This form of analysis is necessary to establish what the actual availability of manpower will be at a given time for specified types of work. Secondly, the analysis may concentrate

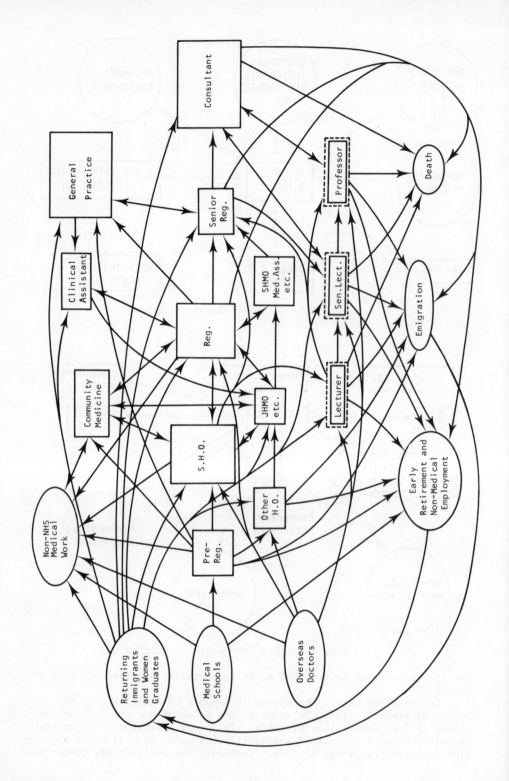

118

on <u>flows</u> along the various lines depicting possible movement. This form of analysis is important in order to understand recruitment and promotion prospects. The mathematical probabilities assignable to movements for different classes of doctors in different directions will vary from time to time, or can be assumed to vary in order to determine the consequences of this.

In general, prediction of what the state of the system will be at a given future date depends on what will happen in each of the intervening years (for most purposes the year being the appropriate unit of time). Calculation therefore has to build the effect of each year on the effect of the preceding ones, taking into account the influence of change within one cell on all other relevant cells and sub-cells. To give a detailed example, a change in the number of British graduates becoming registrars will not immediately alter the promotion rate from registrar to senior registrar, since the composition of the second year registrar and third year registrar sub-cells will be unaltered for twelve and twenty-four months respectively. But outflow from the first year registrar sub-cell to other locations such as general practice (relocation) and overseas (loss) may well change. These outflow changes may equal the inflow change, but if not then either the size of the first year registrar sub-cell must change or the rate of movement into the second year registrar sub-cell must change. This is a fairly complex exercise in micro-planning but it may well be relevant to certain questions about the probable future state of affairs.

Availability of data

To establish a comprehensive data base for the whole system would require the placing of an exact number in each cell and sub-cell of the system (and for each class of doctor) and the assigning of a probability to movement along each arrow in the diagram. To be able to use this basic data it would also be necessary to know the probable error of each of these numerical values, and the rate of change or likelihood of change for each of them. There are many deficiencies in the existing data, which comes nowhere near to fulfilling these criteria. Available data can be used for simplified analysis, in which a number of cells or classes of doctors are grouped together and treated as single entities. Also, individual parts of the system can to some extent be analysed.

It nevertheless remains true that the major limitation in modelling, for the immediate future, is lack of sufficient data. The necessary mathematical and statistical techniques have been worked out in considerable detail (Bartholomew, 1976) and there is very little limitation from this point of view to the amount of sophistication that can be applied. It is a much more difficult problem, however, to test the validity and relevance of the conclusions derived from a model calculation by comparing them with what happens in real life. This is because the real-life data are usually not available in sufficient detail, or with sufficient promptness, to make it possible to see at what stage the modelling process has departed from reality. The end result may become known in terms of a crude overall number of doctors, but this leaves the modeller in a 'black box' situation, in which he is faced with the possibility of making an almost infinite number of modifications to the assumptions about movement within the 'box' in order to achieve a better fit with what comes out at the other end, and without any means of knowing which of the modifications are more likely to be appropriate. This gives a gloomy view of the situation. There are mitigating circumstances, but the need for better data remains.

A particular problem concerns trends. Much forecasting depends on the discernment of trends and their projection. With medical manpower data it is often difficult to know if there are genuine trends, and it may be highly dangerous to assume their existence. Changes in immigration and emigration requirements and possibilities, relative remuneration of different types of work, changes in promotion prospects due to national economic problems and many other factors can profoundly affect the movement and distribution of doctors. These changes can occur very suddenly with a result that 'trends' in particular directions, which perhaps never existed in the first place, become grossly misleading indicators of the immediate future. For these reasons a flair for stockmarket speculation may be more useful in medical manpower forecasting than detailed knowledge of trend analysis.

Problems may also arise in the interpretation of data, and this again emphasises the importance of understanding what a model is meant to do, and what information is expected from it. An example, which is important in relation to promotion rates in the junior hospital grades and also to the question of retirement and replacement of consultants and general practitioners, is length of tenure. The D.H.S.S. publishes tables showing the age distribution of consultants and general practitioners, in 10 and 5 year bands (see Chapter 3 - 'Retirement'), and showing the numbers of junior hospital doctors who have spent varying numbers of years since 'first entry into the grade'. In the latter case, some inference can be drawn about length of tenure allowing for the fact that the given figures are premature and hence incomplete. The fact that a registrar has currently been in the grade for two years but less than three does not give any indication of when he is likely to leave; his true length of tenure can never be known until he has actually moved to some other grade. There is an important distinction between the data for successive cohorts of junior doctors, and for successive calendar years.

Some figures for senior registrars in England and Wales, derived from the D.H.S.S. tables 12.1, are given in Table 8.1, in which cohort data are represented by the diagonal movement of individual doctors through the matrix (as shown by arrows) and census data are derived from the separate vertical columns for individual years.

Unfortunately, in the D.H.S.S. tables, all senior registrars in post for five years or more are grouped together. For purposes of calculation it could be assumed that those remaining five years or more have a mean tenure of six years, but alternative calculations (shown in brackets in the table) assume that those over five years have a mean tenure of seven years. On this basis, it can be seen that the average length of tenure for the three successive cohorts of senior registrars who joined the grade in 1968, 1969 and 1970 was fairly constant, at about 2.6 years. In contrast, the census data, for the average tenure of all senior registrars in post in the successive calendar years between 1970 and 1973 revealed much lower figures, varying from 1.76 to 1.87. It can be shown empirically that appreciable differences of this kind are likely to arise in some circumstances, for example where there is a progressive shortening of the true cohort tenure with a consequent fall in the number of people in the grade. In terms of model building and forecasting, there are some circumstances in which it is important to know the expectations of discrete cohorts in terms of average tenure: a flow exercise. The individual senior registrar, in assessing his prospects, needs most of all to have an insight into the factors influencing the situation. He may feel that he is not very interested in the average length of tenure of senior

Table 8.1

Years since first entry to the grade	Calendar Year							
	1968	1969	1970	1971	1972	1973	1974	1975
Under 1	457	508	559	513	654	658	700	629
1 but under 2	361	391	421	478	414	541	523	589
2 but under 3	245	255	238	308	325	294	343	356
3 but under 4	122	134	148	144	191	181	168	211
4 but under 5	54	54	77	84	72	80	82	69
5 or over 5	36	41	39	57	53	58	62	65
			1.76	1.87	1.80	1.78		2.58 (2.70)
			(1.78)	(1.91)	(1.83)	(1.81)		2.65 (2.77)
								2.54 (2.67)

registrars for the year in which he joins the grade, since he will be looking for promotion two or three years later and, as the above table shows, a single year (such as 1971) may be misleading: he may feel even less interested in the mean lengths of tenure of senior registrars who joined the grade four or five years previously but this is the only 'complete' information about individuals that he can have.

The importance of differences between 'census' and 'cohort' data is discussed by Forbes (1976), and the problem of calculating lengths of tenure for junior hospital doctors was at least partially explored by the Platt (1961) Report (paragraph 95 and Appendix 4). It has been pointed out (Bartholomew, 1971) that there is some advantage in using the median rather than the mean in cohort analysis.

PARTIAL AND SIMPLIFIED MODELS

Partial models have been used to examine the junior hospital grades, both on a stock basis to examine the feasibility of proposed changes such as the Todd proposals (Parkhouse and McLaughlin, 1975a) and on a flow basis, in order to estimate promotion patterns and future prospects in this respect (Parkhouse and McLaughlin, 1975b). Beyond a certain point, these analyses tend to break down through lack of sufficiently detailed data - for example concerning movement of women doctors as opposed to men or overseas doctors as opposed to British doctors. The D.H.S.S. classification of place of birth does not distinguish between doctors born in the older commonwealth countries such as Australia and New Zealand, and those

born in India, Pakistan and elsewhere; but success rates in postgraduate
examinations and prospects of promotion are greatly different for the two
categories, and it is misleading to group them together.

Simplified models of the system as a whole have considerable possibilities. As far as the National Health Service is concerned, the entire
system can be regarded as made up of four cells into which there are two
sources of entry and from which the losses can be pooled (Fig. 8.4).

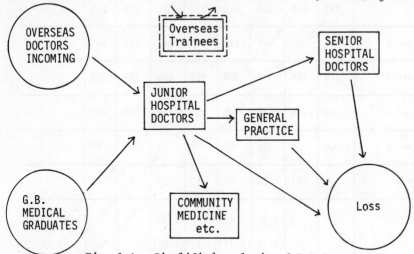

Fig. 8.4   *Simplified analysis of N.H.S. system*

All doctors in the N.H.S., including those with honorary appointments, can be embraced within the above scheme. The junior hospital doctor 'cell' may be taken to include pre-registration and other house officers, and doctors in university and other posts holding honorary N.H.S.
grading up to and including senior registrar. The senior hospital doctor
'cell' may be taken to include consultants, S.H.M.O.s, locums, and university and other staff with senior hospital grading. The general practitioner 'cell' can include principals, trainees and assistants. The
cell for 'community medicine etc.' may be regarded as including doctors
with various appointments not otherwise included, for example ophthalmic
medical practitioners and those with paragraph 94 and 87 appointments
only. The losses from the system will include retirement, death and premature retirement, complete, partial or temporary loss of women and
others leaving the system from time to time, and emigration. For simplicity, it may be convenient to treat the system as if all losses from
death and retirement and losses of women doctors are from the three career grade 'cells', and that all losses from emigration are from the junior hospital doctors 'cell'; this is an adequate representation of the
true state of affairs for most practical purposes, but more detailed
apportionment can be made if necessary. It is also convenient to think
of emigration as the sum of the gross annual loss of overseas doctors together with the net annual loss of British doctors; this is because the
inflow of overseas doctors is shown separately (and is important to take
into account) whereas the return flow of British doctors from abroad is
not.

Input to the system from the British medical schools can be calculated, for future years, on the basis of medical school intake figures

with an allowance of about 6% a year for wastage during the undergraduate course, and with a small additional discount for the few graduates who do not take up pre-registration posts and enter the system (about 20 a year). With these allowances, the input from this source can be based on the medical school output for the year in question. In fact, N.H.S. stock data relate to 30 September of any one year; by 30 September not all the graduates for the calendar year in question will have left medical school and entered the system, but the approximation is trivial compared to other sources of error.

Fig. 8.4 also includes a dotted cell for 'overseas trainees'. This is referred to subsequently in relation to the possibility of arranging, at some time in the future, specified postgraduate training programmes, for overseas graduates, perhaps on the basis of three-years tenure in the United Kingdom.

The total stock of doctors in the system is the sum of the contents of the constituent cells:

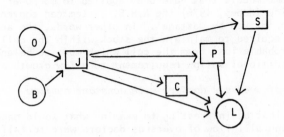

```
O = Overseas immigrants
B = British graduates
J = Junior hospital
S = Senior hospital
P = General Practice
C = Community medicine, etc.
L = Loss
```

Total number of doctors in starting year (Y_o) = J_o + S_o + P_o + C_o

The growth of the system between two points in time will be the sum of the increase in content of each cell, and this will be equal to the total input to the system minus the total loss during the same period of time:

Growth in one year:

$$(Y_1 - Y_o) = (J_1 - J_o) + (S_1 - S_o) + (P_1 - P_o) + (C_1 - C_o)$$

$$= (O_1 + B_1) - L_1$$

The advantage of a simplified model of this kind is that it is readily comprehensible, self-contained and comprehensive. Enough data are available to make it useful, and it gives enough information to enable developments in each of the major sectors of the service to be examined. It is a fair approximation to the real-life situation; for most purposes no serious error is introduced by assuming that the only possible movements within the system are along the few arrows indicated. The model enables a variety of options to be examined relatively simply, and also enables continuous adjustment to be made. This is an important consideration, since with more elaborate models it is necessary to have access to interactive computing facilities, or else to depend upon a predetermined computer programme and obtain a print-out of the resulting data for perhaps 20 or 30 years into the future. It may become apparent on inspection that after the first few years the results become unrealistic because some of the assumptions incorporated in the programme need to be modified. This requires re-programming and examination of a further print-out. To decide in advance that progressive changes should take place - for example that the senior hospital staff grade should grow at 2% a year for five years, then 3% for three/four years and thereafter at 4% a year is difficult. With the simplified model here described year-by-year analysis of events can be simulated by hand, so that the progress of events can be continually inspected and the effect of what appear to be appropriate adjustments can be assessed.

EXAMPLES OF FUTURE ESTIMATES

As with some models that have been applied to manpower planning in the Civil Service (Hopes, 1976) the N.H.S. system can conveniently be regarded as being 'driven by wastage'. In other words, the annual inflow to each cell, required to maintain the stock within the cell, is determined by the probable loss from the cell which must be balanced. To this is added any additional inflow requirement to allow growth of the cell.

Reduced inflow of overseas doctors with constant outflow

It might first be interesting to examine what would happen to the system if the annual inflow of overseas doctors were to fall to 2,000 a year in 1976 and thereafter to 1,000 a year by 1978, while at the same time the annual loss of overseas doctors continued at approximately the present rate of at least 2,500 a year.

The starting point for this and subsequent predictions is the N.H.S. staffing figures for Great Britain in 1975:

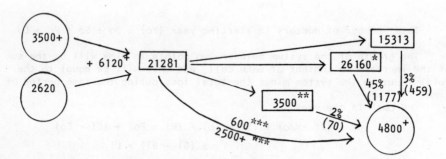

*   the more accurate figure of 26,128 became available after calculations were made, but the difference would be insignificant.

**   this is an estimate based on approximately 2,900 w.t.e. in England and Wales and 590 w.t.e. in Scotland.

*** in this and subsequent diagrams the figure above the line represents net loss of British graduates and the figure below the line represents gross loss of overseas doctors.

Some wastage rates from the four cells of the system are shown
alongside the relevant arrows. For the career grade 'cells' these are
estimates of the allowance to be made in order to replenish the existing
stock, without allowance for increase in the size of the grade. The estimate for general practice is derived from the following figures for unrestricted principals in Great Britain (Table 8.2):

Table 8.2

Year	1. No. of admissions	2. Increase in total number of Principals	3. Admissions to maintain exis- ting stock 1 - 2	4. 3 as a percentage of stock
1970-71	1159	291	868	3.78
1971-72	1298	470	828	3.56
1972-73	1365	243	1122	4.73
1973-74	1479	290	1189	4.96
1974-75	1346	209	1137	4.69

This indicates that there was an increase in the number of new principals required to maintain the existing stock after 1971-72. For the
last three years for which figures are available it appears that losses
from all causes have represented a little over 4.5% of the existing stock.
For senior hospital staff estimates are more difficult to obtain
since the available figures relate to numbers of paid consultants appointed (i.e. excluding honorary appointments). In the year 1973-74 in
England and Wales, 675 such appointments were made; when the increase in
the total number of paid consultants is allowed for this represents the
making good of a loss of about 340 (3.5% of the relevant stock). The
number of comparable appointments in 1974-76 was 592, representing the
making good of about 305 losses (3.0%). It is difficult to assess whether the same relationships would apply to honorary appointments; some of
these 'losses' would of course be to paid posts (e.g. from university
appointments to N.H.S. consultant posts) while the considerable increase
in the number of honorary posts over recent years would suggest a different age stratification and therefore perhaps a lower proportionate loss.
Altogether, however, it seems reasonable to assume that losses from the
senior hospital staff 'cell' will be at about the rate of 3% a year. The
estimate of 2% a year for losses from the community medicine and other
groups is based on the assumption that most of the fairly recently appointed people in this class will not be due for retirement for some time.
The 'cell' is a small one in relation to the whole system, and small variations in this estimate of loss would not be critical.
The figure of 600 above the arrow showing loss from the junior hospital 'cell' is a generous estimate for net emigration of British graduates. This is based on recent evidence (see Chapter 3 - 'Emigration and

125

Immigration'), but should also be regarded as making some allowance for relative loss due to the increasing proportion of women graduates. In fact, the appointments to the senior hospital and general practitioner grades include the replacement of losses from all causes; some loss of women doctors and loss due to emigration is therefore included in these percentages.

Altogether, the input of 6120+ doctors exceeds the total loss of 4800+, implying a gain of 1320 to the system (2%). This is consistent with the behaviour of the N.H.S. in the few years up to 1975.

However, assuming an inflow of only 2000 overseas doctors after 1975, the position in 1976 would be as shown below:

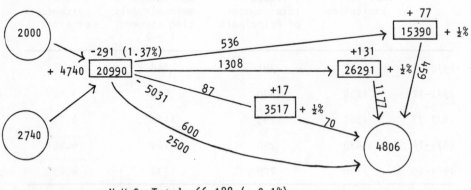

<u>N.H.S. Total</u> 66,188 (- 0.1%)

Here it has been assumed that it would be desirable to try and increase the size of the career grade, and a growth of one-half per cent a year has been allowed in these 'cells'. The number of additional people in each case is shown above the cell and the new total within. The number leaving the cell from the junior hospital staff 'cell' is also shown on the appropriate arrow, being the sum of the increase in cell size and the loss. The total loss from the junior hospital grade 'cell', shown at its bottom right hand corner, exceeds the combined gain from overseas doctors and British graduates by 291. There is thus a 1.37% decrease in the size of this 'cell'. The figure of 2500 below the arrow showing loss from the junior hospital staff 'cell' represents the continuing loss from the system of overseas doctors, at about the current rate (see Chapter 3 - 'Emigration and Immigration'). The N.H.S. total of doctors has diminished by 0.1%.

Following the sequence of events to 1977 gives the result as depicted in Fig. 8.5, and to 1978 the result depicted in Fig. 8.6.

It can now be seen that attempted expansion of the career grades, at even one half per cent a year, has resulted in a reduction in the number of junior hospital staff by almost 2,000 since 1975. The total N.H.S. staff has fallen to 65,014, a reduction of 1.31% from 1977-78, or 1.88% from 1975.

Pursuing the analysis beyond 1978 merely emphasises that the total number of doctors in the N.H.S. would have to continue falling until the British medical schools could supply enough doctors to balance the total losses from the system. With a continuing inflow of overseas doctors at about 1,000 a year, this would not be until after 1984. The small inc-

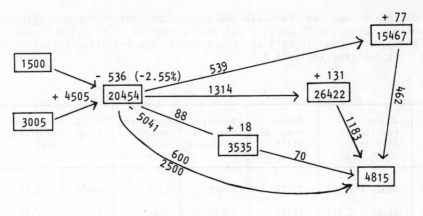

N.H.S. Total   65878   (- 0.47%)

Fig. 8.5   Sequence of events to 1977

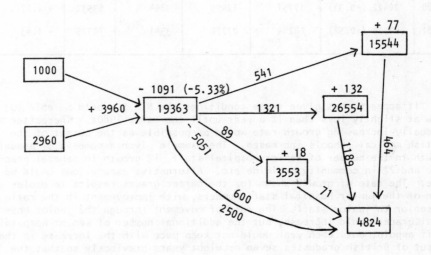

N.H.S. Total   65014   (- 1.31%)

Fig. 8.6   Sequence of events to 1978

rease in size of the career grades would lead to slightly accelerated promotion through the junior hospital grades. This would be required, or expected, as the proportion of British graduates in the junior hospital posts would gradually rise.

Reduced inflow of overseas doctors with correspondingly reduced outflow

It has been argued that if the inflow of overseas doctors falls there will be a tendency for more of those already working in the N.H.S. to seek permanent appointments in this country. The same analysis as outlined can be applied, but with the assumption that inflow and outflow of overseas doctors will balance at 2,000 a year in 1976, 1,500 a year in 1977 and 1,000 a year in 1978 and thereafter. The resulting situation up to 1981 is depicted in Table 8.3.

Table 8.3

	Junior Hospital Staff	Senior Hospital Staff 3% growth	General Practice 1% growth	Community Medicine etc. 2% growth	N.H.S. Total	% change on previous year
1976	20924 (-1.7%)	15772	26422	3570	66688	+ 0.66
1977	20788 (-0.6%)	16245	26686	3641	67360	+ 1.00
1978	20560 (-1.1%)	16732	26953	3714	67959	+ 0.89
1979	20480 (-0.4%)	17234	27223	3788	68725	+ 1.13
1980	20422 (-0.3%)	17751	17495	3864	69532	+ 1.17
1981	20530 (+0.5%)	18284	27770	3941	70525	+ 1.43

It appears that given these conditions the N.H.S. would be able to grow at slightly less than 1% a year until the early 1980s. Thereafter a gradually increasing growth rate would be possible as the output of the British medical schools increased. The example given assumes a 3% annual growth in the number of senior hospital staff, 1% growth in general practice and 2% in community medicine etc. Alternative assumptions could be made. The rate of growth shown for the career grades results in depletion of the junior hospital staff numbers, with improvement in the ratio of senior to junior staff. The rate of movement through the junior hospital grades would increase, but the additional number of senior hospital staff appointments each year would not keep pace with the increase in the output of British graduates seven or eight years previously so that the probability of a given British graduate obtaining a consultant appointment would be slightly reduced by 1981. Although the annual input and loss of overseas doctors is given as equal, it should be noted in this and subsequent analyses that the retirement and other losses from the career 'cells' would include some additional overseas doctors, so that the total number in the system would be expected to fall slightly.

Reduced inflow and correspondingly reduced outflow of overseas doctors, with no N.H.S. growth

The gloomier economic prognostications suggest that it may be impossible for the total medical staff of the N.H.S. to increase in the immediate future, and it has been suggested that the resulting fall in demand for additional medical manpower may compensate for the probable reduced inflow of overseas doctors.

If the inflow and outflow of overseas doctors in 1976 were to fall to 2,000, the resulting situation could be depicted as follows:

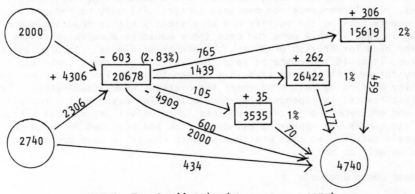

N.H.S. Total 66,254 (the same as 1975)

This is an extreme illustration, showing the effect of attempting to increase the size of the career grades at the expense of the junior hospital grade, while maintaining the total number of doctors without change. A 2% growth in senior hospital staff, with 1% growth in general practice and community medicine would result in a reduction of 603 in the number of junior hospital posts. If all the 2,000 incoming overseas graduates were to be accommodated, there would not be 'room' for all the British graduates, 434 of whom are shown as proceeding directly to the loss 'cell'. This should not be taken as a mathematically exact representation, since all the junior hospital grades are grouped together; in practice, the reduced total size of the junior hospital staff population would largely be due to the creaming off of more senior trainees to fill additional career posts. Some redistribution of posts between junior hospital grades could also, at least theoretically, be arranged in order to accommodate more graduates in the early stages. Nevertheless, this would still imply growth of the total number of doctors in the system, unless losses from the system could in some way be increased to balance the increasing input. This underlines the fact that virtually all the calculations for the future have assumed that the N.H.S. will continue to grow. There is little point in extending the above example beyond 1976; it merely illustrates the point that if the N.H.S. is not to grow the critical factor determining the capacity to accommodate British graduates in the immediate future is the number of overseas doctors seeking to enter the system and allowed to do so. In the longer term, the need for British graduates in a no-growth situation remains constant at roughly 2,350 a year.

Two points are particularly worth emphasising in relation to this analysis. Firstly, the enormous influence of even relatively small degrees of N.H.S. expansion should be noted. A growth of 1% requires almost an additional 700 doctors every year. Somewhere between this figure and the completely no-growth situation is a knife-edge, on either side of which lie the potential dangers of having either far too much or disastrously too little which were eloquently described, in another context, by Mr. Micawber. In fact, the N.H.S. growth rate needed to accommodate British graduates over the next decade, assuming reduced inflow and outflow of overseas doctors, is shown in the preceding analysis to be slightly less than 1% a year. Secondly, although the inflow <u>rate</u> of overseas doctors is assumed to fall, the correspondingly reduced exit <u>rate</u> implies that the actual <u>number</u> who remain in the country, and on whom the N.H.S. is dependent, will not fall except through retirement losses. Our 'dependence' on overseas doctors will only be reduced if the numbers leaving the country are consistently higher than the numbers coming in; and if this were the case there would be a correspondingly greater need for British graduates to take their places. Insofar as this is true, it could therefore be said that any anxiety about inability to employ future British graduates in a no-growth situation would stem from a policy of finding full employment for overseas graduates instead. In the last resort, it depends on whether policy in regard to the recruitment and employment of overseas doctors is to be active, so that the appropriate quotas are approximately determined and provided for each year, or purely passive, so that whatever numbers choose to come are accommodated as well as may be.

Overseas quota analysis

Since there is general agreement that the aim should be to reduce the dependence of the N.H.S. on overseas graduates, it is perhaps more valuable to examine an alternative approach to that given immediately above.

The assumption could be made that posts will be found in the N.H.S. for all British graduates who seek them, and that any residual posts will be made available to overseas graduates. In more emotive but less categorical terms it might be said that when a job is available the tendency will be to give first preference to a British graduate.

It might further be postulated that the rate of progression of future British graduates through the training grades, and the ultimate prospects of achieving a given career, should be no less favourable than they are at present and have been in the immediate past.

In order to construct a model on this basis, it is necessary to know something about the current rate of progress and the promotion prospects of British graduates.

Estimates can be made, from a transition matrix similar to that illustrated on page 121 (Table 8.1), and using data available from D.H.S.S. tables. The available information suggests that each year about 95% of pre-registration house officers are promoted to the S.H.O. grade; about 10% of the total stock of British S.H.O.s and registrars are promoted to the senior registrar grade and about 28% of British senior registrars are promoted to the consultant grade. It should be stressed that these are approximations, but they enable a slightly more detailed picture of this particular part of the N.H.S. system to be compiled.

Starting from 1975 data it is possible to show, on the above assumptions, that the demand for promotion to the consultant grade from British graduates would require a slight expansion of the consultant grade in 1976 (0.6% increase). This would leave no room for overseas doctors to be promoted to the consultant grade. On the other hand, there would not be sufficient British graduates seeking entry to general practice to maintain the existing stock, and in order to prevent a fall in the total number of general practitioners it would be necessary for 217 overseas graduates to enter general practice. Altogether, promotion at the existing rates would require an increase in the career grade cells of 99 persons. If the total size of the N.H.S. workforce were to be held constant, this would require the subtraction of 99 from the junior hospital staff 'cell'. It is then possible to see how many overseas doctors could be accommodated; assuming a loss of 2,500 overseas doctors from the system, there would be room to admit 2,058.

The analysis can be pursued in this manner. By 1980, still assuming that the total N.H.S. workforce has remained unchanged, there would be almost exactly enough British graduates seeking entry to general practice to replace vacancies, and enough seeking promotion to the consultant grade to allow a 1.3% expansion. Assuming that the loss of overseas graduates had fallen to 1,000, there would be room to accommodate only 219 newcomers from overseas.

By 1982 the increased output of the British medical schools would have had an appreciable effect, and general practice would have begun to expand in order to accommodate these British graduates. By 1984, with 3,655 British graduates entering the system, the picture could be represented as below:

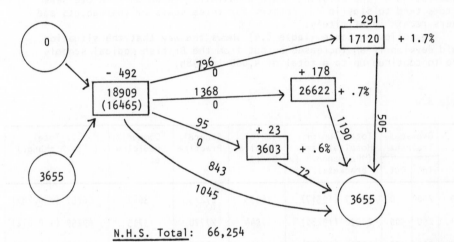

N.H.S. Total: 66,254

In the above diagram the numbers shown above the arrows are in each case numbers of British graduates and the numbers below the arrows represent overseas doctors. It is shown that the consultant grade is growing by 1.7%, and general practice by 0.7%, purely by virtue of the promotion of British graduates alone. The needs of community medicine are also satisfied. If the total size of the N.H.S. workforce is still limited to its 1975 level, there is no room for any newly entering overseas doctors; indeed, the loss of overseas doctors must rise from 1,000 to 1,045 in order to balance the equation.

This illustration is almost certainly entirely hypothetical, since it is a virtual certainty that, despite any temporary economic difficulties that may exist, the number of doctors in the N.H.S. will have risen appreciably by 1984. However, the purpose of the example is to illustrate how redistribution in favour of the career grades could be brought about, together with a progressive reduction of dependence on overseas doctors. It can be calculated on the basis of the above analysis that there would have been a net loss of over 7,100 overseas doctors from the N.H.S. between 1975 and 1984. At the same time, the ratio of junior hospital staff to senior staff would have changed from 1.37 : 1 to 1.1 : 1, and the proportion of British graduates in the junior hospital grades would have risen from 55% to 87%.

Limited-tenure training for overseas graduates to support N.H.S. growth

As a final example, it is interesting to see what would happen if there were to be a reduced intake of overseas graduates for permanent absorption into the N.H.S. workforce, together with some reduction in the annual loss of overseas doctors, but with extra posts at S.H.O./registrar levels specifically provided for overseas graduates seeking postgraduate training for a limited period of three years before returning home. This would represent the introduction of an additional 'cell' into the model for 'overseas trainees' (see Fig. 8.4, page

It is assumed that limited expansion of the N.H.S. workforce would occur, with some shift in distribution from junior to senior hospital posts. The analysis therefore represents a more effective use of our residual capacity to train (Parkhouse, 1972); the tidying-up and improved organisation of the existing state of affairs, in which some overseas doctors tend to stay in the country for three years or thereabouts and others remain indefinitely.

The following table (Table 8.4) shows the way that the situation would develop if an increased output from the British medical schools were to continue up to a total of 4,000 in 1988:

Table 8.4

	Overseas Trainees		Total Junior Hospital Staff ("Permanent" in brackets)	Senior Hospital Staff	General Practice	Community Medicine etc.	N.H.S. Total (with % change)*
	In	Out					
1979	250	0	20817 (19317)	16575	27223	3642	68257 (+ 0.78%)
1981	250	500	20530 (19280)	17244	27770	3715	69259 (+ 0.61%)
1983	500	750	20558 (19808)	17941	28328	3790	70617 (+ 0.96%)
1985	0	0	21259 (20759)	18666	28897	3868	72690 (+ 1.76%)
1987	0	0	21758	19803	29478	3946	74985 (+ 1.95%)
1989	0	0	22232	21419	30071	4025	77747 (+ 1.78%)

* change from previous year

In this example, the annual intake of 'overseas trainees' has been adjusted from year to year in order to maintain a fairly even total number of doctors in the junior hospital staff grades. On this basis, there would be no additional capacity to accept 'overseas trainees' after 1983, but the last of the 'overseas trainees' already present would not have left until after 1985. It can be seen that all the career grades have progressively expanded, with resultant redistribution, and that the N.H.S. total for medical staff begins to rise at more than 1% after 1984 (but

132

never reaches the levels that have actually occurred in recent years).

In these calculations it has been assumed that in addition to the 'overseas trainees' there would be a continuing 'permanent' inflow of overseas doctors at 1,000 a year throughout, with a gradually diminishing annual loss of foreign doctors other than the 'overseas trainees'. Altogether, there would therefore be some reduction in the N.H.S. dependence on permanently resident overseas doctors, but by no means so great a reduction as in the previous example.

Many variations of the above scheme are possible, but it demonstrates the feasibility and potential advantage of identifying residual training capacity and using it for 'overseas trainees' in this way.

Simple models of the above type can be applied to other estimates, for example those of the Willink Report (1957) and the British Medical Association's Evidence to the Royal Commission (B.M.A., 1977). However, enough illustrations have been given to illustrate the ways in which such models can be used. The inherent advantages of year-by-year analysis, with nothing more than the use of a simple pocket calculator, are obvious. The introduction of additional factors, however, soon creates problems, and this is exemplified by the 'overseas quota' analysis above, requiring estimation of promotion rates; the basis for the estimates is given in more detail in a separate paper (Parkhouse, 1978). For more detailed and sophisticated manpower estimates, therefore, it is necessary to have access to interactive computing facilities.

STRATEGY

The evolution of a medical manpower strategy requires an examination of the question of how not merely to predict the future state of affairs, but to influence it.

Comments have frequently been made, (e.g. W.H.O., 1973; Maynard, 1976) about the need for long-term, medium-term and short-term plans and about the necessity to look for alternative methods of control other than manipulation of undergraduate numbers in the medical schools. The length of medical training and the uncertainty of the future make it inherently unsatisfactory to try and achieve precise regulation by control of medical school intake; the effort is rather like trying to add the fine touches to a delicate painting by means of a brush attached to the end of a 12 foot cane.

The development of an appropriate strategy can be envisaged in three stages, representing long-term, medium-term and short-term plans (Fig.8.7).

Coarse control

This is the stage at which medical school numbers are mainly concerned. It requires a minimum cycle of 7 - 8 years to allow for the planning of an increased or reduced intake to the medical schools at one end, and the completion of the pre-registration year at the other.

Medium control

Control over the available number of doctors over a cycle of 3 - 5

133

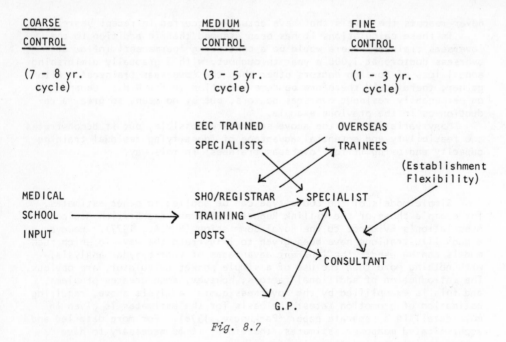

COARSE CONTROL	MEDIUM CONTROL	FINE CONTROL
(7 - 8 yr. cycle)	(3 - 5 yr. cycle)	(1 - 3 yr. cycle)

EEC TRAINED SPECIALISTS

OVERSEAS TRAINEES

(Establishment Flexibility)

MEDICAL SCHOOL INPUT

SHO/REGISTRAR TRAINING POSTS

SPECIALIST

CONSULTANT

G.P.

Fig. 8.7

years must be mainly concerned with the numbers of doctors in non-permanent appointments. Flexibility in the number of training posts is necessary for this, and a particular advantage would be the establishment of
positive arrangements whereby trainees could be accepted from overseas
for defined programmes of postgraduate training. The numbers accepted in
each specialty could then be regulated according to the needs of the
N.H.S. and the available training capacity. Reciprocal arrangements with
the E.E.C. countries might also be important in this phase; for example,
doctors eligible to occupy posts in a 'specialist' grade might wish to
move between countries on a non-permanent basis.

Fine control

This is clearly the most difficult to achieve, and must depend largely on the flexibility of staffing arrangements at local level, with
appropriate adjustment of work commitments. Again, the acceptance of
short-term postgraduate trainees from abroad might well be helpful.

With regard to the career structure in general, there would be great
advantages from the planning point of view in having more than one level
of specialisation, without posts in any of the relevant grades being necessarily regarded as permanent. If the number of suitable candidates for
consultant or 'senior specialist' appointments were sufficient then the
necessary posts could be filled on this basis. If not, rather than lowering the standard of the consultant grade by appointing less suitable
candidates on a permanent basis it would be more satisfactory to provide
the necessary workforce by appointing specialists than by exploiting a

floating population of 'trainees'. But the great advantage of 'trainees' from this point of view is the non-permanence of their appointments; the danger of the alternative would be the blocking of posts for many years by specialists when in fact the shortage of eligible consultants was only temporary. In order to meet the variable and often unpredictable demands of the service adequately, both in terms of quantity and quality of staff, there is no doubt that as much flexibility as possible is needed in the career structure.

A good deal of knowledge would be required, on a continuing basis, to make strategic planning effective. The necessary information would concern both demand and supply. Some of the requirements for a comprehensive and continuing strategy development would be as follows:

Information concerning demand

Course control (long-term planning)

Long-term N.H.S. strategy, including priorities, etc.
Long-term policy concerning immigration and emigration.
Long-term university plans (career and research posts for medical graduates.
Long-term policy on substitution of non-medical for medical manpower.
Long-term population trends.

Medium control (medium-term planning)

Anticipated deaths and retirements, by Region and specialty.
Anticipated growth, by Region and specialty.
Outcome of pilot studies - e.g. concerning work patterns of doctors, G.P./hospital relationships, substitution studies, etc.
Policy changes - e.g. educational requirements for postgraduate training, etc.
Medical progress and developments.
Changes actually developing in the pattern of delivery of health care.

Fine control (short-term planning)

Short-term and immediate needs.
Local opportunities - e.g. increased training potential, etc.
Local problems - e.g. illness, etc.
Application of short-term pilot studies on deployment of medical staff, etc.

Information concerning supply

Coarse control (long-term planning)

University plans - e.g. potentially available medical school places, etc.
Long-term economic trends.
Demography of school population.
International trends in education, etc.
International trends in training of medical auxiliaries, etc.

Medium control (medium-term planning)

Career choice and movement of doctors.
Migration data.
International supply of doctors and freedom of movement.
International supply of medical auxiliaries and freedom of movement.

Fine control (short-term planning)

'Elasticity' in medical workloads.
Arrangement of commitments in relation to local working capacity.

In addition to positive and negative forms of <u>control</u> over total
numbers of doctors, any adequate manpower strategy must also consider
positive and negative <u>inducement</u> in order to ensure better distribution
of the available medical manpower between grades, regions and specialties.
Positive inducement may be by means of better remuneration and better
working conditions in the areas and specialties that require better staffing. As indicated in previous chapters the existing pattern of working
conditions and financial rewards has tended to operate, as would be expected, against the less favoured regions and specialties. The present
economic relationship between junior and senior hospital posts does not
encourage redistribution between grades. Increasing the workload on already heavily over-burdened support specialties by allowing an increase
in demand from the primary specialties also operates against recruitment
in the support fields. Another important factor in positive inducement
would be the prospect of increased ease of movement within the career
grades. For example, an increasing tendency for consultants to move into
a teaching hospital or large centre after a period of time spent in the
periphery, and vice versa, would appear advantageous to many potential
applicants for consultant posts.
'Negative' control over distribution mainly depends on limiting the
available numbers of 'training' posts in over-subscribed specialties and
areas, on the basis that as long as a surplus of these posts exists they
will be filled, to the detriment of relatively deprived regions and specialties. The introduction of planned training programmes, to cater for
defined numbers of British trainees, with the allocation of residual training capacity to quotas of 'overseas trainees' could provide a basis for
this form of control.
The problems of developing an adequate manpower strategy, to ensure
not only the right trends in overall numbers of doctors and others but
also an appropriate geographical and specialty distribution, are not exclusive to Great Britain. The United States established its National
Health Service Corps in 1970, to improve health care in underserved areas.
One part of this plan was to finance the medical education of N.H.S.C.
scholars in return for one year of service with the Corps for each year of
educational support. There seems no reason why an imaginative extension
to the civilian scene of the schemes offered by the Armed Forces in Great
Britain should not be considered along these lines. United States legislation in 1971 provided, among other forms of assistance to medical education, shortage-area scholarship programmes with priority assistance to
low-income students living in underserved areas and agreeing to practise
in such areas after graduation, student loans with 'forgiveness' provis-

ions for students subsequently practising in underserved areas, and grants
to help the setting up of graduate training programmes in primary care or
in any other area of health care with a shortage of qualified doctors.
Much attention has also been given in the United States, in recent years,
to training of physicians' assistants, shortening of the undergraduate
curriculum, integration of internship with residency programmes, designation of specialties such as paediatrics and in some cases internal medicine and obstetrics and gynaecology as primary care rather than referral
specialties, and positive control over the inflow of overseas doctors.
At least one of these trends, for the future provision of paediatric services, has some parallels in the recommendations of the Court Report
(1976). All of them are potentially important mechanisms for increasing
the flexibility of the system and regulating the availability of health
care at the point of delivery, without being dependent exclusively on
attempts at an unattainable precision and speed in the adjustment of medical school numbers. As outlined in the above section, the exploration
of such possibilities increases the range of options available for strategy development.

The progress of events in the United States has been reviewed by the
Carnegie Council (1976) who made further recommendations. Their plea was
for federal support rather than federal control, for example, 'the geographic disparities in the supply of health manpower will be overcome only
with great difficulty and through a combination of policies that provide
positive incentives for physicians, dentists and other health professionals to practise in underserved areas'. The Council made other important
points, for instance the need for close cooperation between central and
regional policy and the destructive effect of 'stop and go' federal support on the attempted development of effective training programmes. The
need for 'stable and consistent' policies was therefore stressed with adequate notice of intending change. To what extent these United States
initiatives will be successful, and their degree of relevance to the British situation must remain to be seen.

The free nations that have now developed elaborate and expensive
systems of health care share many concerns about medical manpower, and
may have much to learn from each other about strategy. This is perhaps
particularly important for Great Britain at a time of changing economic
allegiances and altered flow relationships for doctors with other countries.

CONCLUSIONS

Better work on medical manpower planning, and on the development of
appropriate strategies, must depend first of all on the better use of
existing data and the compilation of better and more up to date infor-
mationa where this is needed. This activity requires some form of permanent medical manpower unit with the necessary range of expertise and facilities to apply statistical analysis and modelling techniques, while having the depth of understanding that is needed to apply these techniques
intelligently to the real world situation. Such a unit must have access
to all currently available data, and must be in a position to demand the
information it needs without fear of delay or prevarication. It should
be independent of Government and, while in a position to supply analyses
and reports to official bodies on request, should also be free to pursue
its enquiries and publish its conclusions independently. There is also a
need for many more studies on the use of doctors and the ways in which
medical care can best be provided. Such studies need to be both well-

137

informed and open-minded; they need to represent a coming together for experimental purposes, outside the strait-jacket of existing professional practices and conventions, of doctors, nurses and others concerned with the welfare of patients.

REFERENCES

Australian Universities Commission (Chairman: P. Karmel) (1973) *Expansion of Medical Education*. Canberra: Australian Government Publishing Service.

Bartholomew, D.J. (1971) The statistical approach to manpower planning. *The Statistician*, 20, 3-26.

Bartholomew, D.J. (1976) *Manpower Planning*. Middlesex: Penguin Books.

Bevan, J.M. (1972) Some studies of the consequences of reallocation and relocation of function within the Community Health Services. In *The Economics of Medical Care*. Edited by M.M.Hauser, London: George Allen & Unwin, 119-142.

Bogatyrev, I.D. (1969) In *Methods of Estimating Health Manpower*. Report on a Symposium, Budapest, 15-19 October, 1968. Copenhagen: World Health Organization, 101-109.

British Medical Association (1977) Submission of evidence to the Royal Commission on the National Health Service. *British Medical Journal*, 1, 299-334.

Bunker, J.P. (1970) Surgical manpower: a comparison of operations and surgeons in the United States and in England and Wales. *The New England Journal of Medicine*, 282, No. 3, 135-144.

Carnegie Council (1976) *Progress and Problems in Medical and Dental Education*. San Francisco: Jossey-Bass.

Court Report (1976) *Fit for the Future*. Report of the Committee on Child Health Services. Cmnd. 684. London: H.M.S.O.

Crombie, D.L. (1972) A model of the medical care system. In *The Economics of Medical Care*. Edited by M.M.Hauser, London: George Allen & Unwin, 61-85.

Forbes, A.F. (1976) Non-parametric methods of estimating the survivor function. In *Manpower Planning*, by D.J. Bartholomew, Middlesex: Penguin Books, 91-117.

Hiestand, D.L. (1966) Research into manpower for health service. *Milbank Memorial Fund Quarterly*, 44, 146.

Hopes, R.F.A. (1976) Some statistical aspects of manpower planning in the Civil Service. In *Manpower Planning* by D.J.Bartholomew, Middlesex: Penguin Books, 190-210.

Hospital Junior Staffs Committee (1977) Present and projected numbers of medical students and doctors. *British Medical Journal*, 1, 659-660.

Judek, S. (1964) *Medical Manpower in Canada*, Royal Commission on Health Services, Ottawa: The Queen's Printer.

Klarman, H.E. (1969) In *Methods of Estimating Health Manpower*. Report on a Symposium, Budapest, 15-19 October, 1968. Copenhagen: World Health Organization, 62-81.

Lee, R.I. & Jones, L.W. (1933) *The Fundamentals of Good Medical Care*. Chicago: University of Chicago Press.

Maynard, A. (1976) Medical manpower planning in Britain: a critical appraisal. Unpublished working paper.

Maynard, A. (1977) Doctor manpower. *The Times*, 17 March.

Parkhouse, J. (1972) The economics of medical education - national and international. *British Journal of Medical Education*, 6, 84-86.

Parkhouse, J. (1978) Medical manpower in Britain, Part 5. *Medical Education*, 12, 230-252.

Parkhouse, J. and McLaughlin, C. (1975a) *Feasibility Study on Postgraduate Medical Education.* London: The Institute of Mathematics.

Parkhouse, J. and McLaughlin, C. (1975b) Future prospects for British graduates and the Health Service. *Lancet*, 1, 211-214.

Platt Report (1961) *Medical Staffing Structure in the Hospital Service.* London: H.M.S.O.

Popov, G.A. (1971) *Principles of Health Planning in the U.S.S.R.* Public Health Papers No. 43. Geneva: World Health Organization.

Reinhardt, U.E. (1975) *Physician Productivity and the Demand for Health Manpower.* Cambridge, Mass: Bollinger.

Reinhold, H. (1976) Anaesthesia in Belgium. In *Anaesthesia in the European Economic Community.* Conference organised by the Royal Society of Medicine, London, 10 December.

Surgeon General's Consultant Group in Medical Education (1959) *Physicians for a Growing America.* Washington, D.C.: Government Printing Office.

U.S.A. Manpower Commission (1974) *The Supply of Health Manpower: 1970 Profiles and Projections to 1990.* Washington: U.S. Department of Health, Education and Welfare.

Vandewater, S.L. (1975) *Report of the Working Party in Anaesthesia to the Requirements Committee on Physician Manpower 1974/75.* Canada: Canadian Anaesthetists' Society.

Willink Report (1957) *Report of the Committee to Consider the Future Numbers of Medical Practitioners and the Appropriate Intake of Medical Students.* London: H.M.S.O.

World Health Organization, Regional Office for Europe (1969) *Methods of Estimating Health Manpower, Report on a Symposium, Budapest, 15-19 October 1968,* Copenhagen.

World Health Organization (1971) *The Development of Studies in Health Manpower: Report of a WHO Scientific Group,* Geneva (W.H.O. technical Report Series, 481).

World Health Organization, Regional Office for Europe (1973) *Health Planning in National Development, Report on a Working Group, Stockholm, 19-22 June 1972,* Copenhagen.

World Health Organization, Regional Office for Europe (1974a) *The Application of Epidemiology to the Planning and Evaluation of Health Services, Report on a Working Group, Copenhagen, 19-23 November 1973,* Copenhagen.

World Health Organization, Regional Office for Europe (1974b) *European Conference on National Health Planning, Report, Bucharest, 12-16 March 1974,* Copenhagen.

9. The Reckoning

For most people money is not all, but a lot; life is not much, but everything. Good health, when it is desperatley desired, is beyond price; and it may be extremely expensive even when it is not. Medical care is always ultimately concerned with individuals, because it is individual people who constitute the community. The aims of the health service as a whole must be to promote, safeguard and maintain health, to treat curable illness as efficiently as possible, to relieve suffering and to provide for the needs of those who must remain chronically sick or disabled. The assignment of priorities within this framework is inevitable, at whatever levels and in whatever ways it is carried out. It involves the inescapable examination of moral, philosophical, political, ethical and economic issues of extreme difficulty, and even the most superficial attempt at such an examination would be far outside the scope of a text on medical manpower.

International comparisons can be misleading, as Klein (1977) has pointed out. The fact that a given country spends less of its resources on health than others does not necessarily imply a poorer standard of care. It depends what can be got for the money. This applies also to relative allocation as between labour and capital; the incomes of British doctors are low by Western European standards, and this makes medical manpower a 'good buy' so long as its availability is not threatened by emigration or disillusionment. Sudden changes may, however, take place; the improved pay of nurses during the last few years has cost a great deal of extra money and the new junior doctors' contract has been prodigiously expensive. Very often changes of this kind are not a matter of policy but of negotiation, and cannot adequately be allowed for in forecasts and planning models.

A number of aspects of the quality and effectiveness of medical practice have been discussed in recent publications (e.g. Donabedian, 1966; Bunker, Barnes and Mosteller, 1977) and the problems of 'audit' are much in the air. More particularly concerning priorities, Mooney (1977) and Card and Mooney (1977) have stimulated discussion through their analyses of the monitary value of human life. Card and Mooney (1977) gave some illustrations of the 'implied value' of human lives as they would be derived from policy decisions. The cost of preventing stillbirth by screening of maternal oestradiol concentrations yielded a maximum value of £50, while recommended changes in building standards following the collapse of a high-rise block of flats implied the valuation of each life saved at about twenty million pounds. A number of relevant aspects of decision

140

theory were discussed by Card and Mooney, but the main usefulness of the paper was perhaps to draw attention to the lack of coherent thinking about this side of the health care problem that underlies most recommendations.

The D.H.S.S. (1977) document on priorities in the health and social services, 'The Way Forward' outlined a broad approach based on the desire to redistribute resources geographically and achieve a 'national pattern'. Slightly more specifically, the main aims were stated as emphasis on prevention, remedy of past neglect of services (particularly those for the mentally ill and mentally handicapped) and provision for the continuing increase in the elderly population and the increasing number of children in local authority care. Some of the implications of this in relation to manpower have been discussed in previous chapters. For example the geographical redistribution of resources, including manpower, can mean various things. That some regions should be better supplied with doctors than others is iniquitous, but the reasons need to be looked at before the best prescription can be given for treatment. Inequality within the region is often worse, but taking registrars away from first-class teaching hospitals and good university training programmes in order to use them as pairs of hands in understaffed district hospitals is no proper solution. Altered priorities and greater emphasis need larger numbers of specially trained people, and the generation of these people requires a time scale that is incompatible with sudden changes in the priorities.

The first major question is whether there can ever be a rational basis for assigning priorities. There would have to be, presumably, some acceptable and agreed means of identifying and quantifying various 'needs', and of measuring the relative efficiency of meeting them in different ways. Such a basis seems a long way off. In practice, there may be much to be said for accepting the fact that all needs cannot possibly be met and that a little stimulus applied here and there, from time to time, within the allowable budget, is as good a way as any of bringing to light deficiencies and ensuring a progressive rise in standards. The potentially disastrous consequences of this attitude for long-term manpower planning have been emphasised enough already. What is needed, perhaps, is a 'stop-go' policy without any 'stop' - or, rather, with a realistic appreciation of the fact that both the build-up and the tailing off of the necessary medical manpower must occur either over a period of a decade or more, or as a result of deliberate policies concerning the control of international movement of trained or nearly-trained doctors.

The relative costs of different parts of the health service are very different. What is proportionately a very small reduction in expenditure on advanced hospital treatment may buy a great deal of primary, geriatric or terminal care. But emphasis on this aspect of geriatrics reveals an important fallacy: nothing is to be gained by cutting back on acute services if this merely leaves more chronically sick people, for longer periods of time, in the community. A large part of good geriatric work is acute medicine and surgery, and 'geriatric' patients are among the main users of acute hospital beds and operating theatres. It is important to realise, therefore, in relation to medical manpower, that although some aspects of geriatric care may have been neglected, the best medical care of old people in general leans very heavily upon surgeons, anaesthetists, radiologists and other specialists. The hitherto neglected aspects may have relatively small medical costs attached to them, but enormous 'social' costs in terms of housing and other amenities. One certain thing is that before making any too-dogmatic pronouncements about the cost-benefit aspects of relative allocations to different parts of the health service, it would be worth looking at how far we are from getting the 'best buy' at

present. Relative costs of different services, as judged by existing
bills, may be heavily distorted by inefficiency and wastage, for example
on unnecessary or low-priority surgical procedures, reduplicated or unnecessary investigations, waste of general practitioners' time, excessive
prescribing, inefficient use of hospital beds and of ambulance services.
     The second major question is whether there is any discernible relat-
ionship between numbers of doctors and standards of health care. This has
been a much debated question (see e.g. Reinhardt, 1975) but the issue is
too broad to allow simple conculsions to be drawn. For example in a primitive community, where the aim is to provide basic standards of health
care, there may be little relationship; 500 doctors may achieve no more
than 50 doctors working with 450 nursing aides. The same may be true, to
a more limited extent, in the community and some other health services of
developed countries. Better provision for the mentally handicapped does
not necessarily need a vastly greater number of medical specialists. In
the highly complex branches of specialised hospital medicine, although
delegation to skilled technicians and other trained ancillary staff may
be an increasing necessity, this is more often a form of augmentation than
of substitution, and it seems inevitable that more doctors are needed if
further improvement in patient management is to be achieved. This is
where the health service really begins to hurt from the economic point of
view - where a very large outlay will often result in a marginal improvement in outcome. Yet a high standard of health care, acceptable to an
affluent society, implies that the expensive minority will be catered for
in their need; medical progress depends on the exploration of advanced
techniques, and their benefits may unexpectedly prove to be colossal.
Some comments have already been made on productivity in relation to medical manpower (see Chapter 8); a particular aspect of this is 'substitution'.
     Although it is fashionable to talk of substitution as though it were
an unexplored field in the economics of medical manpower, it should be
noted that a great deal of substitution already takes place. The doctor
who qualified thirty years ago must often be amazed to recall how much he
used to do for himself that is now done by others. The patient who visits
a cardiologist privately will find this highly trained expert doing his
own note-taking, his own E.C.G. recording and his own X-ray screening without the retinue of housemen, cardiographers and radiographers that attend
him in the hospital. Perhaps we assume too readily that the development
of highly skilled and intensively manned supplementary services is always
worthwhile. The question bears examination before we proceed too much
further with substitution. There are, in fact, two components to the substitution process, although they usually overlap. Firstly, there is the
mere saving of doctors' time. It is rightly argued that doctors are expensive to produce and employ, and that they will lose job satisfaction if
put to do menial tasks. Certainly if they do nothing else there training
is wasted and their employment unjustified; but few people enjoy working
at full pressure for every minute of the day and even fewer retain their
efficiency while doing so. There must be a limit to how much we are prepared to pay to save a doctor ten minutes of relative relaxation. Secondly, there is the improvement of the service. It is now recognised almost
universally that there are jobs which a skilled technician or physiother-
apist can do better than a doctor. It is right to accept this fact actively rather than passively; it should be a recognition of the particular
skills of the people concerned and not an excuse for the doctor to let
slip his understanding of things relevant to his practice. The growth of
the supplementary professions is now leading to serious debate on the

142

question of clinical responsiblity and the right to action independent of medical control (see, for example the British Medical Association symposium on 'Clinical Responsibility': *B.M.J.*, 1977). The obvious relevance to the theme of this book is the need always to look at medical manpower in relation to other available staff, and the need to examine the potential costs and savings of various forms of substitution in terms of the saving of doctors' time - true substitution - and the improvement of the service.

Substitution always implies a suspicion of over-training and raises the question of how far down the scale it is possible or reasonable to go. A job done by a doctor could be done by a nurse or a technician. But nurses and technicians are themselves more highly trained than used to be the case, and increasingly often have university degrees. Their jobs could in turn be delegated, but perhaps only to people who will sooner or later seek their own place in the sun. Public spending can theoretically be cut by employing cheap labour, but how does this measure up to the professional or semi-professional aspirations of the people employed? It may be argued that many nurses, and indeed many doctors, are now over-trained for much of the work that has to be done; it could equally well be argued that the aim of an advanced society should be to give everybody the chance of self-fulfillment and escape from the serfdom of unskilled labour. Again there are deep philosophical problems, but the practical fact is that no profession and no country is entirely its own master in these matters. To amplify the point made by Peacock and Shannon (1968), the Health Service as an employer must ensure in order to obtain the best secretaries, technicians and all other staff (as it is not always successful in doing in competition with industry) that its careers and salaries compare favourably in the short run with those of other countries and in the long run with other forms of employment.

A particular problem for the Health Service, although not a unique one, is the relationship between labour and capital. In part, the Health Service is like any other industry; in terms of such things as laundry services, catering and data processing the concept of 'labour saving' - the substitution of capital equipment for manpower - can be applied. At the point of contact with the patient, however, a different relationship exists. The development of more advanced and specialised manpower provision almost invariably brings additional capital costs. Elaborate machinery for laboratory investigation, patient monitoring, clinical screening and research usually requires additional technical staff and often more doctors. It is also true that the fields such as general practice, where labour substitution may be particularly feasible, are not heavily dependent on capital investment and have little to gain from 'labour saving' in this sense. It certainly seems to be the case, for the forseeable future, that in the rapidly advancing fields of hospital medicine, demands for more manpower and for more capital investment will go hand in hand.

A Health Service costs a great deal of money. A good service costs more than a bad one and a modern service more than an old-fashioned one. The struggle to achieve maximum efficiency is long and hard, but essential. Meanwhile, there is little point in pretending that great improvements will result from the development of some aspects of the service if this has to be done at the expense of other aspects. There is no point at all in clinging to the hope of achieving an ideal service that is entirely free and Government-provided if the balance of evidence points to a need for more money than the Government can supply. There is then a choice between lower standards and alternative methods of supplementary funding.

The public will get what it is prepared to pay for and there seems no
reluctance to pay for good medical care. There is a willingness here
that needs to be, not exploited in the commercial sense, but put to the
best use in the common interest. The job of planners and research workers is to try and ensure that the best value for money is obtained by
both the individual and the community as a whole. To this end, a variety
of models of health care financing clearly need to be studied, independently of political dogma or professional vested interest.

How, then, can economic considerations be incorporated into medical
manpower plans and models? It is clear enough that, leaving aside economics, manpower models can be constructed with varying degrees of sophistication. There is almost no limit to the questions that can be asked of
such models, and hence to the answers they can provide. No further purpose can be served by developing such models beyond the present point, or
inventing new ones, until the appropriate questions have been formulated.
The models stand ready to be used; they await policy decisions and data
worthy of their powers. Such models need not be confined to doctors;
further studies could accommodate other types of health manpower. The in-
corporation of economic factors, however, brings in a whole range of additional elements for which adequate data would be lacking. Indeed, much
of the data would be inherently unascertainable in advance, as has been
said about changes in salary structure. Any attempt at a model would
need to incorporate alternative estimates based on assumptions concerning
substitution not only of labour for labour but capital for labour, and
allowing both for revenue consequences of capital development and capital
consequences of additional employment. No economic model confined to medical manpower would seem to be practicable; the economist's aim would
have to be a model of the Health Service as a whole, in which medical manpower featured as one factor. Such a model, if it were feasible and could
be continuously brought up to date, would be valuable to set alongside
more specific manpower models such as those described in Chapter 8, in
order to enable planners and policy makers to draw and progressively modify their conclusions about the place of the doctor, or any other professional worker, amid the numerous 'priorities' demanding their attention.

REFERENCES

B.M.J. (1977) Clinical Responsibility. *British Medical Journal,* 2,
    1584-1589 & 1637-1642.
Bunker, J.P., Barnes, B.A., & Mosteller, F. (1977) *Costs, Risks, and*
    Benefits of Surgery. New York: Oxford University Press.
Card, W.I. & Mooney, G.H. (1977) What is the monitary value of a human
    life? *British Medical Journal,* 2, 1627-1629.
D.H.S.S. (1977) *The Way Forward: Priorities in the Health and Social*
    Services. London: H.M.S.O.
Donabedian, A. (1966) Evaluating the quality of medical care. *Milbank*
    Memorial Fund Quarterly, 44, 166-206.
Klein, R. (1977) International perspectives on the National Health Service.
    British Medical Journal, 2, 1492-1493.
Mooney, G.H. (1977) *The Valuation of Human Life.* London: Macmillan.
Peacock, A. & Shannon, R. (1968) The new doctors' dilemma. *Lloyds Bank*
    Review, January, 26-38.
Reinhardt, U.E. (1975) *Physician Productivity and the Demand for Health*
    Manpower: An Economic Analysis. Cambridge, Mass: Bollinger.

WBI DEVELOPMENT STUDIES

Principles
of Health Economics
for Developing Countries

William Jack

The World Bank
Washington, D. C.

The World Bank Institute (formerly the Economic Development Institute) was established by the World Bank in 1955 to train officials concerned with development planning, policymaking, investment analysis, and project implementation in member developing countries. At present the substance of WBI's work emphasizes macroeconomic and sectoral economic policy analysis. Through a variety of courses, seminars, and workshops, most of which are given overseas in cooperation with local institutions, WBI seeks to sharpen analytical skills used in policy analysis and to broaden understanding of the experience of individual countries with economic development. Although WBI's publications are designed to support its training activities, many are of interest to a much broader audience.

This report has been prepared by the staff of the World Bank. The judgments expressed do not necessarily reflect the views of the Board of Executive Directors or of the governments they represent.

The material in this publication is copyrighted. The World Bank encourages dissemination of its work and will normally grant permission promptly.

Permission to photocopy items for internal or personal use , for the internal or personal use of specific clients, or for educational classroom use, is granted by the World Bank, provided that the appropriate fee is paid directly to the Copyright Clearance Center, Inc., 222 Rosewood Drive, Danvers, MA 01923, U.S.A., telephone 978-750-8400, fax 978-750-4470. Please contact the Copyright Clearance Center before photocopying items.

For permission to reprint individual articles or chapters, please fax your request with complete information to the Republication Department, Copyright Clearance Center, fax 978-750-4470.

All other queries on rights and licenses should be addressed to the World Bank at the address above or faxed to 202-522-2422.

The backlist of publications by the World Bank is shown in the annual *Index of Publications*, which is available from the Office of the Publisher.

William Jack is currently a consultant in the World Bank's Development Economics Research Group. At the time of writing, he was a research fellow at the Australian National University.

Library of Congress Cataloging-in-Publication Data

Jack, William, 1964–
        Principles of health economics for developing countries / William
Jack.
            p.   cm.—(WBI development studies)
        Includes bibliographical references and index.
        ISBN 0-8213-4571-0
        1. Medical economics—Developing countries.   2. Medical care
—Developing countries. 3. Public health—Economic aspects
—Developing countries   I. Title.   II. Series.
RA410.5.J33   1999
338.4'33621'091724—dc21   99-40975
                                                                               CIP

Contents

Foreword

The efficient and equitable provision of health care has been at the center of public debate in recent years, and many countries in the developing world have adopted health sector reforms and implemented new health policies and programs. Until now, most health economics textbooks and training materials have dealt with industrial country experience. However, as universities, as well as public and professional bodies, in the developing world have begun to equip students and practitioners with the analytical tools to help inform policy decisions and improve research methods, the need for an appropriate text has become apparent.

In its efforts to build capacity among its clients, the World Bank Institute recognizes the importance of building strong foundations in analytical skills. This volume addresses that need, providing a modern treatment of health economics for developing and industrial countries. It addresses both positive and normative issues in the economics of health care and health insurance, drawing on agency theory, welfare economics, econometrics, and development economics. While rigorous in its approach, it presents intuitive expositions of the underlying ideas and draws them together in its discussion of policy objectives and design.

The book is intended for use by advanced undergraduate and first-year graduate students of economics and international development, researchers, health policy professional, and policymakers in industrial and developing countries alike.

I believe this book to be a valuable contribution to the health sector, and hope that it will be widely read and adopted by training institutes and university faculties around the world.

Vinod Thomas, Director
World Bank Institute

1

Introduction

Health indicators in developing countries have shown impressive improvements in the past 50 years—people live longer, fewer children and their mothers die in childbirth, and many serious diseases have been controlled, and some eliminated. But the health status of individuals in these countries remains well below its potential level, and many people lack access to suitable health care and health-promoting services. Life expectancy at birth in Sub-Saharan Africa is still only two-thirds the average level in the West, and the average child mortality rate there is more than 15 times that in the developed market economies.

There is thus much still to be achieved in the promotion of the health and well-being of individuals in the developing world. Not surprisingly, however, where the needs are greatest, the means tend to be least, and the relative poverty of many developing countries constrains their attempts to improve health status indicators. It is imperative that the available resources be used equitably and efficiently, and to this end, an economic approach to the analysis of health and health care is required.

This book attempts to provide a suitable economic framework that will foster an understanding of the allocation of broadly defined health care resources, and to aid the design and analysis of policies that affect health outcomes. It addresses both positive and normative issues in the economics of health, and in this sense is similar in approach, if not in scope, to public finance texts such as Atkinson and Stiglitz (1980). Indeed, in many respects, the book represents an application of public economics, including developments in the past 20 years in the economics of information and incentives, to the analysis of health care resource allocations.

This approach is by no means novel—for example, externalities and the public good aspects of health care have long been acknowledged, and most modern treatments of physician behavior are within a principle-agent framework. However, it helps to explain the attention devoted in some chapters to general issues of equity and efficiency, market failure, and project appraisal that initially may appear to be outside the purview of health policy choices. This focus on general principles, supplemented by examples, represents a deliberate attempt to provide students and practitioners with the tools they need to address particular problems that might not have been covered specifically in the text. It is also meant to help avoid problems that sometimes arise, because health is treated as being "different" from other commodities. While certain differences undeniably exist—for example, in social attitudes toward the distribution of health care resources as opposed to income in general, and in the relationship between consumer (patient) and producer (physician) in some markets—well-established tools of economic analysis are available to accommodate these peculiarities. Indeed, treating every issue as a special case tends to impede the fundamental understanding that is necessary in order to develop good applied analysis.

The examples used to motivate and illustrate the economic techniques presented here have a developing country focus. At the same time, significantly more empirical and theoretical work has been pursued for industrial countries, and this literature is also used. While the health issues and the design of health policy in developing countries often present qualitatively different problems to those in more advanced economies, there is a similarity to the underlying forces at work in both settings that determine individual behavior, the evolution of social institutions, and the incentive constraints that policy interventions must accommodate. Examples from more advanced economies are thus by no means irrelevant to developing country analyses, although additional constraints, particularly with respect to institutional capacity, need to be acknowledged. For example, in the presence of insufficient administrative capacity, otherwise optimal user fees for medical care may turn out to be undesirable, if revenue collection leads to theft attempts at local clinics.

The text can be usefully divided into three parts. Part I focuses on health outcomes—mortality, morbidity, and the like—and the relationships between such outcomes and orthodox variables that measure macroeconomic performance. Chapter 2 documents the types of health indicators that are often used in practice, with the aim of providing some precision to otherwise naturally understood concepts. It also presents information on historical trends in mortality by age and gender, and by cause of death, and reviews issues that arise in the measurement of the prevalence, incidence, and severity of morbidity.

Chapter 3 examines the links between health outcomes, as measured using the tools of the preceding chapter, and orthodox measures of economic performance, including output measures such as gross domestic product (GDP). The channels that may lead higher incomes to yield better health status are investigated, as well as the specific impact of more and/or better medical care. The chapter also addresses the idea that not only may higher incomes result in better health, but that better health may also improve the productivity of individuals, and hence lead to higher incomes. The final section presents empirical evidence and econometric techniques that help to disentangle these two directions of causation. It reports research that suggests that the net effect is in the direction from income to health, which implies that an important strategy in health improvement is the adoption of policies that foster economic growth in general, as well as direct health interventions. Finally, the example of AIDS in Africa is used to illustrate the potentially large impact of health on income associated with an epidemic that primarily victimizes individuals of prime working age.

Following the examination of measurement and linkages of macro level data—population health status measures and GDP—Part II adopts a more microeconomic focus in analyzing demand and supply in health care markets. Chapter 4 begins by presenting a theoretical framework for specifying the effects of income, prices, and illness on the demand for health care and other health-related goods. While the use of health care can be seen as fulfilling either (or both) a consumption or an investment function, for the most part the analysis is strictly within the bounds of orthodox consumer demand theory. The final section of chapter 4 examines the empirical estimation of demand functions based on the underlying theory of the earlier sections, and introduces the reader to some econometric issues characteristic of health care demand estimation, particularly with respect to the limitations of the data generally available in developing countries. It provides a summary of empirical results suggesting that the demand for health care is affected by the price, but that the elasticity is relatively low, on the order of 0.2. This has implications for, among other things, the distortionary costs of subsidizing health care and the impact of user fees on revenue collection, to be examined later in the book.

One of the important ways in which medical care differs from other goods and services is that consumer needs are uncertain. The range of variation in uncertain medical care expenditures (or other costs, such as lost wages) can be very large, exposing individuals to substantial risks. Under the widely held belief that individuals tend to be averse to risk, chapter 5 examines the issue of medical insurance. After illustrating the standard argument in favor of full insurance (in which the individual is exposed to no idiosyncratic risk), section 3 of the chapter identifies three sources of inefficiency in insurance markets. The basic adverse selection model is presented, illustrating how insurance markets may fail to provide full insurance when information about risks is privately held. Adverse selection may actually cause insurance markets to fail completely, with very little insurance coverage observed in equilibrium. Two further information-based sources of incomplete insurance are also presented: hidden action moral hazard and hidden information moral hazard. In these situations, insurance providers are unable to observe either the preventive actions of individuals or what their health needs really are (that is, how sick they are), and each of these constraints leads to overconsumption of medical care. The optimal response then is to reduce the level of coverage, exposing the individual to some risk in order to control the overconsumption of care. These observations are important, because they mean that user fees and other prices, as well as raising revenue to pay for medical care, may also be part of an optimal risk-sharing arrangement.

The chapter then goes on to consider more institutional features of insurance markets, such as group insurance wherein individuals purchase insurance as a group (through their employer or union, for example), and the impact of administrative costs. Alternative organizational forms are also examined that represent attempts to minimize the moral hazard costs identified earlier in the chapter. While these organizational forms have been adopted in the West, their design is important for developing countries if health risks are to be efficiently pooled, while containing budgetary and other expenditures. Finally, we briefly address informal and traditional insurance mechanisms.

Chapter 6 presents an analysis of the supply side of the medical care market. It examines the use of physicians, other medical personnel, and nonlabor inputs in the production of medical care, with particular emphasis on relating such production to standard microeconomic production theory. While the production possibilities of hospitals and doctors can be accommodated within standard microeconomic theory, the incentives of producers in these markets may not necessarily conform to orthodox profit maximization. Thus, we examine in some detail the objectives that physicians might have, and the implications for resource allocation. Separate sections on the supply of drugs and hospital services identify other departures from the standard model of a profit-maximizing firm. Finally, given these peculiarities of incentives on the supply side, we analyze the equilibrium of supply and demand, with particular attention given to the supplier-induced demand (SID) hypothesis and policy responses.

The focus of the text shifts from a descriptive one to a normative one in Part III. Chapter 7 provides a review of the theory of market failures and policy interventions, mostly from an efficiency standpoint. It provides both a general exposition of externalities and public goods and specific examples of these elements in health and health care markets. It is argued in the chapter that most market failures in the health sector derive from the presence of externalities. However, one of the more fundamental public goods in any market, including that for health care, is information, and we examine so-called merit good arguments linking these to issues of information as a public good.

Having established how markets may fail to provide efficient levels of goods and services, the chapter goes on to examine alternative policy interventions that might be used to correct these distortions. For expositional purposes, such policy interventions are divided into market-improving instruments (establishing property rights, adjusting prices with taxes and subsidies, and the like) and direct public provision. When policy interventions result in a net budgetary expenditure by the government, either because of subsidies or public provision, the government must also choose appropriate financing instruments. The chapter provides an overview of issues in optimal taxation that are relevant to the issue of health care financing. Within this framework, user fees, earmarked funds, and decentralization of expenditure and revenue collection can be addressed.

Chapters 8 and 9 continue the normative investigation of Part III, but with a focus on projects instead of policies. Chapter 8 provides an overview of the methods of project appraisal or cost-benefit analysis and their variants. It begins with a review of some standard social choice criteria and argues in support of a "welfarist" approach to making social decisions. The use of welfare functions is seen as a convenient way of integrating both the efficiency objectives central to the analysis in chapter 7 and distributional concerns. This is particularly important in the health sector, because equity considerations tend to be given relatively more weight there than in some other policy spheres. The practical application of welfare-based social choice is cost-benefit analysis, and its principles are presented. Two alternative social choice mechanisms that are often used in the analysis of health projects—cost-effectiveness analysis and cost-utility analysis—are also exhibited, and they are compared with the standard approach. It is argued that, given the welfarist approach, cost-effectiveness measures can be misleading, and that cost-benefit analyses should be preferred. Indeed, the confusion that tends to surround the validity of cost-effectiveness and cost-utility analyses led to the inclusion of a short but rigorous review of welfare economics at the beginning of the chapter.

Chapter 9 goes on to provide more in-depth analyses of project appraisal in the health sector. We examine issues in the valuation of costs, and, more specifically to health projects, benefits, including willingness to pay. Again, given the welfare-based approach to project appraisal, willingness to pay, despite its likely positive correlation with income, is shown to be the appropriate measure of benefits when distributional weights derived from the welfare function are incorporated in the aggregation across individuals. A more thorough review of cost-effectiveness and cost-utility analyses in the health sector is then presented, with a final section that illustrates application of associated measurements to the estimation of the burden of disease, as conducted by the World Health Organization and the World Bank. These applications are included to expose the reader to tools that are often used in health project analysis, but they are not necessarily advocated as conceptually well founded.

The final chapter is an attempt to draw together the strands of the earlier material to address some big-picture issues in the design and implementation of national health systems. We begin by presenting some evidence on the extent of public intervention in the health sector and relate this to the theory of public intervention in chapter 7. The important role of government observed in many countries suggests that efficiency criteria are only part of the motivation for public intervention. Equity of access to health care and health insurance seem to be equally, or more, important, and we examine the potential of public provision to facilitate redistribution. We then present a number of specific issues in the provision of public insurance, including the distinction between providing insurance and medical care, the use of both demand- and supply-side controls to ensure efficient implementation of government policies, the choice of the share of public and private provision in a mixed system, and the use of prices and other rationing mechanisms. A thorough guide to designing and running a public health system would obviously constitute a book in itself, so perhaps more than anything this chapter provides examples of applying the theory and evidence of earlier chapters to specific questions that will need to be addressed by ministries of health and finance in the operation of a national health system. Far from being comprehensive, it should be seen as providing examples of the kind of approach that might be used in addressing these and other problems in health policy.

Reference

Atkinson, Anthony, and Joseph Stiglitz. 1980. *Lectures on Public Economics.* New York: McGraw-Hill.

Part I

Health Outcomes and Economic Linkages

2

Health Status and Trends

In this chapter we examine the measurement of health status and trends in health outcomes over time, across regions, and across demographic groups. The measures we define and use are those of the traditional "public health" school, focusing on mortality rates, life expectancy, and morbidity measures. We disaggregate these measures according to age, sex, cause of death or illness, and region. A key observation is that the pattern and nature of mortality and morbidity has changed over the past 100 years and continues to change in developing countries today. This so-called epidemiological transition is linked with the concurrent demographic transition, wherein population age structures also undergo significant changes as societies develop. We begin, however, by discussing the measurement of traditional population health status measures and move on to present detailed descriptions of mortality and morbidity developments.

Mortality, Life Expectancy, and Other Epidemiological Statistics

Later we will discuss ways to measure the economic burden of disease and death, but for now we are interested in measuring crude rates of illness and death, without imposing value judgments about relative costs and benefits. The traditional measures of health status are life expectancy, mortality rates, and morbidity rates. We first spend a few moments making some formal definitions for clarity (see Selvin 1991 for a more thorough analysis of epidemiologic data), then examine practical measurement of health status.

Formal Definitions

In order to distinguish between the mortality rates of different age groups and different times, the following definition can be used:

Definition: *The age- and time-specific annual probability of death,* π_a^t, is the probability that an individual of age a at time t will die within a year.

As long as the population under study is large enough, the *ex post* ratio of the number of deaths to the number of individuals of age a alive at the beginning of the year is a good approximation to the average *ex ante* probability faced by each individual. The probabilities can be calculated for specific population groups—for example, men versus women, urban versus rural dwellers, and so on. When the probability is expressed as a rate per 100,000 individuals (instead of as a rate per individual), it is approximately equal to the mortality rate.[1]

For presentation purposes and empirical convenience, we usually confine ourselves to mortality rates over longer periods. Thus, we use the following definition:

Definition: The *"cohort" n-year probability of death at age a and time* t, $\pi_{a,c}^t(n)$ is the probability that an individual of age a at time t will die within n years. That is,

$$\pi_{a,c}^t(n) = \pi_a^t + (1 - \pi_a^t)\, \pi_{a+1}^{t+1} + (1 - \pi_{a+1}^{t+1})(1 - \pi_a^t)\, \pi_{a+2}^{t+2} +$$

$$\ldots + (1 - \pi_{a+n-1}^{t+n-1}) \ldots (1 - \pi_a^t)\, \pi_{a+n}^{t+n}$$

(2.1)
$$= \pi_a^t + \sum_{i=1}^{n} \left(\prod_{j=0}^{i-1} (1 - \pi_{a+j}^{t+j}) \right) \pi_{a+i}^{t+i}$$

$$= \pi_a^t + \sum_{i=1}^{n} S_{a,c}^t(i)\, \pi_{a+i}^{t+i}$$

---

1. The mortality rate allows for time spent alive during the period (one year) by individuals who die by the end of the year. Thus, if individuals die at a uniform rate over the course of the year, so that the average length of time spent alive by individuals who die is 0.5 years, then the total life years lived between the beginning and end of the year, per individual alive at the beginning of the year, is $(1 - \pi_a^t) + \pi_a^t / 2 = 1 - \pi_a^t / 2$. The mortality rate is then calculated as the ratio of the number of deaths to total life years lived, which is $\pi_a^t / (1 - \pi_a^t / 2)$. When π_a^t is small, the mortality rate is approximately equal to the probability of death, π_a^t. Note that when $a = 0$, the discrepancy between the two measures is increased somewhat, because the distribution of deaths in the first year of life is skewed toward the first month. Despite this difference, we will tend to use probability of death and mortality rate interchangeably.

where $S_a^t(i) = \prod_{j=0}^{i-1}(1-\pi_{a+j}^{t+j})$ is the probability that a person of age a at time t will survive until age $a + i$, and is referred to as the cohort survival function (or survival curve).

This mortality rate is equal to the proportion of the population aged a at time t who die by the time they reach the age of $a + n$. Such a rate is difficult to estimate empirically, because the probabilities at distant future dates are unknown. An alternative measure is calculated on the basis of annual mortality rates of currently older individuals. This cross-sectional or "period" approach substitutes π_{a+j}^t for π_{a+j}^{t+j} in 2.1 to yield:

Definition: The *"period" n-year probability of death at age a and time* t, $\pi_{a,p}^t(n)$ is the probability that an individual of age a at time t will die within n years, assuming no change in current age- and time-specific annual mortality rates. That is,

$$\pi_{a,p}^t(n) = \pi_a^t + (1-\pi_a^t)\,\pi_{a+1}^t + (1-\pi_{a+1}^t)(1-\pi_a^t)\,\pi_{a+2}^t +$$

$$\cdots + (1-\pi_{a+n-1}^t)\cdots(1-\pi_a^t)\,\pi_{a+n}^t$$

(2.2)
$$= \pi_a^t + \sum_{i=1}^{n}\left(\prod_{j=0}^{i-1}(1-\pi_{a+j}^t)\right)\pi_{a+i}^t$$

$$= \pi_a^t + \sum_{i=1}^{n} S_{a,p}^t(i)\,\pi_{a+i}^t$$

where $S_{a,p}^t(i)$ is the period survival function.

The period mortality rate, otherwise known as the mortality risk, measures the probability of death between the ages of a and $a + n$ *based on the annual mortality rates of individuals currently alive* and between the ages of a and $a + n$. If health conditions—particularly death probabilities—are not expected to change much over the n-year horizon, then the two measures will be close. However, if the population concerned is expected to experience improvements in health, brought about by economic growth, medical discoveries, and the like, π_{a+j}^{t+j} will be expected to fall with j, and the cohort n-year mortality rate will generally be lower than the period n-year rate. That is, $\pi_{a,c}^t(n) \le \pi_{a,p}^t(n)$.

Life expectancy, which is also defined for a given age a and date t, is inversely related to the probability of death and the mortality rate.

Definition: The *cohort life expectancy of an individual of age a at time t*, $\lambda_{a,c}^t$, is the expected value of the number of years until death, calculated on the basis of the age- and time-specific annual mortality rates. That is, if t_d denotes the random variable that is the time of death, then

(2.3)
$$\lambda_{a,c}^t = E_c\left[(t_d - a)\,|\,a,\,t\right]$$
$$= \sum_{i=1}^{\infty} i\pi_{a+i}^{t+i}\left(\prod_{j=0}^{i-1}(1 - \pi_{a+j}^{t+j})\right)$$
$$= \sum_{i=1}^{\infty} i\pi_{a+i}^{t+i}\, S_{a,c}^t\,(i),$$

where E_c is the expectations operator using cohort mortality probablities.

Once again, this can be approximated by the period life expectancy, using annual mortality rates of currently living individuals of all ages greater than, or equal to, a.

Definition: The *period life expectancy of an individual of age a at time t*, $\lambda_{a,p}^t$, is the expected value of the number of years until death, calculated on the basis of the age- and time-specific annual mortality rates at time t. That is, if t_d denotes the random variable that is the time of death, then

(2.4)
$$\lambda_{a,p}^t = E_p\left[(t_d - a)\,|\,a,\,t\right]$$
$$= \sum_{i=1}^{\infty} i\pi_{a+i}^t\left(\prod_{j=0}^{i-1}(1 - \pi_{a+j}^t)\right)$$
$$= \sum_{i=1}^{\infty} i\pi_{a+i}^t\, S_{a,p}^t\,(i),$$

where E_p is the expectations operator using period mortality probabilities.

Because life expectancy is inversely related to mortality rates, it is clear that the cohort life expectancy is greater than the period life expectancy if it is anticipated that π_{a+j}^{t+j} will fall over time—that is, $\lambda_{a,c}^t \geq \lambda_{a,p}^t$. Such a relationship is dramatically seen during wartime, when the cohort life expectancy of young men, which abstracts from short-term fluctuations in death rates, is much higher than the period measure. Similarly, during a severe epidemic, such as the influenza epidemic following the First World War, period life expectancy can plummet compared with the cohort measure. This is depicted in figure 2.1, adapted from Murray and Lopez (1994).

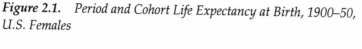

Figure 2.1. *Period and Cohort Life Expectancy at Birth, 1900–50, U.S. Females*

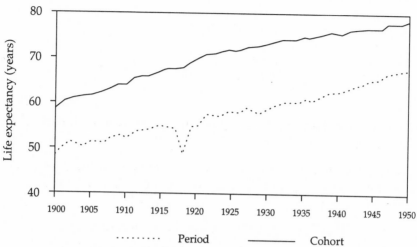

.... Period   ———— Cohort

Source: Murray and Lopez (1994, figure 1, p. 7).

A final statistic useful in the analysis of epidemiological data is the hazard rate. Again, for completeness, this can be defined for an individual of a given age at a particular time, and on a cohort or period basis:

Definition: The *cohort hazard rate for an individual of age a at time t* is a function $\eta^t_{a,c}(x)$, which gives the probability that such an individual will die between the ages of x and $x + 1$, conditional on him or her being alive at age x. That is,

$$(2.5) \qquad \eta^t_{a,c}(x) = \frac{\pi^{t+x-a}_x}{S^t_{a,c}(x-a)} .$$

The cohort hazard rate at birth is thus $\eta^t_{0,c}(x) = \pi^{t+x}_x / S^t_{0,c}(x)$, which is the probability that an individual born at date t will survive until age x, and subsequently die within a year. As usual, the estimate of the hazard rate using cross-sectional data is often employed, defined as follows:

Definition: The *period hazard rate for an individual of age a at time t* is a function $\eta^t_{a,p}(x)$, given by

(2.6)
$$\eta_{a,p}^{t}(x) = \frac{\pi_{x}^{t}}{S_{a,p}^{t}(x-a)}$$

where we have just substituted cross-sectional probabilities of death and used the period-based survival rates.

Examples of survival curves and hazard functions are shown in figure 2.2, drawn from Selvin (1991).

The measures described above concentrate on death as a defining characteristic. But, similar rates and probabilities can be calculated using illness or incapacity as the underlying event of interest. For example, the rate of malaria infection in a population is usually expressed per 1,000 population, and it is essentially identical to the mortality rate or probability of death, defined above.

Measuring Mortality Rates in Practice

The most widely reported mortality rates are the period measures for infants (aged zero to one year), children (aged zero to five), and adults (aged

Figure 2.2. Survival Curves and Hazard Rates

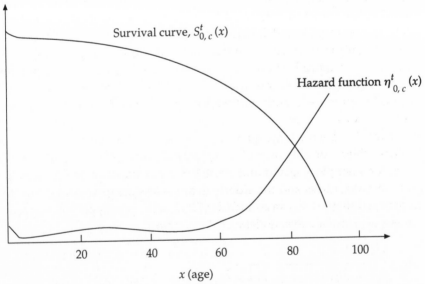

Survival curve, $S_{0,c}^{t}(x)$

Hazard function $\eta_{0,c}^{t}(x)$

x (age)

Source: Adapted from Selvin (1991, figure 9–1, p. 250).

16 to 59). These measures are sometimes denoted by 1Q0, 5Q0, and 45Q15, respectively, where

$$nQa = \pi_{a,p}^{t}(n)$$

is the probability of death between ages a and $a + n$, or the percentage of a-year-olds who will die before their $(a + n)$th birthdays.[2] Subcategories of the adult mortality rate measure can also be calculated, such as 25Q15 (the percentage of 15-year-olds who will not reach their 40th birthdays), and 20Q40 (the probability of a 40-year-old not reaching 60), as can the mortality rates for elderly individuals.

When comparing mortality rates across countries, it is necessary to use *age-standardized* measures. To illustrate this idea, suppose that we wish to compare the child mortality rates, 5Q0, in two countries. Suppose also that a high proportion of child deaths occur before age one, and that one country, country A, has relatively more 3-, 4-, and 5-year-olds than the other, country B. In this case, country B, with a younger group of children, will record more deaths per child under 5 than will country A, even if the two countries have the same age- and time-specific annual mortality rates for children of each age. Thus the raw mortality data must be adjusted to reflect the possibly different demographic structures of the two countries.

As an empirical matter, if good-quality vital registration data are available, period mortality rates can be measured straightforwardly on the basis of π_a^t estimates, for $a = 1, 2,...$ Such measures, calculated using equation 2.2, are sometimes referred to as "empirical" estimates. When the data are less reliable and are incomplete, which is often the case in developing countries (particularly in Sub-Saharan Africa), "model-based" estimates are required. These estimates essentially make use of mortality information from other countries with comparable economic and health-related environments and conditions in order to make statistical estimates of local mortality rates.

There has been a large quantity of resources directed to the measurement of child mortality rates in developing countries over the past 30 years (see, for example, Cleland and Scott 1987), but information on mortality rates among adults and the elderly is much less comprehensive. For this reason, adult mortality rates such as 45Q15 in the poorer developing countries are almost always model-based estimates.

---

2. Note that we are not differentiating between probability of death and mortality rate here. See footnote 1.

Historical Trends in Mortality Rates

The World Bank (1993, table A.5) presents mortality rates by demographic region for individuals in different age groups, particularly for children (0–4), schoolchildren (5–14), adults (15–59), and the elderly (60–75). These are period mortality rates, because they are estimated on the basis of the (projected) number of deaths in each age group as a proportion of that age group's population. A summary of the table is presented in the first panel of table 2.1.

Mortality Rates of School-Age Children

The data presented in table 2.1 are derived from both empirical estimates and model-based projections, especially the 1950 figures. The first thing to

Table 2.1. *Historical Trends in Mortality Rates and Life Expectancy by Region and Age*

Demographic region and age group	Probability of dying (percent)			Life expectancy (years) at beginning of age group		
	1950	*1980*	*1990*	*1950*	*1980*	*1990*
Developing countries						
0–4	28.6	13.5	10.6	40	59	63
5–14	5.7	2.6	2.2	50	62	64
15–59	46.7	26.7	23.5	43	53	55
60–75	60.3	46.7	43.8	13	16	17
Established market economies and former socialist economies of Europe						
0–4	8.4	2.1	1.5	64	73	75
5–14	1.5	0.4	0.3	65	70	71
15–59	21.2	15.0	13.7	55	60	61
60–75	47.0	33.7	30.4	17	19	19
World						
0–4	24.8	12.0	9.6	48	62	65
5–14	4.7	2.1	1.9	55	64	66
15–59	40.6	24.7	20.7	47	55	56
60–75	56.0	40.1	40.1	14	17	17

Source: World Bank (1993).

note from the table is that school-age children consistently have the lowest mortality rates. Having survived exposure to early childhood diseases, they have selected themselves as the relatively strong (or privileged) but have yet to develop the chronic illnesses associated with aging and adult practices (including sexual activity, smoking, and drinking), or to encounter especially dangerous environments on a regular basis (for example, at work or in war).

Child Mortality Rates

There were large drops in child mortality rates between 1950 and 1990: in developing countries, the child mortality rate fell from 29 to 11 percent, a reduction of about 60 percent. In the established market economies, the child mortality rate fell from 6 percent in 1950 to about 1 percent in 1990, while in the former socialist economies of Europe, it fell from 13 to 2 percent. Probably the most impressive improvement was in China, where the probability of dying before age 5 was 32 percent in 1950, but it had fallen to just 4 percent in 1990. The performance of Sub-Saharan Africa was much less striking, although the child mortality rate was reduced by about 40 percent over the period, from 29 to 17 percent.

Data for the established market economies are available on a much longer time scale than reported in the table above. In the mid-nineteenth century, these countries were effectively developing countries and had child mortality rates between 25 and 40 percent, which subsequently fell more or less monotonically. For example, the combined child mortality rate for England and Wales fell continuously from just less than 30 percent in 1860 to less than 1 percent in 1990, although there was a quickening in the pace of improvement in the first half of the twentieth century with the discovery and adoption of new drugs and improvements in living environments. A similar pattern was realized in Japan from 1900, and Italy, which registered a relatively high 40 percent child mortality rate in 1880, and enjoyed an uninterrupted decline to negligible rates by 1990 (see Feachem and others 1992 for more details).

Adult Mortality Rates

The worldwide adult mortality rate fell by about half between 1950 and 1990. As mentioned earlier, few developing countries have sufficiently complete records to make empirical estimates of adult mortality rates since 1950, although there are some exceptions. In particular, according to Murray, Yang, and Qiao (1992), Chile, Costa Rica, Cuba, Singapore, and Sri Lanka have suitable data for the performance of reliable analyses. These authors report that the adult mortality rate for males has fallen over the past 40 years in Chile, Costa Rica, and Singapore, but it has remained relatively stagnant in Cuba and Sri Lanka. However, it should be noted that, except for the period since 1980, Cuba exhibited the lowest adult mortality rate, of about 15 percent. The adult mortality rates for women had fallen in all five countries to about 10 percent in 1990, although least noticeably in Cuba.

Adult mortality rates in the established market economies fell continuously over the past 100 years, from rates of 40 to 45 percent at the turn of the century to an average of 14 percent in 1990. One notable exception was Japan, where the adult mortality rate remained at about 40 percent until 1940, but dropped precipitously following the end of World War II. Sweden was also an outlier, with an adult mortality rate in 1910 of a somewhat lower than average 30 percent.

Gender Differences

Adult mortality rates in 1990 by gender are presented in table 2.2 by demographic region. The mortality rates for men are consistently higher than those for women, despite the presumption that childbearing imposes significant risks on women in their early adult lives. For some countries, notably India and Sri Lanka during the 1950s and 1960s, the early adult mortality rates of women were greater that those of men, but improvements in maternal care have altered this pattern. There are no countries in which the female mortality rate is higher than the male rate for older adults, aged 40 to 60.

Table 2.2.   Adult Mortality Rates by Gender, 1990

Demographic region	Male rate	Female rate
Sub-Saharan Africa	38.1	32.2
India	27.2	22.9
China	20.1	15.0
Other Asian economies and islands	24.3	17.7
Latin America and the Caribbean	22.8	16.3
Middle Eastern Crescent	22.8	17.4
Former socialist economies	28.1	11.2
Established market economies	14.7	7.3
Developing countries	25.0	19.9
World	23.4	16.9

Source: World Bank (1993).

Life Expectancy

The trends in mortality rates discussed above translate directly into changes in life expectancy at different ages, as detailed in the second panel of table 2.1. Just as there has been a steady decline in overall mortality rates since 1950, life expectancy rates across regions have also risen, albeit at different rates. Figure 2.3 shows the range of dynamics for life expectancy at birth for eight regions of the world, as estimated by the World Bank (1993). Life expectancy in the established market economies increased steadily, but slowly, over the period, reflecting the large gains made earlier in the century and the likely existence of some kind of natural upper limit to the

Figure 2.3. Trends in Life Expectancy by Demographic Region, 1950–90

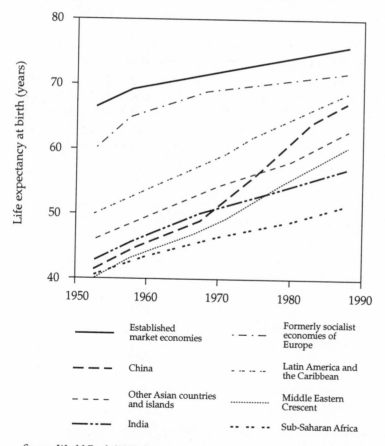

Source: World Bank (1993, figure 1–2, p. 23).

length of life. One can think of the production of life expectancy as exhibiting increasing marginal costs, so that additional improvements for the market economies can now come only by incurring large resource costs.

Other regions, particularly Latin America and the Caribbean and China, have shown a great propensity to "catch up" to the market and former socialist economies of Europe over the period, while other developing countries have made somewhat slower progress. Since the early 1970s, coincident with the large increase in oil prices and living standards, the increase in life expectancy in the Middle Eastern countries has accelerated. It is tempting to suggest that, given sufficient financial resources, the improvement in life expectancy of the late developers should be relatively faster, once it begins, compared to that of the early developers. This pattern would occur to the extent that the late developers could adopt technological and process innovations (both medical and other) relatively quickly from the early developers but may require significant international wealth transfers.

Causes of Death and the Dynamics of Mortality

Some of the changes in mortality rates over the past 40 years can be attributed to changes in the causes of death. Deaths are typically classified by cause into three main categories: communicable diseases, noncommunicable diseases, and injuries. Communicable diseases include most viral, bacterial, and parasitic infections; examples of noncommunicable diseases include diseases of the circulatory and respiratory systems; and injuries result mainly from motor vehicle accidents, workplace accidents, and violence (including domestic violence). Table 2.3 (from Murray, Yang, and Qiao 1992) presents a more complete list.

Table 2.3.   Categories of Causes of Death

Communicable and reproductive diseases	Noncommunicable diseases	Injuries
Diarrhea	Neoplasms	Unintentional
Tuberculosis	Endocrine	Motor vehicle transport
Malaria	Cardiovascular	Intentional
Venereal diseases	Respiratory	Suicide
Respiratory infections	Digestive	Homicide
	Senile and ill-defined	Undetermined

Source: Murray, Yang, and Qiao (1992).

The bulk of the decline in mortality can be explained by improvements in the control of communicable diseases. For example, while deaths from communicable diseases fell by over 95 percent in England and Wales from 1891 to 1990, deaths from noncommunicable diseases fell by just over 50 percent. This pattern has also been exhibited by developing countries over the past 40 years. It has generally been associated with improvements in environmental conditions, including sanitation, mosquito control, vaccinations, and the like, and medical advances in the treatment of infectious diseases. Improvements in the treatment of noncommunicable diseases have been less dramatic.

This change in the structure of the causes of death has also led to a change in the composition of deaths by age, because children are affected disproportionately by communicable diseases. Thus, as these diseases have been controlled, mortality rates of adults have grown relative to those of children.

Not all cause-of-death categories have seen reductions in mortality rates as the overall mortality rate has fallen. As a matter of principle, this is not surprising—everyone must die at some age, and reductions in particular causes of death inevitably show up as increases in other causes. However, even for age groups that have seen decreases in mortality rates in absolute terms—that is, for young ages—deaths from certain causes have increased. For example, among women, there is evidence that deaths from breast cancer, motor vehicle injuries, and intentional injuries (homicide and suicide) have increased for 15- to 60-year olds. Similarly, mortality caused by certain cancers has increased for men in the same age group.

Some of these changes are consequences of development itself, either directly or indirectly. Motor vehicle accidents may increase as a cause of death as the number of individuals using motor transport increases, and as speeds increase beyond the capacity of local roads. Also, improvements in medical technology may enable medical personnel to identify given conditions more readily, thus increasing their measured prevalence as causes of death.

Intranational Comparisons of Mortality Rates

The information presented so far has been largely at the national or regional level. It is useful, however, to examine some trends within countries to identify particular groups that face higher than average risks of death. One example is that of minority racial groups within some of the industrial market economies, such as the United States. In the United

States, the adult mortality rate (45Q15) among black men is 30 percent, and for black women it is 16 percent. The corresponding figures for whites are 16 and 9 percent, respectively, so that blacks face about twice as much risk of dying between the ages of 15 and 60 as whites.

In a developing country context, studies have shown that individuals with lower socioeconomic status often have higher mortality rates. For example, a World Bank (1989) study found that individuals with lower incomes and education levels in Brazil face higher risks of certain noncommunicable diseases, and they also engage in higher levels of risky behavior, such as smoking, alcohol consumption, and obesity.

Not only may poorer and less well-educated individuals face greater exogenous and behavior-related risks, but medical treatment may also be less effective. This may be because such individuals face greater access costs to care or are slower to seek medical care for some other reason (say because the opportunity cost of their time is too high), so that when medical care is sought, the illness or condition is more advanced. Also there is evidence that such individuals are less likely to follow medical advice and treatment schedules as closely as higher income individuals (again, for a variety of reasons), so the effectiveness of such treatment is reduced.

These divergent intranational health status measures indicate that socioeconomic factors are likely to be highly correlated with health risks and outcomes. We will examine these potential links and the possible causal correlations in greater detail in the next chapter.

AIDS: An Emerging Cause of Death

The HIV/AIDS epidemic has spread quickly across western, central, and eastern Africa. As it is transmitted primarily by sexual contact, it affects mainly young adults. Unlike the experience in North America and other industrial market economies, the disease has affected both the heterosexual and homosexual communities, and infection rates are approximately equal for women and men.

The disease began to reach epidemic proportions in Sub-Saharan Africa in the late 1970s and early 1980s. In mid-1993 about 8 million people were infected, and by 1996 this number had risen to about 14 million, representing more than 60 percent of the total infected world population. As the disease strikes individuals in the prime of their working lives and without fail results in death at some stage, the economic and social impact is proving enormous. (The economic impact of AIDS will be discussed at greater length in the next chapter.)

Morbidity

As well as dying, people get sick. It is clearly gross mismeasurement to identify population health status solely with mortality rates, while ignoring the
disability, impairment, and discomfort caused by illnesses that do not cause
death, or that do so with a lag. This would not be a severe problem if morbidity rates were related to mortality rates in a systematic and stable fashion, so that we could say, for example, that a population with certain child
and adult mortality rates would have a predictable number of individuals
suffering from illnesses that do not cause death. Partly because of the difficulties in obtaining objective measures of morbidity, however, such relationships have not been established with any degree of robustness.

Prevalence and Incidence Measures of Illness

Issues related to the measurement of the objective and subjective extent of
illness will be detailed below, but it is useful to first define the concepts of
prevalence and incidence of a disease. In a population, the number of people
with a given disease may change over time. In general, we can let the number of people with the disease at time t be denoted by $n(t)$. This number is
known as the *prevalence* of the disease. The prevalence of the disease can
change either because new individuals become infected (in which case,
$n(t)$ increases), or because infected individuals are cured or die (in which
case, $n(t)$ falls). The rate of infection of new individuals is known as the
incidence of the disease.[3] Note that the incidence is measured as the number of cases per unit of time, and it will generally differ according to the
unit used (month, year, and so forth). Prevalence is unit-free.

   A typical pattern of a disease's prevalence may look like that shown in
figure 2.4. Initially a small number of individuals is infected, but this number grows at an increasing rate (perhaps exponentially) until a large fraction of the susceptible population is infected. At that stage, the number of
new cases may be generally offset by the number of deaths or cures, so the
prevalence of the disease flattens out. If a cure if found or if some other
disease takes over, then the incidence falls, potentially very quickly. The

---

   3. The number of cases at time $t + 1$ as a function of the number at time t can
be written $n(t + 1) = n(t) + i(t) - d(t)$, where $i(t)$ is the number of new cases between
t and $t + 1$, and $d(t)$ is the number of deaths (or cures) between the same two dates.
In this case, $i(t)$ is the incidence of the disease, or the gross rate of increase.

Figure 2.4.   Dynamics of Disease

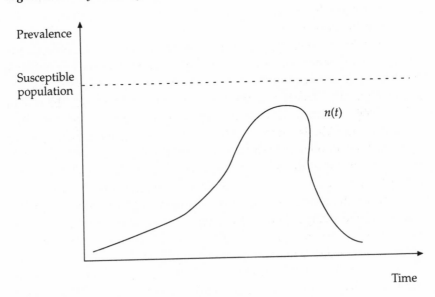

Source: Author.

duration of the disease—the time between infection and death or between infection and recovery—clearly determines the time it takes for the prevalence rate to flatten. If the duration is the same as the unit of time measuring incidence, the incidence and prevalence rates will be about equal (the number of new cases will closely match the number of existing cases).

The dynamics of disease can exhibit far more complicated behavior than that suggested by figure 2.4. In particular, incidence and prevalence rates may oscillate in either regular or apparently unpredictable (chaotic) ways, depending on the environmental, economic, and behavioral conditions. The description and analysis of such dynamics are the subjects of epidemiological studies such as Anderson and May (1991), but they are beyond the scope of this text.

Measuring Morbidity in Practice

One of the defining differences between mortality and morbidity measures of health status is the ease with which the first can be measured (assuming available survey and statistical resources) against the difficulties that surround measurement of the second. Death is a binary variable—you are

either dead or you are not—but morbidity is a continuous and multidi-
mensional variable, with both objective and subjective components that
make quantification difficult.

Nonetheless, attempts have been made to measure national morbidity
rates. These measures fall into two main categories: "observed" or objective
rates, based on clinical tests or medical examinations, and "self-perceived"
or subjective rates, based on reports by individuals of how sick they are or
feel. The objective measures include, for example, antibody concentrations
in infected individuals, analysis of functional capacity, and expert opinions
of medical practitioners. These rates of morbidity respond to changes in the
nature and extent of disease in a community—for example, malaria cases
increase when mosquito populations thrive. Subjective measures, based on
interviews with patients, tend to respond not only to the underlying pathology, but also to changes in the perceptions and expectations of individuals.
As reported by Murray, Yang, and Qiao (1992), this may explain why the
United States records a higher rate of self-perceived morbidity than does India. Such an observation is anecdotal evidence that cross-sectional analyses
using self-perceived measures of morbidity are likely to be unreliable, unless
the subjects have very similar socioeconomic and cultural characteristics.

Time series data provide a somewhat more reliable basis for analysis
but still suffer from changes in expectations and other nonpathological
determinants of illness (such as income, and the like). One approach is to
assume that sharp changes in morbidity rates stem from changes in the
characteristics of underlying diseases and their treatments, but that slow
changes reflect changing subjective criteria.

It is interesting to compare the objective and subjective measures of
illness for certain conditions. For example, a survey conducted in Ghana
(Belcher and others 1976) found that while only 0.2 percent of individuals
thought they had intestinal parasites, examinations revealed that fully 55
percent were infected. Similarly, while 0.8 percent of respondents considered themselves to be undernourished, objective measures found 32 percent to be so. At the same time, while 4.5 percent reported lower-back pain,
only 1 in 15 of these cases were confirmed on an objective basis.

These figures do not necessarily suggest that individuals overestimate
their health status or are hypochondriacs. Some medical conditions may
be objectively measurable but have relatively limited effects on functional
capacity or general wellness, at least in the short run. Also, if individuals
have lived all their lives with a given disease (such as parasitic infections),
subjectively they may feel reasonably well. Conversely, the report that 15
times as many people thought they had lower-back pain than actually did

suggests that objective measures of morbidity may fail to capture relevant aspects of ill health.

From this discussion one can infer that, given the subjective nature of health, the output of health care services—that is, better health—is likely to be very difficult to measure in practice. We shall see in later chapters of this book that this has far-reaching implications for the organization and delivery of health care services. It is one of the principal practical reasons that health is "different" from other goods.[4]

References

Anderson, Roy, and Robert May. 1991. *Infectious Diseases of Humans: Dynamics and Control.* Oxford, U.K.: Oxford University Press.

Belcher, D. W., A. K. Neumann, F. K. Wurapa, and I. M. Lourie. 1976. "Comparison of Mortality Interviews with a Health Examination Survey in Rural Africa." *American Journal of Tropical Medicine and Hygiene* 25(5): 751–58.

Cleland, J., and C. Scott. 1987. *The World Fertility Survey: An Assessment.* Oxford, U.K.: Oxford University Press.

Feachem, Richard, Tord Kjellstrom, Christopher Murray, Mead Over, and Margaret Phillips. 1992. *The Health of Adults in the Developing World.* New York: Oxford University Press.

Murray, C. J. L., and A. D. Lopez, eds. 1994. *Global Comparative Assessments in the Health Sector: Disease Burden, Expenditures, and Intervention Packages.* Geneva: World Health Organization.

Murray, Christopher, Richard Feachem, Margaret Phillips, and Carla Willis. 1992. "Adult Morbidity: Limited Data and Methodological Uncertainty." In Richard Feachem and others, eds., *The Health of Adults in the Developing World.* New York: Oxford University Press.

Murray, Christopher, Gonghuan Yang, and Xinjian Qiao. 1992. "Adult Mortality: Levels, Patterns, and Causes." In Richard Feachem and others, eds., *The Health of Adults in the Developing World.* New York: Oxford University Press.

Selvin, Steve. 1991. *Statistical Analysis of Epidemiologic Data.* Oxford, U.K.: Oxford University Press.

World Bank. 1989. *Adult Health in Brazil: Adjusting to New Challenges.* Report No. 7807-BR. Washington, D.C.

_____. 1993. *World Development Report, 1993: Investing in Health.* New York: Oxford University Press.

4. There are undoubtedly other reasons to consider health as being different from other goods that take into consideration moral or ethical arguments. It seems prudent to leave the development of such arguments to moral philosophers.

3

The Determinants of Health

In this chapter we investigate the factors that affect the health of individuals and populations. An important correlate with health outcomes is income, both at the disaggregated (individual or household) and at the aggregate (regional or national) level. This general pattern is observed over time and across countries and suggests that an important part of any strategy to improve health is broad-based economic development. Recognizing that healthier people are likely to be more productive, the link from health to income can also be important, as evidenced by the economic impact of AIDS in Africa. We report one study, however, that shows that the net direction of causation is likely to be from income to health.

Health and Development

As countries develop economically, the structure of economic and social organizations changes. At first, the industrial sector tends to grow at the expense of the agriculture sector (both in employment and value added), and subsequently the service sector increases as a share of the economy. As the population becomes more urbanized, traditional social structures may become less important, and the distribution of income may change. The effects of these changes in social structure on health outcomes are ambiguous (see Lee and Mills 1983). While the nature of health problems may change, the effect on the overall health status of the population is difficult to ascertain. For example, a switch from agriculture to industrial production may reduce the incidence of some infectious diseases found primarily in rural areas, such as schistosomiasis, but such a decrease may be associated with an increase in diseases related to pollution, including lung cancer.

Similar ambiguity surrounds the direct effects of rural-urban migration. Urban populations have lower transportation costs and generally greater access to health care providers and other public goods, but they must deal concurrently with the health effects of overcrowding, including the greater chance of contracting infectious diseases such as tuberculosis and increased stress levels.

Despite these ambiguous effects of development on health, increases in income, and hence in the consumption of health-improving goods and services, mean that there is a generally positive relationship between health status and stage of development. This relationship will be examined in more detail below, but it is useful to note two important consequences of the improvements in health.

First, as populations become healthier, they also age. This is known as the *demographic transition,* and it occurs for two reasons. There is a direct effect—as the health of individuals improves, they live longer. In this case, at a given birth rate, the net addition to the population each year increases, as does the share of older people in the population. In addition, the fertility rate (the average number of children born to a representative woman in her life) tends to decline. This is a somewhat more indirect effect of the change in health status on the population structure, because it stems from individual choices about the desired number of children. If the behavior of individuals were unaffected by improvements in health, then we would expect to see birth rates increase as the number of deaths at birth fell. The channels through which better health, and more generally greater economic security, determine fertility rates are diverse and interconnected, but if it is assumed that at least one reason for bearing children is for their use as a productive resource, reduced child mortality rates mean that fewer births are required to sustain a desired level of income security.[1]

---

1. A formal analysis of the determinants of fertility rates is beyond the scope of this text. It is interesting to note, however, that the effects of fertility rates on the age structure of the population are subtle. For example, consider a simple two-period model of the life-cycle, in which children are those alive in the first period and adults are those alive in the second. Adults have preferences for children as a productive resource, and children born have a certain probability of being productive (that is, remaining alive) in their youth. As this probability increases (that is, as the child mortality rate falls), the number of births may be expected to fall in line with such a reduction, with the net number of children living remaining unchanged. However, if there are costs associated with birth (and, in practice, with rearing an unproductive child until age 5 or 6), then as the survival rate increases, the average cost of obtaining a productive child falls, and the optimal number could increase, suggesting that the average age of the population could fall. However, an additional factor to consider is the risk faced by adults. When the probability of

The pattern of the demographic transition over time depends on the timing of both the mortality effect and the fertility effect. In currently high-income countries, these effects generally occurred simultaneously, in the late nineteenth century, so that while the age structure shifted, net population growth rates remained stable, rarely reaching 2 percent yearly. However, in developing countries, declines in mortality rates have preceded declines in fertility rates, leading to bursts of high population growth rates of up to 4 percent. This divergent experience is likely the product of the origin of changes in mortality rates. Mortality improvements in high-income countries occurred, at least in part, because of the *discovery* of medical interventions and causes of ill-health, which necessarily took time, while the reduction in mortality rates in developing countries was, at least in the early stages, driven by *adoption* of the existing techniques and knowledge. Assuming that the effects of better health on fertility rates, which required cultural and behavioral responses to changing environments, occurred at similar rates, then high transitional population growth rates in developing countries can be explained.

The demographic transition can be visualized using population structure diagrams, as shown in figure 3.1. These figures represent the populations of England and Wales and are reproduced from World Bank work (1993). The first diagram in the figure shows information for 1891, and the second contains the same numbers for 1966. The left-hand side of each diagram shows the proportion of the population that falls in each age group. Thus, in 1891, the largest age group was children between the ages of zero and 4, and the size of each successive age group fell, with those aged over 75 making up less than 2 percent of the population. By 1966, however, older generations made up a much larger share of the population, with the over-75 group making up about 5 percent. The share of the population over the age of 65 (retirement age) grew from about 4 percent in 1891 to about 12 percent in 1966.

On the right-hand side of the diagrams the proportion of deaths that befell members of each age group is shown. Thus, in 1891 fully 35 percent of all deaths occurred in the 0–4 age group, and the shares for other age groups were lower. By 1966, however, the over-75 age group accounted for nearly 45 percent of deaths, reflecting both their larger share of the population and the lower mortality rates in younger age groups.

---

survival increases, the risk of having no surviving children from a given number of births falls, so the number of births may fall more than proportionately.

Figure 3.1. Population Structure Diagrams for England and Wales, 1891 and 1966

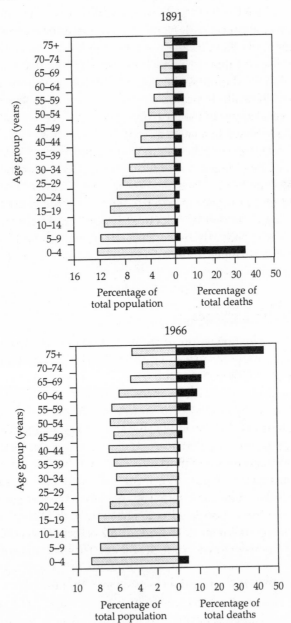

Source: World Bank (1993, box 1.4, p. 31).

The second consequence of improved health is that the pattern of disease changes as development proceeds. This is known as the *epidemiological transition*, and it can be thought of as resulting from two effects. First, as some diseases and causes of ill-health are eliminated or controlled, the relative importance of other diseases rises, as a matter of arithmetic. In all likelihood, the diseases that are controlled early are relatively less costly to combat, so that we should not be surprised to see reductions in the rate of improvement in health indicators such as life expectancy over the development process (issues in the measurement of productivity in health production are addressed in a later section).

The second effect contributing to the epidemiological transition is that as individuals live longer, diseases that only affect older individuals increase in absolute terms. Thus, because the prevalence of heart disease is low in children but higher in adults over 50, if more children live to be adults, the population-wide incidence of heart-attack-related deaths necessarily increases. Similarly, reductions in maternal mortality lead to larger numbers of older women and to a greater prevalence of post-menopausal health problems.

Income-Health Linkages

Many studies have shown a positive correlation between income and health status, both on cross-sectional and longitudinal bases. For example, Gertler and van der Gaag (1990) report cross-sectional analysis of the links between per capita gross national product (GNP) and health status for a sample of 34 countries in 1975. The highest per capita income, in the United States, is 20 times the lowest, in Malawi, and the variance explains between 74 and 79 percent of the variation in life expectancy at birth, the infant mortality rate, and the child mortality rate. In their study, the only health status variable for which per capita income does not provide such explanatory power is the crude death rate. They find that, on average, a 10 percent increase in income is associated with one extra year of life expectancy, an 8.3 percent lower infant mortality rate, a 14.2 percent lower child mortality rate, and a 1.5 percent lower crude death rate. These results are reproduced in table 3.1.

The structural relationship between income and health status has shifted over time. This is most clearly seen from an examination of figure 3.2. While there continued to be a positive correlation between health status measured by life expectancy and income on a cross-sectional basis throughout the twentieth century, this relationship shifted over time. Thus, in 1930, a

Table 3.1. *Health Indicators and Economic Development, Selected Countries, 1975*

Item	Life expectancy at birth	Infant mortality	Child mortality	Crude death rate
Constant	2.951	10.024	11.851	3.510
	(26.84)	(14.96)	(11.52)	(8.75)
GNP per capita	0.157	–0.833	–1.415	–0.151
	(11.09)	(9.65)	(10.68)	(2.91)
$\bar{R}^2$	0.787	0.737	0.774	0.185

Note: Figures in parentheses are *t*-values.
Source: Gertler and van der Gaag (1990, table 2.2, p. 9).

Figure 3.2. *Life Expectancy and Income Per Capita, Selected Countries and Periods*

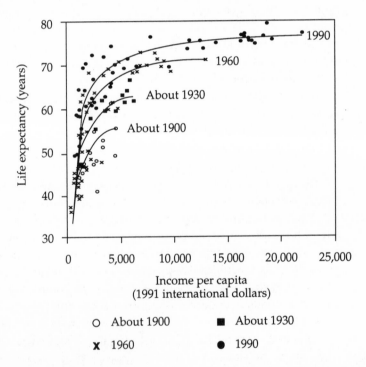

Note: International dollars are derived from national currencies not by use of exchange rates, but by assessment of purchasing power. The effect is to raise the relative incomes of poorer countries, often substantially.
Source: Adapted from World Bank (1993, figure 1.9, p. 34).

country with a per capita income of $2,500 (in 1991 international dollars) experienced a life expectancy at birth of around 50 years, while a second country, with twice the per capita income, had, on average, a life expectancy of 55 years. However, if it took the first country 30 years to double its per capita income, it would find its life expectancy had increased not to 55, but to 60 years.

There are two basic explanations for this shifting relationship between income and health. The first is that it has become easier, or cheaper, to attain and maintain given levels of health over time because of technological innovations (such as scientific discoveries of the causes and treatment of disease) and investment in public infrastructure (such as sanitation systems, and the like). Not only does health increase with income because people are better-off, but it also increases because it is more affordable.

The second possible explanation for the shift in the relationship is that individuals' preferences have changed over time, and that, for a given level of income, individuals have become more concerned about health. Although the escalation in the number of sports clubs, fitness magazines, and health-food stores in rich countries suggests that there may be some truth to the idea that people have become more health conscious, such an effect would not appear to be of great importance in explaining broad structural trends across a wide range of income levels.

The technological advances that have allowed improvements in health—particularly advances in scientific and technical knowledge—have both public good and capital good characteristics. This means that it is inadvisable to use cross-sectional relationships, even if augmented by longitudinal information, to make direct inferences about possible effects of income changes on health. This is particularly true when considering the effects of short-term downturns in economic performance, characterized by falls in real GNP. While health status is unlikely to improve during such episodes, any deterioration will be relatively small, compared with that predicted by direct use of regression elasticities. Only when economic downturns are of sufficient duration to accommodate significant depreciation of health-related physical and institutional infrastructure will health status decline commensurately. Unfortunately, the economic underperformance of some Sub-Saharan African nations over the past two decades has been sufficient to give rise to serious concerns over long-term health trends (Cornia, Jolly, and Stewart 1987).

The discussion so far has concerned the general association between income and health but has not examined the specific linkages, apart from technological innovations, that allow rising incomes to improve health status. An extra 100 schillings does not in itself make an individual healthier or increase his or her life expectancy. It is even possible to argue that the direct effect of an increase in measured income would be, if anything, to reduce health, if it requires the exertion of greater physical effort (leading directly to exhaustion), the operation of more dangerous machinery (increasing the chance of injury), or the cultivation of more marginal land (and hence deterioration of the environment). However, when more income is generated by greater physical and technological endowments— either naturally occurring or created by previous savings and investment decisions—then there is little reason to assume that the direct effects on health of the higher income will be significant.[2,3]

Clearly then, it is the use of income that is of importance in the determination of health status. As a general rule, we would expect that, as income increases, consumption of health-improving goods and services also increases. But health improvement is not the only objective of individuals, and consumption of certain health-reducing goods and services may also depend on the level of income. A useful way of examining the link between income and health is to look first at the way certain broad classes of consumption goods and services affect health, and to then ask how the use of these goods and services is usually related to income.

Perhaps the most obvious input into good health is medical services, including both curative and preventive treatments. Such services, however, particularly curative care, can be less important when other goods and services—including clean water, nutrition, effective and safe shelter, and so on— are also available and used effectively. It is important to take note of the qualification that these consumption goods must be used *effectively*. Simple improvements in behavior, such as washing of hands with clean water and appropriate use of mosquito nets, can have substantial impacts on health

---

2. The argument here is simply that income is determined by available resources and technologies and by production choices—that is, the uses made of those resources. A country with more iron ore can produce more steel with the same inputs of other goods and services than one with less iron ore. The income of the first country will be higher, but, assuming the same levels of other inputs, its health status, as a function of income, is unlikely to differ. If both countries were to have the same income—that is, to produce the same amount of steel—then we would expect the first to have better health, other things being held constant, than the second.

3. We have spoken so far of the ability of income to cause health improvements. But clearly one input into production, and thus the determination of income, is a healthy work force; it is thus conceivable that health causes increases in income. We will address this issue later in the chapter.

status. Some studies have found that the level of education of individuals is a significant determinant of health status, and particularly that improvements in parents' literacy are correlated with improvements in children's health (see, for example, Cochrane, O'Hara, and Leslie 1980; Strauss 1987). Again, education, an investment in human capital, should not be expected to increase health status by itself. But as a proxy for effective use of other health-improving goods and services, it has been found to be significant.

Consumption of some other goods and services has potentially negative effects on health status. These effects include exposure to pollution, increased likelihood of motor vehicle accidents, overconsumption of alcohol, smoking, indulgence in unsafe sex, and consumption of unhealthy foods (such as those with high fat content). Some of these items, particularly pollution and road accidents, are at issue only to the extent that they are an unavoidable (or at least costly to reduce) by-product of available production processes. Sometimes these economic activities constitute home production in the sense that the output is not marketed but consumed directly. For example, burning of dried cow dung or cheap, high-sulphur coal for household cooking and heating can result in high pollution levels at night and during winter in urban areas, and use of poorly maintained cars for private transport on deteriorating roads can increase road accidents.[4]

Other goods that negatively affect health, such as alcohol, cigarettes, and high-fat foods, may only become affordable at certain levels of income. This is particularly true if consumption of sufficient quantities of the goods is required before significant negative health effects are observed. At the same time, some goods may become less affordable as income increases, because the opportunity cost associated with their consumption increases. Perhaps the most striking example of such an activity is the sexual practices of individuals. These are clearly determined in part by cultural and social norms, but in the presence of potentially disastrous consequences arising from infection with sexually transmitted diseases—particularly the HIV virus—current and future income may be significant determinants of the price of unsafe sex. A wealthy businessman and a well-educated teenager with good prospects are likely to impute a higher price to unsafe sex than a prostitute with no alternative employment or an unemployed twenty-five-year-old with little training in a region in long-term economic decline (Philipson and Posner 1995). Thus, while most goods become more affordable as income rises, if

---

4. Of greater concern, perhaps, given the low rate of private car ownership in developing countries, is the use of poorly maintained buses and taxis.

consumption entails a potential loss of income (in the extreme case, through death), the opportunity cost of consumption may increase sufficiently for the net price to increase significantly.[5]

The discussion of the previous paragraph highlights the likely importance of cultural norms in determining consumption patterns and health outcomes. It has been found, for example, that the social status of women is positively correlated with both their health status and that of their children. Access by women to prenatal care and the extent of their heavy household and agricultural work (such as carrying water) are likely to have significant impacts on their health but are often determined within social strictures that are unresponsive, especially in the short run, to economic interventions.

The final point to note with regard to this discussion of the production of health is that, despite the existence of some externalities (for example, related to immunization), one's health depends primarily on one's own consumption of medical care, food, shelter, clothing, water, sanitation, and so forth. Thus, when aggregate data are used to analyze the correlations between health and these factors, it is not surprising that the distribution of income also matters. This is not a normative argument for a more egalitarian distribution of income (which may well be a highly commendable objective in itself), but solely a realization that an individual's health status is unlikely to be strictly proportional (in some ill-defined sense) to income, and relatively small transfers to the poor from the rich, perhaps in the form of in-kind transfers of health-improving services such as health clinics, can be expected to improve overall health levels.[6]

A simple illustration of this point is provided by examining figure 3.3, which is drawn from Anand and Ravallion (1993), and shows actual and fitted values of life expectancy and private consumption per capita for 86 developing countries. Assuming that such a relationship also exists within countries, it is clear that the average life expectancy across incomes is much less than the life expectancy of those with average incomes (because the fitted relationship is concave).[7] The flatness of the relationship at incomes

---

5. As we shall see below, AIDS may not be a good example in some developing countries where higher income and socioeconomic status are associated with larger numbers of sexual partners (for men), and thus a greater chance of HIV infection.

6. That is, the health status of the poor will increase while that of the rich will not fall. The rich may even see their health status increase if they were previously using their high incomes to consume health-reducing goods, such as unhealthy foods and alcohol.

7. This is a consequence (more accurately, a restatement of) Jensen's inequality, which states that if x is a real valued random variable with cumulative distribution

above the (unweighted) average suggests that redistribution from the rich to the poor would have a significant impact on average life expectancy, with little if any negative effect on the health status of the rich.[8]

Health Care as an Input into the Production of Health

Some goods and services have the sole purpose of improving health. The most obvious of these are services provided by medical personnel such as

Figure 3.3.   *Life Expectancy at Birth and Private Consumption Per Capita for 86 Developing Countries, 1985*

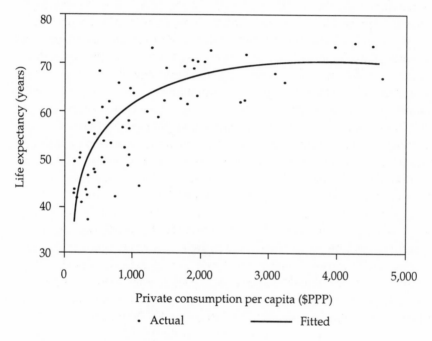

Source: Anand and Ravallion (1993, figure 1, p. 139).

---

function F, and if $g : \mathbb{R} \to \mathbb{R}$ is increasing and concave, then $g(\int xdF) \geq \int g(x)dF$. That is, $g(\bar{x}) \geq \overline{g(x)}$, or the value of g at the average of x is greater than or equal to the average value of g.

8. Clearly, the absolute number of rich individuals, or more specifically, the amount of resources available for redistribution, determines the actual increase in average health status (as measured here by life expectancy at birth). If most income

physicians, nurses, clinicians, and the like, although another important source of such services is the household itself (in the form of nursing services provided by parents for children, and vice versa, for example). Extra-household medical services can be provided in a number of institutional and physical environments, from state-run hospitals, to private doctors' surgeries, to community-based village cooperative health centers. The organization of health care delivery can have potentially large effects on its effectiveness and cost, and we will address many related issues in later chapters. Here, however, we are interested in the basic technological constraints that determine the way resources can be transformed into health care, and subsequently, to better health status.

Because data are limited, it is often necessary to analyze the effects of medical care on health outcomes at highly aggregated levels, usually relying on gross medical care expenditures per capita and a few other variables (such as the number of clinics, hospital beds, and physicians per capita) as explanators. Upon reflection, however, it is apparent that the direct outputs of medical care are both multiple and diverse, and such aggregation might hide important microeconomic effects, both in terms of efficiency and equity.[9]

In basic microeconomic theory models, we describe the alternative production possibilities available to a production unit (usually a firm) by a production function $y = f(x)$, which gives the output y produced for a given combination of inputs, $x = (x_1, \ldots, x_n)$ (a vector). This permits one to derive a cost function, $c(w, y)$, that gives the minimum cost of producing y units of output when the vector of prices of the inputs is set at $w = (w_1, \ldots, w_n)$.

There are a number of complications introduced when considering the production of medical care. First, hospitals, physicians, clinics, and other facilities clearly serve different purposes and thus can be thought of as producing different goods. And within each of these units, multiple goods are produced, such as immunizations, family planning services, emergency surgery, treatment of on-going chronic diseases, and so forth. A second and fundamental way in which these institutions produce different products is that the product or service produced is usually patient-specific. Thus,

---

is generated by the poor, because they are so abundant, then redistribution will have little effect on average health status.

9. It should be noted that empirical studies generally attempt to use the most detailed information available, but, particularly in developing countries, appropriate data can be quite thin on the ground.

the same service rendered to different individuals may cost different amounts, depending on the health of the individual, his willingness and ability to respond to treatment, and the like.

Not only may some patients be more costly to treat than others, but the production and delivery (or marketing) of the services are more intimately connected than with the standard consumption goods of undergraduate textbooks. In ordinary production theory, the production decision is more or less independent of the marketing decision. Widgets can be produced first, and then sold to consumers at a price and in a fashion that best suits the firm or managers. Health care, in contrast, is produced and consumed coincidentally. In addition, once allocated to a patient, it is not possible for that individual to transfer the good to another individual, as can be done with a standard widget. This last point means that, because good health is a fundamental input of an individual's capacity to work and live, the government may not be able to correct for a poor distribution of health care by redistributing income through the tax and transfer system, even in the unlikely event that a sufficiently sophisticated system exists.

These observations lead us to consider explicitly so-called intensive and extensive margins in the production of health care. Production is increased on the intensive margin if the inputs used in the treatment of a particular individual, or group of individuals, are increased. Alternatively, production is increased on the extensive margin when the number of patients and types of cases increase. Thus, some measures of the extent of health care production on the extensive margin include hospital admission rates, number of women provided with birth control services, and the rate of immunization. At the same time, measures of production on the intensive margin include such things as the average length of hospital stay per person admitted, the number of drugs per person treated, and the number of booster shots received by immunized children after the first shot.

As in many other economic production processes, increases in output along these intensive and extensive margins can be expected first to exhibit decreasing and then increasing marginal and average costs. A simple example is the production of hospital admissions: the first of these is very costly, because it requires the construction of the hospital, but the additional costs of further patients are relatively low, and only when crowding starts to make individuals' hospital stays ineffectual does the economic cost of admissions again increase. Similarly, the education of women about birth control may initially be costly as a program is set up, but then in urban areas the marginal cost of providing the information and services might be quite low. When much of the urban population has been covered, extension to the rural population becomes more expensive, and the marginal and average costs of increasing production on this extensive margin increase. Examples on the intensive margin include the length of a hospital stay—there may be administrative costs associated with the initial admission, but these diminish until, for a given admission rate (that is, for a given extensive margin choice), longer stays increase crowding sufficiently that marginal and average costs begin to increase. Similarly, the costs of drugs per person may be expected to rise as increasingly expensive therapies are tried in succession.

A good example of the decreasing returns associated with medical care in developing countries is provided by Over's (1991) discussion of Preston's (1975, 1980, 1985) analyses of the possible effects of medical care on life expectancy. Fully 50 percent of the improvement in life expectancy in developing countries from 1940 to 1970 (when life expectancy rose by 17.6 years on average) was potentially the product of improvements in health care. Between 1965–69 and 1975–79, however, life expectancy grew by only 3.9 years on average, and improvements in medical care could account for only 1.1 years, or 28 percent of this increase. Of course, when discussing marginal and average productivity and costs, it is important to keep other inputs constant. It is plausible that the underlying productivity of health care did not change between the first and second periods of Preston's studies, but that increases in other inputs, such as income, education, and nutrition, may have reduced the effect of medical care.[10] Despite this possibility, it seems reasonable to assume that at some stage, all else being equal, it becomes increasingly costly to expand life expectancy. This result would appear to be generally descriptive of a wide range of medical interventions.

Indeed, some cross-country analyses have difficulty finding much of a link between medical care and health outcomes, suggesting that at an aggregate level, medical care has a low marginal productivity. Controlling for income and education, Filmer and Pritchett (1997) and Filmer, Pritchett, and Hammer (1998) find little effect of public medical care on health.[11]

---

10. For example, if I have little chance of guarding against infection because of lack of sanitation, then the productivity of medical care may be very high, because I become ill very often. But if I have clean water and good sewerage, then the productivity of medical care may be somewhat lower, because I do not need it as much. Technically, medical care (x_1) and other inputs (x_2) may be substitutes in the production of life expectancy (y), so that $d^2y/dx_1 dx_2 < 0$.

11. Anand and Ravallion (1993) find a positive effect between public medical care and health, but do not control for education.

Before we leave this general discussion of the production of medical care, it should be noted that another aspect of the process that distinguishes medical care from our standard widget is that highly trained producers (physicians) differ widely on their opinions about the most effective or efficient means of production.[12] Usually we assume that firms know the technological possibilities available to them, but this cannot be true of physician services in some countries where, having had high levels of training and having passed uniform examinations and other requirements to enter the profession, they differ by wide margins on their approaches to the treatment of given conditions. These differences are seen on both the intensive and extensive margins (see Phelps 1992b, chapter 3, for some examples). That so many individuals, exposed to similar training, undertake different production procedures suggests that there is a lot of discretion in choice of production technique and also great potential for variation in the quality of the product (or, equivalently, a lot of variation in the true productivity of the producers).

Health-Income Linkages

So far we have examined the potential effects of income on health status. We argued that the main effects were transmitted through the general level of consumption that was made possible by higher incomes, and specifically through greater access to medical care. But empirical analyses of the linkages between income and health must also account for the possibility that health improvements lead to increases in income. In this section we discuss the possible effects, and in the next section we review some empirical techniques and evidence on the direction of causality.

The share of labor in national income is about two-thirds in most countries. Labor thus constitutes the most important factor of production, and changes in its productivity can significantly affect total income. In turn, the productivity of labor is a function of two types of factors: the skills of individuals, derived from their innate physical and mental capabilities, and education, training, and other investments in their human capital; and the efficiency of labor organization and management. Improvements in health can affect labor productivity through both of these channels.

It is not difficult to imagine that healthier people tend to be fitter, stronger, and more energetic than unhealthy individuals, so that time spent on

---

12. Phelps (1992a) presents a useful survey of the evidence and policy implications of widely varying medical practices.

the job is more productive, although the extent of this effect on labor productivity clearly depends on the type of work involved. Perhaps more important, the greater amount of time spent on sick leave or away from work for other reasons by less-healthy individuals has a detrimental effect on their total annual output.[13]

The direct costs of absenteeism arise from the worker in question not being available to engage in productive activities. An additional cost is incurred when organizational structures adapt in the direction of otherwise inefficient forms in response to absences. For example, overstaffing may result as an insurance mechanism against the possibility that key workers are absent on a given day. If the labor services in question are firm-specific, relying on an outside spot labor market will be dominated by overstaffing, although this is likely to be socially inefficient.

The need to care for sick relatives can mean that the productivity of healthy individuals is also reduced as a direct consequence of ill health. One should be careful when using this argument, however, because it applies well to the definition of productivity that one may derive from national accounts data, but may be less persuasive on purely economic grounds. In the national accounts, income is reduced when a healthy relative stays home from work to look after a sick member of the family. However, if some other outsider had left his or her job in order to attend to the sick person on a commercial basis, national income would change by the difference between the wage given up and the payment for the nursing services. Assuming that the worker switched because the wage for looking after the sick person was higher than in the earlier occupation, and ignoring possible market failures and distortionary government taxes and other interventions, national income would increase because of the switch in jobs of the new nurse.[14]

A possibly more significant effect of illness on family members, especially over the long term, derives from the need for children and others to

---

13. It may be tempting to suggest that time spent away from work because of sickness should not be counted in the denominator of any output per person calculation of labor productivity, so that absences from the workplace should not have a direct impact on productivity measures. However, if such time would have been spent at work if not for the ill-health of the worker, productivity can be said to have fallen.

14. National income has still fallen due to the fact that the sick individual is not at work. We are just concentrating here on the effect of the change in formal labor force participation of relatives.

forego vital years of schooling if one or both of their parents are chronically ill. Although this cost may appear similar to the somewhat discounted cost in the previous paragraph, it is differentiated by its dynamic nature, particularly when capital markets do not function well. If children could effectively borrow against their future returns to current investment in education, they would be able to pay the wages of a live-in nurse or similar health worker, instead of foregoing the whole of their additional future earnings (which may outweigh the cost of a nurse manyfold).[15]

Finally, improvements in health, to the extent that they increase life expectancy, will have positive effects on the experience level of the active labor force. While some commentators argue that a young labor force is necessarily productive, a more mature worker pool has the advantage of benefiting from greater experience and more time learning by doing. The significance of this effect is not well established, particularly in times of rapid technological growth, when skills soon become redundant. Nevertheless, virtually all empirical studies of wage determination within a human capital framework find positive and significant coefficients on variables that measure experience (Mincer 1974). Of course, taking account of the institutional structure is important in making inferences from these empirical studies. For example, if promotions and pay increases are based rigidly on years of experience, with no close relationship to individual productivity, the positive returns to experience do not necessarily indicate a positive relationship between national output and the experience of the labor force.

A further point to note with regard to the effect of an older population on labor productivity is that there may be indirect effects stemming from induced changes in savings and investment incentives. Put simply, the basic argument is that if an aging population relies on taxes on current wages to finance consumption of the elderly nonworking population (for example, through a pay-as-you-go social security system), there may be significant negative effects on the steady-state level of capital per worker in the economy. This in itself will reduce the labor productivity of future generations, controlling for their health and other factors. Whether such an effect

---

15. In the example of the previous paragraph, in which current market labor income was given up in order to perform home nursing services, there is no obvious market failure that drives a wedge between the value of nursing services provided and the foregone wage (in a direction that makes the latter greater than the former). However, due to well-documented capital market imperfections, foregone future income may well exceed the value of current nursing services, which nonetheless have to be provided in kind by relatives.

should be attributed to the improvement in health status of current generations or to the distribution of resources across generations (through the social security system) is debatable.

Empirical Studies of the Health-Income Nexus

We made the point earlier that it is not income per se that improves health, but how that income is used, and that average incomes do not necessarily capture the availability of resources to all members of a society if the distribution of income is uneven. The implications of that discussion for empirical work are straightforward. For example, some studies have found that equations of the form

$$h_i = \beta_0 + \beta_1 y_i$$

where h_i is a health status observation and y_i is income, deliver a positive and significant income coefficient, β_1. Unsurprisingly, however, as more terms are added to the right-hand side, such as the poverty rate (a proxy for the distribution of income or for the number of individuals with very low incomes) and public health expenditure per capita, the coefficient on income becomes insignificant (see, for example, Anand and Ravallion 1993, footnote 20, p. 141).

This is not to say that the uses of measured household income are the only determinants of health. For example, if public services received are not captured in the income term, including them will not necessarily remove the influence of income on health. Also, household health status may well be a function of both household consumption decisions and the general level of health in the community, especially with regard to infectious diseases. Thus, average income may also affect household health, so that including distributional variables need not remove the influence of average income on aggregate health outcomes. Of course, both these concerns would disappear if income were measured perfectly, including both public transfers in kind and the external effects of the individual's living environment and exposure to disease.[16]

---

16. To clarify the last point, an individual with 100 schillings living in a cholera-infested slum is clearly worse-off than another with the same monetary income living in a sulubrious suburb. If their incomes can be adjusted to capture the differences in living environments, average income should cease to be a significant explanator of health status, other things being equal.

Finally, we also noted that some individuals may be able to use a given amount of income more effectively to improve their health than others. Better-educated individuals, in particular, may be expected to transform given quantities of resources into higher levels of health, so that including educational attainment on the right-hand side may improve the explanatory power of a regression. This is essentially the same issue as that of capturing the effects of the individual's living environment. The difference is that the average income term is the same for all individuals, but educational levels will differ.[17]

In the following subsection we discuss one study that attempts to empirically estimate the relationship between income and aggregate health status and to establish the net direction of causality using econometric techniques. While there are plausible links in both directions, the study finds that the net effect is from income to health—that is, higher incomes imply better health. The following subsection examines a more specific health problem of particular importance in Sub-Saharan Africa—AIDS—and explores the possible economic impact of the disease. The focus there is on the link from health to income.

Cross-Country Aggregate Study

Following Pritchett and Summers (1993), a general formulation of the total impact of income on health in a cross-country time-series model is of the form

$$h_{it} = \beta y_{it} + \gamma x_{it} + \alpha_i + \delta_t + \varepsilon_{it}$$

where h_{it} is the health status measure of country i at time t (mortality rate, life expectancy, infant mortality rate, and the like), y_{it} is (log of) per capita income, x_{it} contains other variables that we might think improve the effectiveness of income use in producing health, α_i is a country-specific fixed effect allowing for the influence of local conditions independent of income that affect health (such as climate), and δ_t is a time-specific effect, allowing for exogenous (global) improvements in technology, and so forth. In their analysis, Pritchett and Summers report both regressions that employ the country-specific fixed effects term, α_i, and regressions in which

---

17. When performing cross-country analysis, average world income is unlikely to be a useful proxy for local living conditions (essentially, they are local public goods), although educational attainment will continue to be potentially significant.

the fixed effect is omitted but the data are differenced, eliminating the need to include it.

Within this framework, the authors argue that β represents the *total* effect of income on health. Including additional variables on the right-hand side that are direct functions of income, such as nutrition intake, number of doctors per capita, and the like, would mean that the coefficient on h would represent a *partial* effect of income on health not covered by the additional variables. As discussed above, if enough variables were added to the right-hand side, we would expect the coefficient on y to become statistically insignificant.[18]

The model is then used to establish a structural and causative relationship between income and health, as opposed to a solely associative one. That is, the authors wish to examine first whether income and health are directly related, or whether there is a third, excluded factor (such as cultural values or good government) that jointly determines both, and second, if this is the case, whether higher income leads to better health, or better health causes income to rise.

The question of whether there is a structural link between income and health is addressed by controlling for country-specific fixed effects (either by differencing the data or including the fixed-effects terms) and by using instrumental variable techniques. Instrumental variable techniques are useful in testing to see if there is some third, unobservable variable in addition to country-specific fixed effects that affects both income and health. Examples of possible third variables given by the authors include "good government" and "culture"—variables that are intrinsically difficult to include in a regression analysis. The strategy is then to identify other measurable variables that one might expect to be correlated directly with income, but not with health status, and to use these as instruments for income in separate regressions. To the extent that the estimated coefficients on the instrumental variables are similar in each regression, this suggests a structural relationship between income and health and not one derived from a joint relationship with a third, unobservable variable. Such instruments include measures of the misalignment of the official exchange rate (its deviation from purchasing power parity, PPP, level, and the black market premium) and the ratio of investment to GDP. Each of these is suspected of being associated with income but not

---

18. Alternatively, the coefficient may not become insignificant if there is sufficient multicolinearity among the right-hand side variables. In this case, however, interpretation of the coefficient would not be possible.

directly with health status. A fourth instrument the authors construct for each country is income growth in "similar" countries, which is meant to capture common external shocks that affect income growth but exclude internal variables potentially related directly to health status.

The results of this analysis suggest that there is a structural relationship between income and health and that the direction of causation is from income to health. The elasticity of the infant mortality rate with respect to income is reported as about 0.2, so that a 5 percent increase in income leads to a 1 percent fall in infant mortality. Estimates of the effects of income on child mortality rates are very similar, given the high degree of correlation between the infant and child mortality rates across countries.

Empirical estimates of the links between income and life expectancy are subject to greater uncertainty. This is because some causes of death, such as motor vehicle accidents and smoking, increase with income (as we saw earlier), and because the data on mortality rates among adults are of poor quality. The authors, however, identify an income elasticity of life expectancy equal to 0.015, implying that a 10 percent increase in income raises life expectancy at the mean by about one month, but the estimated coefficient is not significant at the 5 percent level.

The Economic Consequences of AIDS in Africa

Ainsworth and Over (1994) and other authors (see, for example, Cuddington 1993 and Over 1992) have attempted to project the impact that HIV/AIDS is likely to have on African economic development. They identify four factors that make HIV potentially different to other, more common, diseases.[19] First, given the current state of medical technology, AIDS is always fatal. While in some industrial countries new multiple-drug therapies are delaying the onset of AIDS for HIV-infected individuals, such drugs are extremely expensive and are unlikely to be available on a widespread basis in developing countries in the near future. Second, unlike many diseases, AIDS is particularly prevalent among individuals of prime working age who would otherwise be expected to be relatively

---

19. The authors also report World Health Organization estimates of about 1.2 million cumulative deaths caused by AIDS by mid-1993, implying that the total historical infection prevalence was somewhat over 9 million people by that time. For comparison, the number of individuals that contract malaria each year—that is, the annual incidence of malaria—is estimated to be much higher, at about 110 million.

healthy. Third, HIV infection is already widespread, and because there is a long (up to 10 years) incubation period before full-blown AIDS is developed, this creates a large stock of sick individuals. Thus, in addition to the number of people dying of AIDS each year, many more are debilitated by the disease for long periods before death. Finally, unlike many other diseases, AIDS is not more prevalent among those in lower socioeconomic groups. This is of importance both economically and politically. It clearly has direct implications for the economic cost of the disease, but also, given the domination of political institutions by higher-income individuals, it means that there may be more political will to combat the disease.

Estimating the economic effect of AIDS into the future requires epidemiological, demographic, and economic projections. For example, epidemiological information about the current number and distribution of infected individuals in the population needs to be collected and estimated. Based on this initial snapshot, projections must be made about the likely epidemiological dynamics—are infection rates likely to increase, level off, oscillate, or behave in some other manner? Which segments of the population will be more affected than others? Such projections require information about the way in which the disease is spread and the behavior of individuals. Given this epidemiological framework, the demographic consequences can be projected, including the changes in population age, gender, and socioeconomic structure. Finally, based on assumptions about the economic responses (such as savings behavior and labor supply) of individuals faced with AIDS, the effect on economic activity, output, and growth is examined.

Such a projection process is clearly intended to identify the link from health to income, with the reasonable expectation that deteriorations in health, as measured by increases in the extent of HIV/AIDS, will reduce income. An interesting feature of the case though is that, at the individual level, higher incomes can be associated with more severe HIV infection. Because of the nature of the transmission process and cultural norms, men with higher socioeconomic status have higher infection rates than other men. Ainsworth and Over note that in many African countries higher status for men is associated with a greater number of sexual partners and thus a greater chance of becoming infected. The opposite appears to be true for single women—those from backgrounds with higher social status tend to have fewer sexual partners, and thus they have less chance of contracting the disease.

Inferring from these stylized facts that higher income causes greater infection rates among men is obviously problematic. However, the impact of such a pattern of disease on projections of the economic effects in lost output is clear. Under the reasonable—although, in societies with widespread corruption and rent-seeking, not irrefutable—assumption that those with higher incomes have higher economic output, the economic loss is larger than it otherwise would be.[20] This loss is made up of both the reduced output from higher-income individuals when they are infected and sick, plus the loss of all their output when they die from AIDS.

This discussion focuses on the effect of AIDS in per capita output. But what can be said about the impact of the disease on the rate of economic growth? A full discussion of growth dynamics is beyond the scope of this text, but it is sufficient to note here that, to the extent that growth rates depend on the accumulation of capital, AIDS can affect growth by altering domestic savings rates (taking external capital flows as exogenous). For example, if treatment costs for AIDS patients are relatively high and are financed at the expense of capital investment (financed from savings), then growth rates may fall. If the government provides significant resources for AIDS treatment, the question is, if the budget (tax revenue) is fixed, do these funds come at the expense of public investment or public consumption? Or, if extra tax revenues are raised to pay for additional treatment, do these come at the expense of private consumption or investment? Some studies suggest that public spending on AIDS may have increased at the expense of other public health care expenditure, because access to public hospitals by non-AIDS patients has fallen. If such cases were indicative of general responses, the impact on investment, and subsequently on growth rates, may be small.

To the extent that individuals and families foresee the potential to contract HIV, they may adjust their economic (as well as social) behavior to offset some of the possible effects. For example, faced with an increased chance of developing AIDS, individuals may increase their savings rates as a means of self-insuring against future medical expenses. Such increases in savings could also serve to partially protect surviving family members in the absence of life insurance and annuity markets. At the same time, Over and Mujinja (1997) note that if social norms and organizations permit family composition to be adjusted relatively quickly, then the loss of a breadwinner, while a personal tragedy, might impose relatively short-term economic costs on households if remarriage is possible.

---

20. Whether the effect on social welfare is proportionately greater is another question, because this depends on a society's attitudes toward income inequality. See chapter 8.

References

Ainsworth, Martha, and Mead Over. 1994. "AIDS and African Development." *World Bank Research Observer* 9(2): 203–40.

Anand, Sudhir, and Martin Ravallion. 1993. "Human Development in Poor Countries: On the Role of Private Incomes and Public Services." *Journal of Economic Perspectives* 7(1): 133–50.

Cochrane, Susan H., D. J. O'Hara, and J. Leslie. 1980. "The Effects of Education on Health." Staff Working Paper 405. World Bank, Washington, D.C.

Cornia, Giovanni Andrea, Richard Jolly, and Frances Stewart, eds. 1987. *Adjustment with a Human Face*. New York: Oxford University Press.

Cuddington, John T. 1993. "Modeling the Macroeconomic Effects of AIDS, with an Application to Tanzania." *World Bank Economic Review* 7(2): 173–90.

Easterlin, R., ed. 1980. *Population and Economic Change in Developing Countries*. New York: National Bureau of Economic Research.

Filmer, Deon, and Lant Pritchett. 1997. "Child Mortality and Public Spending on Health: How Much Does Money Matter?" Policy Research Working Paper, 1864. Washington, D.C.: World Bank.

Filmer, Deon, Lant Pritchett, and Jeffrey Hammer. 1998. "Health Policy in Poor Countries: Weak Links in the Chain." Policy Research Working Paper, 1874. Washington, D.C.: World Bank.

Gertler, Paul, and Jacques van der Gaag. 1990. *The Willingness to Pay for Medical Care: Evidence from Two Developing Countries*. Baltimore, Maryland: The John Hopkins University Press.

Lee, Kenneth, and Anne Mills, eds. 1983. *The Economics of Health in Developing Countries*. Oxford and New York: Oxford University Press.

Mincer, Jacob. 1974. *Schooling, Experience and Earnings*. New York: Columbia University Press for the National Bureau of Economic Research.

Over, Mead. 1991. *Economics for Health Sector Analysis: Concepts and Cases*. Washington, D.C.: Economic Development Institute, World Bank.

_____. 1992. "The Macroeconomic Impact of AIDS in Sub-Saharan Africa." Population and Human Resources Department, World Bank, Washington, D.C.

Over, Mead, and Phare Mujinja. 1997. "The Economic Impact of Adult Mortality on Consumption in the African Household." World Bank, Washington, D.C.

Phelps, Charles E. 1992a. "Diffusion of Information in Medical Care." *Journal of Economic Perspectives* 6(3): 23–42.

_____. 1992b. *Health Economics*. New York: HarperCollins.

Philipson, Tomas, and Richard Posner. 1995. "A Theoretical and Empirical Investigation of the Effects of Public Health Subsidiaries for STD Testing." *Quarterly Journal of Economics* 110: 445–74.

Preston, S. H. 1975. "The Changing Relationship between Mortality and Level of Economic Development." *Population Studies* 29(2): 2231–48.

_____. 1980. "Causes and Consequences of Mortality in Less Developed Countries During the Twentieth Century." In R. Easterlin, ed., *Population and Economic Change in Developing Countries*. New York: National Bureau of Economic Research.

_____. 1985. "Mortality and Development Revisited." In World Bank, ed., "Quantitative Studies of Mortality Decline in the Developing World." World Bank Staff Working Paper 683. Washington, D.C.

Pritchett, Lant, and Lawrence Summers. 1993. "Wealthier is Healthier." Policy Research Working Paper, WPS 1150. Washington, D.C.: World Bank.

Strauss, John. 1987. "Households, Communities, and Pre-School Children's Nutrition Outcomes: Evidence from Rural Côte d'Ivoire." New Haven, Connecticut: Yale University, Economic Growth Center.

World Bank. 1985. "Quantitative Studies of Mortality Decline in the Developing World." Staff Working Paper 683. World Bank, Washington, D.C.

_____. 1993. *World Development Report 1993: Investing in Health*. New York: Oxford University Press.

Part II

Microeconomics of Health Care and Insurance Markets

4

The Demand for Health Care Services

Individuals make choices about medical care. They decide when to visit a doctor when they feel sick, whether to go ahead with an operation, whether to immunize their children, and how often to have checkups. The process of making such decisions can be complicated, because it may involve accumulating advice from friends, physicians, and others, weighing potential risks and benefits, and foregoing other types of consumption that could be financed with the resources used to purchase medical care. This chapter presents some simple tools for describing these choices and making empirical estimates of the effects of certain factors, such as prices, incomes, and health status.

Economists have employed two alternative models for describing the way individuals make choices regarding health care utilization and related decisions. A simple approach, which we shall follow for the most part, is to treat health as one of the several commodities over which individuals have well-defined individual preferences, and to use orthodox consumer theory to investigate the determinants of demand (see Phelps 1992, chapters 3 and 4, for a similar presentation to that used in this chapter). A question of interpretation then arises as to whether we should think of individuals as having preferences for health, or for health care. One can argue that, in general, health care is only valued to the extent that it improves health, so that health should be primitive in the description of consumers' preferences. Yet, demand for services is more easily observed and quantified, so a mapping between the two concepts is required.

A second approach to analyzing health care choices is to use an intertemporal model of consumption decisions and to treat health as a stock variable within a human capital framework. Health care use can certainly have long-lasting effects, and the idea of health care representing an investment in health has been popular at least since the World Bank's 1993 *World Development Report* (the subtitle of which was *Investing in Health*). In fact, the approach was originally pioneered by Grossman (1972) in a model in which individuals consume health care not because they value health per se, but because it improves their stock of health, which is used as a productive resource. Cropper (1977) extended Grossman's model to account for the disutility that illness may impose on individuals, and to examine differences in the demand for preventive and curative care, and the dynamics of demand over the life cycle. Couched firmly in human capital theory, these models value health care services in terms of their potential to improve productivity. While this is clearly one outcome of better health, the consumption value of improved health status would suggest that such measures are lower bounds.

Thus in this chapter we describe the demand for health care services within an orthodox static utility-maximizing framework. As alluded to above, the first issue we must address regards the appropriate choice of goods that enter the utility function. On the one hand, it is natural to think of individuals as having preferences for health care services directly. Depending on their health needs, these preferences change, so we need to make the utility function state dependent. Alternatively, we might think of individuals as having preferences for health. Health care services would then be demanded only as an input into the production of health, and the level of demand for services would be determined by the extent to which they satisfied the individual's underlying preference for health. Preferences for health would then be independent of health status, and health care demand would change as the onset of illness altered the way in which medical care services could improve health. We adopt the second of these approaches and use it to examine the effects of health status, income, and price on the demand for medical care.

Due to the existence of insurance, many health care services are provided at zero or low monetary prices, and so the standard model would suggest that demand should be infinite, or at least extremely high. Indeed, excess demand by some insured individuals is seen as a problem in many industrial economies, but in the developing country context, underutilization is generally more of a concern. The main reason for this is a lack of supply, especially in rural areas. But even when clinics and services are available, utilization rates can be low, due to both significant nonpecuniary costs of consuming medical services and poor quality. With this in mind, we introduce travel costs into model of demand, as well as quality variations.

Next we recognize that the demand for medical care is not constrained to a choice of how much, but also of what kind. Thus, individuals can choose among visiting a hospital, clinic, or traditional healer, as well as how often to visit. The existence of such discrete choices means that somewhat more elaborate econometric techniques are required to estimate demand curves. Knowledge of such demand patterns may also allow policymakers to target services more effectively.

Finally, we analyze the extent to which information about demand can be used to make judgments about social welfare. These techniques will be of use later when we consider appropriate health care financing mechanisms (chapter 6) and the appraisal of health care projects (chapter 8).

Preferences for Health and Health Care

We start with a very simple representation of preferences for health within a standard utility-maximizing framework: individuals use their available resources to acquire health. To admit a substantive choice, individuals must have alternative uses for their resources. We bundle all of these alternative uses into a generic consumption good, denoted c. Utility is then represented as a function $u(c,h)$, where h is the level of health; h is not the quantity of health care services consumed, but rather the level of health that the individual enjoys. We assume that greater health and higher levels of other consumption make the individual better-off, and that an increase in one coupled with a decrease in the other (of a particular magnitude) leaves the individual's well-being unchanged. Thus we can draw standard indifference curves representing preferences between h and c, as in figure 4.1.

How do we interpret the variable h? Introspection suggests that we know when we are feeling healthy and when we are not, but can we really hope to quantify health levels using a particular unit? This is the subject of a large literature, and we shall have cause to address it more fully in chapter 9, but for now we should at least be keeping such concerns at the back of our minds. In some instances, a natural unit might suggest itself: for example, a person with terminal cancer might measure her health in expected number of years of life, although given the potentially severe health side effects of life-prolonging anti-cancer drugs, such a measure may be woefully inadequate. It is sufficient to leave interpretation of h to one side and to use it only as a vehicle to derive the (observable) demand for medical care services, as we do below. However, if the social welfare implications of the allocation of health among individuals are thought to differ from

Figure 4.1.   *Indifference Curves Representing Preferences over Health and Other Consumption Goods*

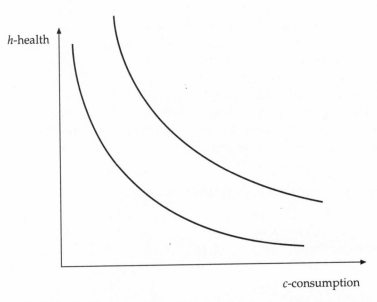

Source: Author.

those associated with the allocation of ordinary goods, a quantifiable measure of h itself is necessary.

Now let us consider how the simple description of preferences can be used to determine the demand for medical care. Consistent with the discussion in the introduction to this chapter, we assume that medical care is desired only for its use in producing health. In general, its effectiveness in this regard depends on the health status of the individual (as well as other factors). We assume for now that the production process is very simple, and that in order to produce an additional unit of health, θ units of medical care are required. θ provides a natural index for the health status of an individual—the higher is θ, the sicker the individual is. Thus h represents the level of health, and θ represents the health status (or the [inverse of the] productivity of health care services in producing health).

One caveat to this representation of the production of health is that it is almost certain that there are decreasing returns to medical care, so that the required inputs of medical care per unit of health improvement increase at the margin. While this is undeniably true—one only has to consider the marginal increase in days lived because of successively more intrusive and costly medical interventions in old age—the assumption of constant returns to scale is convenient for our illustrative purposes.

Given the simple description of the technology of health production, it is straightforward to characterize the set of feasible health-consumption pairs that an individual can choose between—that is, the budget set. For a particular health status, θ, an individual with income m faces a budget constraint $c + \theta h \leq m$, where for now we assume that the prices of consumption and medical care are both unity. When the individual becomes ill, the value of θ increases, and the boundary of the budget set swings inward, as shown in figure 4.2. Notice that the effect of getting sick, in this model, is just the same as having the price of health (not health care) increase.

We would expect people who are sicker to have greater demand for medical services, other things being equal. At the same time, we would expect them to have a lower demand for health, because health has effectively become more expensive. These conditions will be met if we suppose that the (absolute value of the) price elasticity of demand for health is between zero and one: that is, if a proportionate increase in the price of health leads to a less than proportionate decrease in the desired amount of health. Such a case is shown in figure 4.2.

Figure 4.2. *Budget Constraints and Optimal Consumption Bundles for Individuals with Different Health Status*

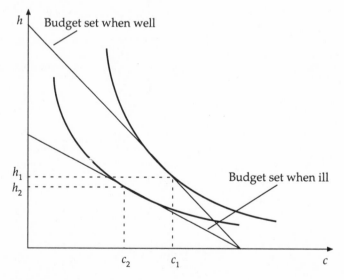

Source: Author.

When the elasticity condition is satisfied, we can draw indifference curves between consumption and health care services in a convenient manner. First consider an individual with a health status characterized by $\theta = 1$. In this case, each unit of health requires one unit of health care, and her preferences between consumption and health are identical to those between consumption and health care. We can directly translate indifference curves from (c,h)-space to (c,s)-space, where s represents health care services. Her budget constraints are also identical in the two spaces, and she consumes at point $x_1 = (c_1, h_1)$ in figure 4.3(a).

Now consider an individual in a health state characterized by $\theta = 2$. This person requires two units of health care to produce one unit of health. Her indifference curves in (c,h)-space are identical to those of the individual in the better health state ($\theta = 1$), although her budget line pivots inward. Suppose this individual chose the same level of consumption as the first person, c_1. This leaves her with the same resources to spend on health care services, but they afford her only half as much health in the sick state, so she will consume at point $y = (c_1, h')$ in figure 4.3(a). Because of the elasticity assumption, we know that the sick person prefers to consume less of the consumption good, and more health, at point $x_2 = (c_2, h_2)$, for example. Her indifference curve in (c,h)-space through y must be less steep than that through point x_2, which is less steep than the indifference curve through x_1.

Figure 4.3.   *Translation of Indifference Curves and Budget Sets from (c, h)-space to (c, s)-space*

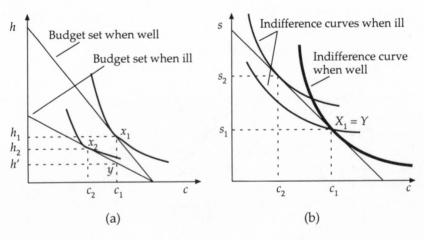

(a)   (b)

Source: Author.

Let us now draw the individuals' preferences in (c,s)-space, where those with different health statuses have different indifference curves but face the same budget constraint. As already mentioned, for the individual with $\theta = 1$, the indifference curves are identical, because one unit of health, h, is the same as one unit of health care, s. One such curve is shown in bold in figure 4.3(b). Consumption at point x_1 in (c,h)-space by this individual corresponds to consumption at point X_1 in (c,s)-space. The slope of the well individual's indifference curve through X_1 is equal to -1, as is the slope of her indifference curve through x_1 in (c,h)-space (equal to the slope of her budget constraint). For the sick individual, with $\theta = 2$, consumption at point y in (c,h)-space corresponds to consumption at point $Y = X_1$ in (c,s)-space, because she enjoys the same level of the consumption good and spends the same amount on health care as the first individual. However, we know that the sick individual's indifference curve at y is relatively flat. Starting from point y, a marginal reduction in c of one unit requires an increase in h of less than half a unit to compensate the individual (we know that at x_2, the slope of the indifference curve is equal to the slope of the budget constraint, $-\frac{1}{2}$, and it is greater than the slope of the indifference curve at y, in absolute value). This means that in (c,s)-space, the slope of the indifference curve for the sick individual that passes through point $Y = X_1$ must be less than 1. Thus, the sick individual has indifference curves in (c,s)-space that cut those of the well individual from below, as shown in figure 4.3(b).

Before we examine the demand for health care services, we should note that the translation we used required the assumption that the elasticity of demand for health was between 0 and 1, or that spending on health care was higher for sicker individuals, other things (such as income, available services, and the like) being equal. If the price elasticity of the demand for health were greater than 1, then indifference curves of sicker individuals would cut those of well individuals from above in (c,s)-space. It is possible to imagine cases where the standard elasticity assumption is unlikely to hold. For example, if someone is sufficiently ill that medical care is essentially ineffective, she might choose to spend less on health than she would in a healthier state. This might be descriptive of someone who has been told that she has terminal cancer and, instead of submitting to intensive chemotherapy, decides to live her remaining life well and spend her resources on non-health-care consumption (such as travel). Clearly, the reasonableness of the elasticity assumption is an empirical matter; we shall return to it later in the chapter.

A final point to note is that we have assumed that the only effect of illness is to increase the effective price of health that an individual faces. It

Figure 4.4.   *The Effects of Illness on Budget Sets When Income Is Reduced as a Consequence of Ill Health*

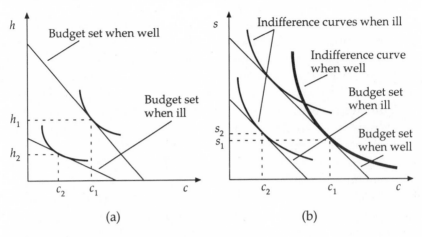

(a)   (b)

Source: Author.

may have other economic effects as well, however, including reducing the ability of the individual to earn income. In (c,h)-space, this would mean that not only does the budget constraint pivot inward, but it also shifts horizontally to the left (figure 4.4[a]). In (c,s)-space, the illness effect shifts an individual's indifference curves as described above, but her budget constraint is also shifted inward in a parallel fashion, as shown in figure 4.4(b).

Income and Price Effects

Now that we have a description of preferences for health care services, we can examine the determinants of demand, following standard microeconomic theory of consumer behavior. First, if health is a normal good, for an individual in a given health state (that is, with a given value of θ), health care will be normal as well. That is, increases in incomes lead to greater demand for health care services, other things being equal. Of course, we may well expect that income and health status as measured by θ are negatively correlated, because those with higher incomes have better access to clean water, housing, sanitation, and the like, so the qualification "other things being equal" is important. The effects of income on the allocation of resources between consumption and health care can be represented by the income expansion curve in (c,s)-space, shown in figure 4.5. If the income expansion curve bends upward as in figure 4.5(a), we say that health care

Figure 4.5.   *Income Expansion Curves When Medical Care Is (a) a Luxury and (b) a Necessity*

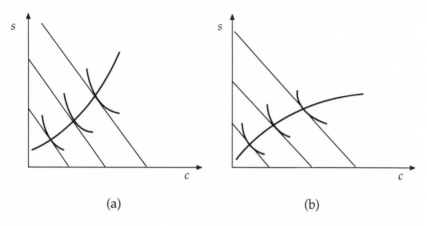

(a)   (b)

Source: Author.

is a luxury good, and as income increases, a higher share is devoted to health care. If the expansion curve bends toward the consumption axis, we say that h is a necessity, and its expenditure share falls as income rises.[1]

For an individual with a particular health status, changes in the price of medical care will affect her demands for c or s, and probably both. An increase in the price of services pivots the budget line inward in (c,s)-space, requiring a reduction in consumption of at least one of the two goods. If medical care use is not responsive to price changes—that is, if it has a price elasticity close to 1—the indifference curves must be like those shown in figure 4.6(a). In this case, an increase in the price of medical care services leads to a relatively large reduction in consumption of non-medical-care services from c_1 to c_2. If the elasticity of demand for medical care is close to zero, then a price increase leads to a proportionate drop in demand from s_1 to s_2, and there is virtually no effect on the demand for other consumption, as in figure 4.6(b). The intermediate case is represented in figure 4.6(c), in

---

1. Care should be taken in interpreting these characterizations. For example, it is natural to think of using medical care when it is needed, so that it might be assumed as a matter of definition that such care is a necessity. Rich countries tend to spend a much larger fraction of national income on health than poor countries, however, so that in economic terms, at the aggregate level at least, health appears to be a luxury good.

Figure 4.6.   *Variations in the Elasticity of Demand for Medical Care: (a) $\varepsilon \approx 1$,*
(b) $\varepsilon \approx 0$, and (c) $\varepsilon \in (0, 1)$

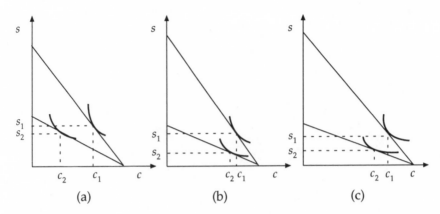

Source: Author.

which the elasticity of demand for medical care is less than 1, and consumption of both goods falls as the price of health care increases. The locus of demanded bundles as price changes, corresponding to the income expansion curve, is called the price offer curve, and is shown in figure 4.7.

The most useful analytical tool of economists in analyzing consumption choices is the demand curve. From our discussion of preferences for health care and the effects on income, price, and health status above, it is now straightforward to construct demand curves for health care. Fixing income and health status, demand will be a downward-sloping function of price. As income increases, we expect that, if health is normal, the demand curve for health care will shift out to the right. Similarly, the demand curve of a sicker individual will most likely be shifted outward because of the higher effective price of health, although this effect will be somewhat tempered by the possible reduction in income that the individual might suffer as a result of her illness. Finally, the price elasticity of demand may vary with income—in particular, we might expect that the demand for health care services by higher-income individuals would be less responsive to changes in prices than that of low-income individuals. If this were so, we would also expect changes in pricing policies to have differential effects on the demand for services by individuals with different incomes. For example, increases in user fees may not have much affect on the demand of individuals with average to high incomes but may result in reduced demand by lower-income individuals. Of course, these issues are empirical matters.

Figure 4.7.   *Price Offer Curve for Health Care Services and Other Consumption*

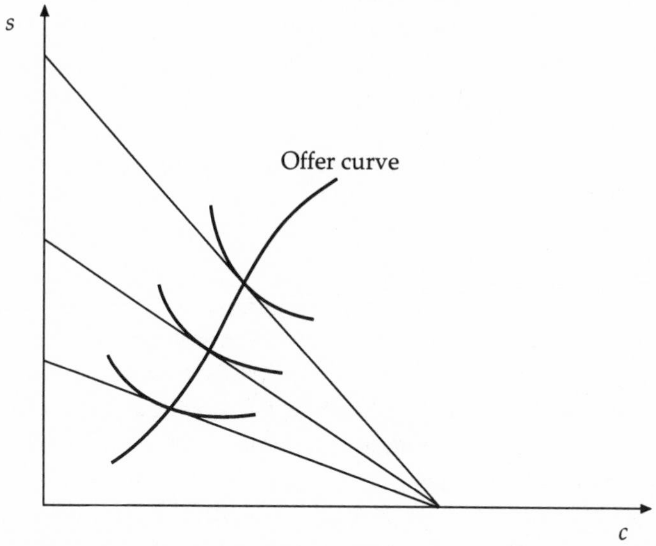

Source: Author.

What Prices?

We are used to thinking of prices as monetary payments for goods and services. But the availability of insurance or government subsidies in many health care markets make the monetary prices paid at the point of service— that is, when the service is rendered by the provider—very low or zero. In such cases, we would expect demand for health care to be very high indeed. This is a concern in some of the more advanced economies where the share of GDP spent on health care is very high, but in many developing countries utilization rates are often low, despite low monetary prices.

There are two related reasons for this. First, the quality of medical care services may be sufficiently low that demand, even at low prices, is discouraged. The second is that consumers may well incur significant additional costs in consuming medical care above any monetary prices charged. These costs include, for example, forgone income and travel costs. While these costs are present in the industrial economies, consumers are sometimes protected from the first by provisions in formal employment contracts that allow them to take time off for medical treatments, while travel costs are usually a relatively small share of income. The large informal labor markets of developing countries mean that forgone income may, on average, constitute a larger relative burden than in the industrial economies, and the large, rural populations mean that travel costs are likely to be greater as well. Generalized travel costs allow economists to estimate demand curves for health care, even when there is little variation in observed money prices. We will see this method used in the empirical analysis later in the chapter.

Multiple Goods

We have spoken of health care as a single good or service, but many inputs are used in the production of health from health services. Doctors' time, hospital beds, X-rays, drugs, and information are all used in the delivery of medical care. The prices of these inputs will not only determine the overall level of medical care sought by individuals but also the mix of services through which it is provided. This multiplicity of inputs means that if governments or insurance companies are involved in setting prices for components of medical care, they must be aware of the potential for the mix of inputs used to change in response to relative price changes. For example, if the government wishes to encourage a given level of health care by subsidizing its use, the pattern of subsidies across inputs should be chosen carefully. Subsidizing a subset of inputs will effectively discourage use of the others, which may or may not be desirable. Similarly, if an insurance company wants to restrain use of expensive technologies, it may find that use of other inputs increases in an offsetting fashion.

The Effects of Quality

The quality of medical care services can vary considerably, and it has numerous dimensions, including the direct effectiveness of the treatment, the costs it imposes on patients (in repeat visits, side effects, and so on), the politeness of providers, the opening hours and cleanliness of facilities, and the waiting times encountered at clinics or hospitals. Phelps (1992, chapter 4) has divided these aspects of quality into two components. The first relates to the underlying productivity of the intervention in producing health, as determined by the training of the doctor, the technology available, and so forth. The second relates more to the amenities aspect of health care, such as the convenience of opening hours, friendliness of staff, and the like.

This characterization of quality suggests that our earlier assumption that individuals consume medical care services only for the purpose of improving their health may be called into question. If going to the doctor is sufficiently enjoyable, demand might be driven as much by enjoyment of the activity as by medical necessity. Some have suggested that high utilization rates by pensioners is as much a product of their need to get out and interact with the world as with their need for medical attention.[2]

Some quality improvements could conceivably reduce the demand for health care by improving the health status of individuals. For example, if higher-quality care reduces the need for repeat visits, the demand for care will fall as quality increases. It is thus necessary to keep in mind that when we are examining demand functions, certain parameters are considered fixed, such as health status (changes that shift the position of the demand curve). Thus, other things being equal, higher quality may shift the demand curve out, but it might also improve health status enough that the demand curve shifts back in even further. This can clearly prove problematic for empirical estimates of the effects of quality on health care demand.

Some authors have examined the link between pricing policies for health care and the effects of quality on demand. The simple argument is that if higher quality shifts the demand curve out, higher prices can be charged, while attaining the same or a greater level of effective health care, thus mobilizing more resources for the health sector. We will discuss this more in later chapters on the role of government intervention, but for now it is necessary to make two points. First, increases in quality are not free, so that while more resources may be mobilized through cost recovery, at least a portion of these resources (and perhaps all of them) will need to be spent to attain and maintain the higher level of quality. Second, there is no particular reason why higher prices will create higher-quality levels. Only if the resources made available through higher charges are channeled into quality provision will this occur. The question then arises as to whether medical care charges represent the most equitable and efficient means of taxation for providing the funds for these quality improvements.

Empirical Analysis of the Demand for Health Care

Our formal discussion of preferences and demand for health indicated that prices, income, and health status are likely to have an effect on the utilization of health services. While the existence of such relationships seems plausible,

---

2. This is not to suggest that the fulfillment of such needs for social interaction are not important. The issue is whether six years of medical school training is needed to provide the service. Other examples of nonmedical quality include the provision of free incidentals, such as coffee in some doctors' surgeries in Australia. Anecdotal evidence suggests that such services had the effect of inducing individuals to visit the doctor each morning, complaining only of a headache (perhaps caused by the previous morning's coffee!).

their magnitudes are both unclear *a priori* and potentially quite important in the design of public policy in the health sector. This section examines econometric techniques used to estimate the size of demand relationships based on the conceptual analysis of the preceding sections.

Economists and policymakers care about the price and income elasticities of demand for health care, because they determine the effects of various pricing and distributional policies on demand. If there is no responsiveness of demand to price, then prices play little role in determining the allocation of health care resources among individuals. In the absence of financing constraints, free provision might be warranted. But, if medical care is responsive to price, some user fees should probably be charged to discourage overuse, but they should not be so high as to force individuals into imprudent decisions about whether to seek medical attention. Similarly, if income has a large, direct effect on demand or on the price responsiveness of demand, some form of targeting of subsidized health care services may be desirable.

This section does not provide an in-depth discussion of the large number of econometric issues that arise in studying the demand for health care; such information is found in texts devoted to econometrics. Instead it provides a brief overview of the types of econometric issues that might be considered particularly important for health care demand analyses and provides a link between these issues and the theoretical treatment discussed earlier in the chapter. We also present a sample of empirical results from the literature.

Two important factors influence the econometric techniques used to study the demand for health care. The first relates to the nature of the dependent variable data that characterizes health demand, and the second to the types of variation in the independent variables, particularly prices.

Health care choices open to consumers are made on a number of dimensions. First, there is the choice of whether to seek medical care or not, and then what kind of facility to visit and how often. Having made these choices, consumers may also face the choice of what kinds of treatments they wish to adopt, including the use of drugs and other remedies. While many of these input decisions will be based on recommendations made by the provider, such recommendations may be altered with variations in prices and incomes.[3]

---

3. For example, if prices of certain drugs increase, physicians may start prescribing alternatives, under the understanding that their patients will not be able to afford the original medications.

Data on Medical Care Use—Continuous and Discrete Choices

The simplest form of data available on individual use of medical care services reports expenditures in a given time period. Because medical care usually is used only when people get sick, the data are characterized by a relatively large number of zero expenditure items, corresponding, in part, to individuals who had no need to visit a clinic or hospital during the time period. Of course, prices and other factors may well deter individuals from using services, and these factors also contribute to the observed density of zero expenditure items. For example, in the RAND health insurance experiment in the United States (to be examined in detail later in this chapter), the probability of an individual not using medical care was positive and ranged from 13 percent for those with generous insurance coverage to 28 percent for those with virtually no insurance.

The second characteristic of the data on medical expenditures is that the positive observations tend to be highly skewed toward zero. Again, this partly reflects the nature of the random process of generation of health needs. It is normally the case that a small number of individuals suffer large health shocks that require significant expenditures, while a much larger number of users of services have relatively small health needs in the given time period. This means that we need to be careful about using simple average expenditures across groups to infer price elasticities and the like, because the elasticities can vary considerably between those with large expenditures and the other, larger, group with moderate medical care use.

Finally, we need to recognize that medical care is not a homogenous commodity, and that there may be interesting and important differences and interactions among the types of service. Indeed, the distribution of expenditures across individuals generally differs for different types of care—such as patient versus outpatient—so that examining data aggregated across types may conceal relevant information on own- and cross-price elasticities.

These three characteristics of medical spending data mean that regressing expenditures on prices and other variables directly may not provide particularly useful information. Instead, multilevel analysis is often employed, in which an attempt is made to separate types of consumption choices, including the decision to use care, the choice of the type of care to use, and finally the intensity of care use, given the type chosen. Such analyses incorporate both discrete and continuous choice econometric modeling techniques, because the choices of whether to consume care and what kind of service to consume are discrete choices, while the decision of how much to consume (of the chosen type) is a continuous choice.

Either because of data availability or the specific focus of the research, some studies examine the determinants of only the discrete choices involved in medical care use. This may be appropriate if we are primarily concerned with ensuring that individuals have "access" to care, meaning that they are not deterred from consulting some kind of provider. It also might provide a useful indicator of the effects of demand-side interventions (user fees and the like) if it is thought that there may be a significant difference between the determinants of demand for initial consultations (which are usually initiated by the consumer) and those of demand for subsequent consultations (which may be more a function of the doctor's advice). The second group of elements may be more responsive to supply-side interventions than those on the demand side.

Many recent studies in developing countries have been based on household survey data. The World Bank has conducted studies of the determinants of health care use in a number of countries, based on analysis of questionnaires completed by households. To avoid requiring respondents to keep detailed records of past decisions and to prevent mismeasurement, the surveys typically pose questions that can be answered either with a yes or no response—for example, "Did you seek medical care outside the home in the last month?"—or with a relatively small integer number—such as, "How many times did you seek medical care outside the home in the last month?" Less often respondents are asked to recall the amount of money spent on care, their foregone income, and so forth. The data derived from such surveys are thus of a discrete nature, and their analysis requires use of the appropriate econometric tools.

Other studies concentrate on demand for a particular type of medical care service, including both the discrete choice of whether to consume and the continuous choice of intensity. When there is little room for substitution among services, such analysis provides useful information not only on the determinants of demand for the particular service, but also on the impact of policy changes on medical care spending in general. However, when substitutions of other types of care are possible, concentration on own-price elasticities may be misleading. This is particularly relevant when the service under consideration is differentiated from others on a purely institutional basis. For example, in studying the price responsiveness of public hospital demand, the effect on total medical care demand will be a function of the existence of private and charity hospital services. A large own-price elasticity may indicate only a switch from one institutional form to another, with little effect on total demand for hospital services.

Assuming sufficient data exist, the discrete and continuous choices can be modeled in an integrated fashion, using a multilevel approach, along the following lines. Let the vector x denote the regressors used to explain medical care use—these may include prices, incomes, and demographic variables such as age, sex, family status, and so on. The demographic variables can be thought of as proxies for health status and taste. Let us also assume that medical care services are categorized into $j = 1\ldots n$ alternatives, including clinics, public hospitals, traditional healers, and so forth. The estimated expected medical care expenditures of individual i are then:[4]

$$(4.1) \qquad \hat{e}(x_i) = \hat{p}_i[\hat{\pi}_{1i}\hat{e}_{1i} + \hat{\pi}_{2i}\hat{e}_{2i} + \ldots + \hat{\pi}_{ni}\hat{e}_{ni}]$$

where $\Sigma_{j=1}^{n}\hat{\pi}_{ji} = 1$, and $\hat{p}_i = \hat{p}(x_i)$ is the estimated probability that individual i will consume some quantity of medical care, $\hat{\pi}_{ji} = \hat{\pi}_j(x_i)$ is the estimated conditional probability that individual i will use medical service j, given that she consumes some medical care, and $\hat{e}_{ji} = \hat{e}_j(x_i)$ is the estimated medical expenditure by individual i, given that she consumes service j.

Given this general framework, the econometric questions revolve around how to best estimate the probabilities of use and the determinants of the intensity of use. Note that $q_{0i} = (1 - \hat{p}_i)$ can be interpreted as the estimated probability that an individual engages in "self-care." Formally, we could multiply $\hat{p}_i$ through in the above equation and estimate the probabilities $\hat{q}_{ji} = \hat{p}_i\hat{\pi}_{ji}$, which would have to satisfy the condition $S_{j=0}^{n}\hat{q}_{ji} = 1$, but it turns out to be more convenient to treat the choices of whether to consume, and from whom, separately in a two-stage process.

First suppose that we are concerned only with the determinants of use of a particular service by those who use it—that is, let us initially ignore the estimation of the probabilities of use. There are many issues that arise regarding the appropriate methodology and interpretation determined by the nature of the regressors; we will turn to these below. For current purposes, the important characteristic of the expenditure (the dependent variable) data is its observed skewedness. Using raw expenditures in a regression would likely lead to asymmetrically, and hence nonnormally, distributed errors, making standard ordinary least-squares regression techniques inappropriate. However, a convenient way to eliminate, or at least reduce, such problems is to use the natural logarithm of expenditures as the dependent variable, because this transformation tends to reduce the skewedness of the distribution of expenditures.

---

4. As is usual in econometric analysis, we use "hats," ^, to denote estimated values of variables.

MODELING DISCRETE CHOICES—LINKS WITH CONSUMER THEORY. Estimation of the probabilities of use of medical care and of a particular type of medical care is performed using discrete choice econometric models. Included among the more common of these are the probit and logit specifications and their extensions. Let us first provide a framework to link the analysis of discrete choices to the theoretical discussion of the first part of this chapter. Recalling our description of indifference curves and budget sets, consider the tradeoff between health and consumption for an individual in a given health state. This person has a budget set defined by θ, and her income, m. In a continuous choice model, she can choose any point along the frontier of her budget set (she can choose any point inside it as well), and does this by purchasing medical care services. In the discrete model, in addition to caring for herself, she can visit one of a fixed number n of health care providers. Let us think of the providers for now as differing only in the quantity of services they provide (per visit), with provider j's level, s_j, greater than provider k's, s_k, if and only if $j > k$. These service levels are fixed. From our definition of θ, the amount of health "purchased" from provider k is thus s_k/θ, because it takes θ units of health care to produce one unit of health. Thus, the available choices open to the individual, including self-care, are given by the $n + 1$ points on the budget line, as shown in figure 4.8.

Figure 4.8.   *Available Health Consumption Bundles for Individuals with Different Health Status*

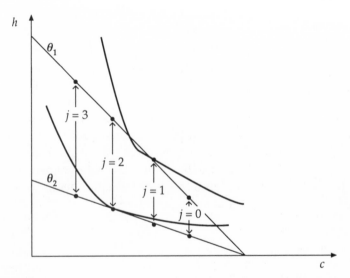

Source: Author.

We have drawn two budget lines, θ_1 responding to a relatively well individual and θ_2 corresponding to an individual with greater health needs. The positions of the $n + 1 (= 4)$ available choices for each individual depend on how one interprets self-care. In the diagram we have shown the self-care point, $j = 0$, as yielding the lowest, although a still strictly positive, level of health in each state. This self-care is achieved at the cost of forgone consumption, which is the same in each state. That is, we have assumed that there is a fixed amount of resources used for self-care, which does not change with the health status of the individual. While this assumption is unrealistic, it captures the idea that individuals might look after themselves if it does not take too much effort, but they will seek external help if the cost of their own time is too high. If the individual chooses to seek medical care outside the home, she chooses one of the points $j = 1, 2,$ or 3. The diagram is drawn under the assumption that the cost of each service (that is, her forgone consumption) is independent of her health status, although the productivity in producing health increases with health status for any given provider. This means that the points representing health-consumption bundles associated with a given provider in the two different states of health are aligned vertically.

In figure 4.8, we have drawn two indifference curves. When health status is labeled by θ_1, the individual's preferred choice of provider is $j = 1$. Her most preferred health-consumption bundle in the budget set is not attainable. When health status is given by θ_2, the individual is sicker and chooses provider $j = 2$, which is close to her most preferred point on the new budget set.

The effects of income on provider choice can be easily seen using the figures presented above. For example, for an individual with a given health status, an increase in income will generally affect her choice of provider. A positive influence of income on choice of provider is illustrated in figure 4.9(a), where health is a normal good. Income does not affect the choice of provider when preferences between health and consumption are quasilinear with respect to the consumption good. Such preferences can be represented by a utility function $u(c, h) = c + \phi(h)$, for some increasing and concave function $\phi(.)$. In this case, exemplified in figure 4.9(b), health is not a normal good.

Note by implication that any empirical specification that attempts to capture income effects on the demand for health cannot be based on a quasilinear specification of utility. This will be important in our discussion of logit and probit models, which rely on the calculation of a utility index (see Gertler and van der Gaag 1990, p. 65 for further discussion of this point).

We can also use the model to examine the effects of price on discrete demand, but in doing so we must be careful about our treatment of self-care.

Figure 4.9.   *Effect of Income on Provider Choice*

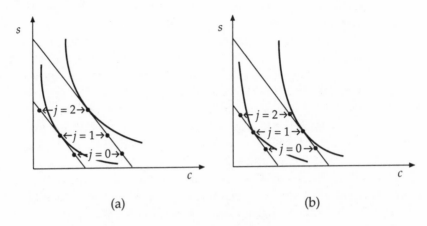

(a)   (b)

Note: (a) when health is a normal good, higher income leads to a change in provider; (b) when preferences are quasilinear with respect to the consumption good, income has no effect on the choice of provider.

Source: Author.

Consider an individual in a given health state, θ, with a given income, m. We have assumed that the available (c,h)-pairs lie on the budget line defined by $c + \theta h = m$, including the self-care option. Suppose now that the price of care increases. The effect of this is to swing the budget line for *purchased* services inward, but there is no effect on the (c,h)-pair that can be attained through self-care. Thus, figure 4.10 shows two alternative sets of attainable (c,h)-pairs, when the price of medical services changes (note that the point $j = 0$ is the same in each set of available choices). Notice that we have assumed that each health service delivers the same improvement in health in the two price regimes, with the only difference that the reduction in consumption is greater in the high-price situation. That is, the positions of the attainable purchased (c,h)-pairs are horizontally displaced, as shown in figure 4.10.

Higher prices now lead to, other things being equal, a choice of the provider offering a lower level of service. Note, however, that because of its special nature, self-care may be preferred when prices increase, not when there is merely a marginal reduction in provider quality. This accounts for the differential treatment of self-care and alternative health care sources in the analysis below.

So far we have described the discrete choices available to consumers as specific points on the budget sets defined in the stylized continuous model. This provides a useful and familiar framework for examining price and

Figure 4.10. *Distinguishing between Purchased Medical Care and Self-Care When Prices Change*

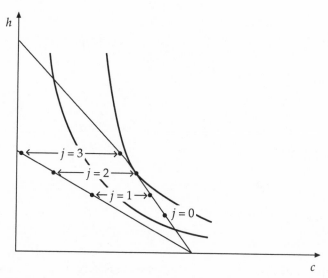

Note: When the price of purchased care increases from p_1 to p_2, the $j = 0$ option (self-care) remains unaffected, and may well be chosen.

Source: Author.

income effects, but is somewhat restrictive empirically. By assuming that available health-consumption bundles associated with the various providers are located on a straight budget line, we are imposing a proportional relationship between health and price that may not necessarily obtain.

A more direct description of the choices available to individuals of a given health status is represented by a list of $n + 1$ pairs of health attainments, h_j, and forgone consumption, or prices, p_j. That is, for a given health status, θ, the pair of vectors $(h_0(\theta), h_1(\theta), \dots , h_n(\theta))$ and $(p_0, p_1, \dots, p_n)$ represent the available choices. For an individual with income m, the price vector defines a consumption vector $(c_0, c_1, \dots, c_n) = (m - p_0, m - p_1, \dots, m - p_n)$. An example of the health-consumption bundles available to individuals with incomes m_L and $m_H > m_L$ is shown in figure 4.11(a). A similar diagram can be drawn to represent the different sets of available choices when health status changes (for a given income). This is shown in figure 4.11(b), with θ_L representing a better health status—that is, lower health needs—than θ_H.

Notice that in figure 4.11(a), the available bundles for those with higher incomes are all shifted to the right by the same amount (equal to the

Figure 4.11. *Discrete Health Consumption Choices with No Budget Constraint*

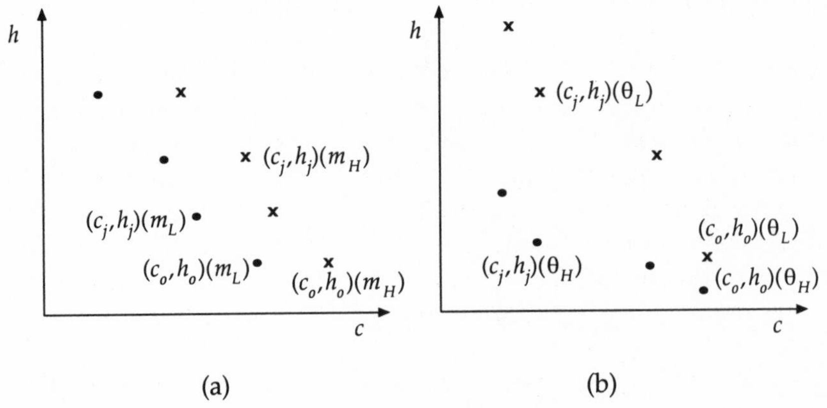

(a)   (b)

Source: Author.

difference in income, $m_H - m_L$). This represents the implicit assumption that, if prices differ at all between individuals, they do so by an additive constant that is independent of the service. That is, if we write p_j^i as the price of service j to individual i, then $p_j^{i'} = p_j^i + k(i, i')$, where $k(i, i')$ is independent of j. When prices reflect only monetary costs, it may be reasonable to expect $k(i, i')$ to be zero, unless prices are set on a progressive (or other income varying) scale.[5] However, a potentially important cost of consuming health care services is that associated with time and travel, which may well vary with income, in which case $k(i, i') \neq 0$, and with service, so k is not independent of j.

In the simplest forms of econometric modeling, the variables to be explained (as well as the explanators) are continuous, and ordinary least-squares (OLS) estimation, or some variation of the approach, is used to identify relationships between them. The coefficients on the independent variables then represent the marginal change in the value of the dependent variable associated with an infinitesimal increase in each of the independent variables.

---

5. In many traditional health systems, prices paid by individuals were linked to their ability to pay. For example, Ikegami and Hasegawa (1995, p. 34) report that nineteenth century Japanese physicians were "… paid what moral obligation dictated…. In theory, the rich paid munificently, to cover the services provided to the indigent."

When the dependent variable is discrete—that is, when it can take on only a finite number of values—the coefficients in regression analysis are interpreted as indicating the marginal change in the probability of a particular choice being made, given an infinitesimal increase in the associated independent variable. The simplest form of discrete choice model is that in which the dependent variable (health care demand, in our case) can take on one of two different values. For example, the only choice faced by a consumer might be to go to a clinic or engage in self-care. These situations are usually analyzed with "probit" or "logit" models. When there are more than two alternatives, these techniques are extended in "multinomial logits," "nested multinomial logits," and "multinomial probits."

DICHOTOMOUS CHOICE—LOGITS AND PROBITS. Let us suppose now that there are just two alternatives—self-care ($j = 0$) and a clinic visit ($j = 1$). The general equation predicting medical care use, equation 4.1, then collapses to

$$(4.2) \qquad \hat{e}(x_i) = \hat{p}_i \hat{\pi}_{1i} \hat{e}_{1i} = \hat{q}_i \hat{e}_i$$

which is composed of the probability that a clinic visit will be chosen, times the expected quantity of services purchased, conditional on use. If we further assume that the quantity conditional on use is fixed, we are interested only in estimating the probability, $\hat{q}_i$. From our description above regarding the effects of income, health status, and price on the available health-consumption bundles, it is clear that the utility gained from choosing a clinic visit over self-care will generally depend on all of these variables. It is reasonable to assume that the utility gained may also vary according to individual characteristics, such as education (if it makes health care services more productive), age (as an additional proxy for health status), type of employment, and so forth. Both the logit and probit models calculate indices of the relative utility of choosing a clinic visit over self-care as a function of these explanatory variables. These indices can range from minus to plus infinity, and they are mapped into the interval $[0, 1]$ using a cumulative probability function. The resulting variable is interpreted as the probability of a clinic visit being chosen over self-care, given the values of the explanatory variables.

For example, consider the utility index associated with the choice of a clinic visit over self-care. First recall from our discussion of figure 4.9 that to identify any effects of income on the demand for health care, utility cannot be linear in c. Thus, there must be nonlinear terms on the right-hand side involving $c = m - p$. For example, Gertler and van der Gaag include squared consumption and a price-income interaction term (see Gertler and van der Gaag 1990, equations (15) and (16), p. 72), to obtain the following index of utility from a clinic visit:

$$u^i_1 = u_1(x^i, p^i_1, m^i) = \alpha'_0 x^i + \beta_1(m^i - p^i_1) + \beta_2(m^i - p^i_1)^2 + \varepsilon.$$

The parameters α_0, β_1, and β_2 are to be estimated. Notice that θ does not appear on the right-hand side. This is because health status is difficult to measure exactly, and so other variables that determine it (such as age) are included in the x vector. The probability that individual i will choose a clinic visit over self-care is then calculated as $\hat{q}_i = F(\hat{u}^i_1)$, where $\hat{u}^i_1$ is the fitted value of u^i_1 and $F: \mathbb{R} \to [0, 1]$ is monotonically increasing. That is, the higher the utility index, the higher the probability that the individual will choose a clinic visit. The two functional forms for F that are most often used are the cumulative normal distribution function and the cumulative distribution function for the logistic random variable. Using the first yields the probit model, and using the second yields the logit model.[6]

Of course, the data we observe are not in the form of probabilities— either an individual goes to a clinic or does not—so the parameters of the model, α_0 and the βs, are estimated using maximum likelihood techniques. For a given set of parameters, the probability of choosing a clinic visit is $q^i = q^i(\alpha_0, \beta_1, \beta_2)$. Therefore, if individual i is observed to have chosen a clinic visit, then the probability of this occurring was q^i. If that individual was observed to have chosen self-care, the probability of this having occurred would have been $(1 - q^i)$. Thus, the probability that we would have observed the existing data given some set of parameters $(\alpha_0, \beta_1, \beta_2)$, otherwise known as the likelihood function, is

$$l(\alpha_0, \beta_1, \beta_2) = \prod_{i \in C} q^i(\alpha_0, \beta_1, \beta_2) \prod_{i \notin C} (1 - q^i(\alpha_0, \beta_1, \beta_2))$$

where C is the set of individuals who chose to visit a clinic. The estimates of the parameters α_0, β_1, and β_2 are then calculated (usually with numerical computer packages) to maximize the likelihood function, and the estimated probabilities are given by

$$\hat{q}^i = \hat{q}(x^i, m^i, p^i_1) = F[\hat{\alpha}'_0 x^i + \hat{\beta}_1(m^i - p^i_1) + \hat{\beta}_2(m^i - p^i_1)^2].$$

If the quantity of services conditional on use of a clinic is not fixed, and if data on actual expenditures are available, a second-stage equation can be used to estimate the relationship between the explanatory variables and the conditional expenditures. The simplest approach is to use a

---

6. For the probit, $F(u) = \frac{1}{\sqrt{2\pi}} \int_{-\infty}^{u} \exp(-z^2/2)dz$, and for the logit, $F(u) = (1 + \exp(-u))^{-1}$.

linear regression of the logarithm of expenditures against the explanators, although some adjustments may be required if the error terms are not normally distributed (see Manning and others 1987). Ignoring these more technical econometric issues, one could estimate the relationship

$$1ne^i = \gamma_0' x^i + \varepsilon^i$$

using ordinary least-squares, with the OLS estimator of γ_0 being denoted as $\hat{\gamma}_0$. Estimated unconditional expenditures of individual i are then given by

$$\hat{e}(x_{\nu}\, m^i - p_1^i) = \hat{q}(x^i, m^i - p_1^i) \times \exp(\hat{\gamma}_0' x^i).$$

POLYCHOTOMOUS CHOICE. When there are more than two alternatives, the probit and logit models briefly discussed above must be extended. There are a number of alternatives that vary in their numerical manageability and their economic realism, that are discussed briefly by Gertler and van der Gaag (1990, p. 73) and at greater length by McFadden (1981).

A straightforward extension of the logit model to the multinomial logit model is relatively easy to implement, but it imposes the restriction that the cross-elasticities of demand between the alternative choices (for example, the effect of an increase in the price of hospital admissions on the responsiveness of clinic visits to price) be constant. Alternatively, the so-called nested multinomial model entails something of a two-step procedure, in which groups of relatively substitutable alternatives are distinguished, allowing the within-group cross-price elasticities to vary across groups.

The natural grouping used by Gertler and van der Gaag is to separate self-care from non-self-care. Calculating utility indices for each alternative, j, for each individual, i, u_j^i as in the dichotomous choice model, the probability of individual i opting for self-care is given by

$$\pi_{0i} = \frac{\exp(u_0^i)}{\exp(u_0^i) + [\,\Sigma_{j=1}^n \exp(u_j^i/\sigma)]^\sigma}$$

and that of opting for alternative j is

$$\pi_{ji} = (1 - \pi_{0i}) \left[\frac{\exp(u_j^i / \sigma)}{\Sigma_{j=1}^n \exp(u_j^i/\sigma)} \right].$$

Maximum likelihood techniques are again employed to estimate the parameters α_0, β_1, β_2, and σ. As in the dichotomous-choice model, conditional expenditure equations can be estimated, and combined with the nested multinomial logit to provide estimates of the effects of explanatory variables on unconditional expenditures.

Dependent Variable Issues—Cross-Sectional Analysis, Natural Experiments, and Randomized Experiments

The discussion of the previous section reviewed the implications of the nature of health utilization data for empirical analyses, particularly the need to incorporate discrete choice techniques. This section briefly examines issues related to the nature of the explanatory variable data used in the regressions. We are particularly interested in examining the effects of changes in prices on demand, and we will focus on information about price variation that can be used in estimating price elasticities. Three kinds of data are distinguished: cross-sectional data, natural experiments, and randomized experimental data.

CROSS-SECTIONAL DATA. To establish a relationship between prices and demand, it is necessary for the econometrician to observe a range of different prices, variations in which are used, potentially, to explain some of the variation in demand. Because of the extensive role of some governments in the provision and allocation of health care services, it is sometimes possible to observe a range of publicly set prices for certain services. Alternatively, private health insurance contracts often require individuals to pay a set proportion of their medical expenses, and variations in insurance coverage then provide variation in effective prices paid for medical care.[7] Finally, in some countries, geographic variations in the price of medical care are large enough to permit estimation of demand relationships based on correlated geographic differences in demand.

However, each of these three sources of price data has its problems, essentially related to the endogeneity of prices and omitted variables that affect both prices and demand. For example, in the case of variations in publicly set prices, suppose the government's policy is to charge individuals with high health needs relatively low prices. Any negative correlation that is observed between prices and utilization could then arise both from the usual impact of price on demand and the lower prices paid by those with higher needs, as determined by the government. If it were possible to accurately account for health needs (as measured by the government) separately in the regression, the price effect would not include the confounded influence of government policy. Without accounting for the differences in health needs, the estimate of the price effect will be biased upward.

---

7. In the next chapter we will examine possible reasons why private health insurance contracts require individuals to pay some of the cost of care.

Alternatively, prices and incomes may be jointly determined, so that an observed correlation between utilization and price cannot be meaningfully interpreted. For example, if travel costs are used as proxies for prices, then as Gertler and Hammer (1997, p. 14) note, "If facilities are located closer to urban areas where individuals are wealthier, then the correlation between travel costs and utilization reflects both the relationship between income on utilization and the effect of travel costs on utilization."

NATURAL EXPERIMENTS. The underlying problem of cross-sectional data identified above was that because the variation in prices is across individuals, there may also be correlated variations in other variables that independently affect demand. If these correlated variations cannot be corrected for, the estimated coefficients are biased. A possible solution to this problem is to use data that exhibit exogenous variations in the prices that given individuals face—usually, but not always, over time. When policy regimes shift, or other exogenous changes to the pricing environment occur, it may be possible to observe changes in the behavior of the affected individuals and to attribute such behavioral responses to the price changes.

A number of these so-called natural experiments have been studied to identify the elasticity of demand for drugs. For example, when the Medicaid program in the United States began to pay for prescription drugs in the southern state of Mississippi (so that the price fell to zero), the number of prescriptions almost doubled, and the expense per prescription increased by 25 percent (Smith and Garner 1974).[8] The arc-elasticity over the range from zero price to full price was about –0.4 (Phelps 1992, p. 135). Another example is from a Canadian insurance plan that offered virtually full insurance coverage for prescription drugs to a section of the population. The effects of the coverage on demand, as compared with that of individuals without insurance, were similar to those in the Mississippi study.

However, problems similar to the cross-sectional studies above may arise with natural experiments. Policy shifts may be in response to changes in other related variables (health status, income, and so on) that also affect demand, and price changes for particular groups of individuals can clearly have confounded effects. Even if policy changes are not explicitly motivated by or related to changes in other endogenous variables, they may be correlated with such changes, making it difficult to interpret the estimated coefficients.

8. Medicaid is the public program in the United States funded jointly by the federal and state governments that provides some medical care for the poor.

RANDOMIZED EXPERIMENTS. To avoid the potential problems of both cross-sectional data and natural experiments, controlled experiments in which prices vary independently of other endogenous variables are required. Such studies tend to be expensive to undertake, and only a few have been implemented. Probably the most famous is the RAND health insurance experiment in the United States in the 1970s, in which individuals were randomly assigned different insurance policies (and hence medical care prices). In addition, district-level data in China have been used to examine the effects of exogenous price variations on demand, and most recently a controlled experiment in Indonesia using variations in provincial pricing schedules has been analyzed. We review each of these studies below.

The RAND health insurance study (see Manning and others 1987) tracked the behavior of a large number of individuals and families who were randomly assigned different health insurance packages. Some participants were fully insured (facing a zero monetary price for health services), others paid 25 percent of the cost of services, a third group paid 50 percent of their medical costs, and a fourth had virtually no insurance, having to pay 95 percent of the cost of care. These percentages are known as coinsurance rates. Thus, US$100 worth of medical care would cost members of the first group nothing, members of the second US$25, those of the third US$50, and those of the fourth US$95. Where the underlying price received by the provider of medical care is constant across groups, the price faced by consumers in each group varies in the obvious way (further details of the experiment can be found in Newhouse 1993, and Phelps 1992, p. 119–33).

Because of the randomized nature of the allocation of the insurance policies, the underlying prices of medical care received by providers who served the different groups were, on average, equal. Also, again because of the randomization, the health status and incomes of the different groups were, on average, equal. Any variations in the use of medical care services among the groups could be attributed to the different prices they faced. Even though, as mentioned above, it is difficult to measure quantities of medical services accurately, proportionate changes in quantities are identical to proportionate changes in medical expenses (including both those paid by the patient and the portion paid by insurance). Similarly, given that the only differences between the groups was in the fractions of costs reimbursed, even though unit prices are difficult to define, proportionate differences in prices among groups were just equal to relative coinsurance rates. Because medical care expenses are easily measured, and coinsurance rates were assigned directly by the experiment, proportionate differences in each among the groups were easy to identify, and price elasticities easy to compute.[9]

The data were collected for types of medical care, including acute, chronic, and well (for example, checkups) outpatient care, hospital care, and dental treatment. The average data for outpatient and inpatient services are reproduced in table 4.1 (from Manning and others 1987), showing a general trend downward in spending on each category of care as the coinsurance rate increases. Also included are quantity data, measured on the basis of the number of physician visits and hospital admissions respectively, which also show corresponding trends with respect to coinsurance rates.

In practice, because only a small number of coinsurance rates were used, the data derived from the study could be used only to calculate so-called arc elasticities.[10] The arc elasticities for both outpatient and inpatient care were 0.17 for those with coinsurance rates of zero and 25 percent. For higher coinsurance rates, the arc elasticity for all care was 0.22, although the arc elasticity of demand for outpatient services (0.31) was significantly higher than that for hospital care (0.14). On average, full insurance increases medical care usage by about 75 percent compared with no insurance.

Table 4.1. *Expenditure and Quantity Data by Insurance Coverage*

Coinsurance rate	Expenditure data		Quantity data	
	Outpatients	Inpatients	Outpatients	Inpatients
zero	340	409	4.55	0.128
25%	260	373	3.33	0.105
50%	224	450	2.73	0.092
95%	203	315	3.02	0.099

Source: Manning and others (1997).

9. Formally, let p_0 be the price of service, x its quantity, and κ the coinsurance rate. Then the elasticity of demand is $\varepsilon = - (\kappa p_0/x)\, dx/d(\kappa p_0) = - \kappa/(p_0 x)\, d\,(p_0 x)/d\kappa = - \kappa/e\,(de/d\kappa)$, where $e = p_0 x$ is medical expenditures.

10. An arc elasticity is equal to the change in one variable as a proportion of its mean, relative to the change in another as a proportion of its mean. For example, given two data points, (p_1, x_1) and (p_2, x_2), the arc elasticity derived from these is $\varepsilon_{arc} = [(x_2 - x_1)/(x_2 + x_1)]/[(p_2 - p_1)/(p_2 + p_1)]$.

The effects of income on medical care usage are likely to be somewhat smaller than the effects of price. Other things being equal, we would expect use of health services with the same price to increase with income. However, some types of medical care, especially those entailing hospital admission, might impose a larger cost in forgone income on individuals with higher money incomes than on others. Indeed, for outpatient care, the income elasticity of the number of visits to a physician (episodes of illness) was about 0.22 for non-well care, but it was not significantly different from zero for hospital care.

Most empirical estimates of demand in developing countries employ discrete choice econometric models, mainly because of the nature of the survey data available. However, one study in rural China (Cretin and others 1988) (see table 4.2) made use of insurance coverage that varied by local district to estimate the effects of prices on demand for services. Fee-for-service medical care was provided by village doctors, with Local Cooperative Medical Funds providing insurance against some of the financial risks. Because coinsurance rates varied by locality, it was possible to make elasticity estimates in a similar fashion to those of the RAND study.

Coinsurance rates (that is, the share of costs paid by the patient) varied from 100 percent to 20 percent, with annual per capita expenditures increasing by a factor of 2.4 from around 15 yuan to nearly 37 yuan. The results are shown in table 4.2, drawn from Phelps' (1992) discussion of the study.

The estimate of elasticity of demand for ambulatory care based on these data is approximately –0.6—somewhat higher than that found in the RAND

Table 4.2.   *Health Expenditure Data by Insurance Coverage in Rural China*
(yuan per year)

Coinsurance rate	Per capita outpatient expenditure
100	15.36
90	17.16
80	18.96
70	21.12
60	23.52
50	26.04
40	29.52
30	33.12
20	36.96

Source: Cretin and others (1988).

study, but comparable nonetheless. Of course, we should not expect exactly similar results in magnitude, because of the different economic environment, particularly the much lower incomes of rural Chinese compared with the United States.

Gertler and Molyneaux (1997) used longitudinal panel data of medical care use in two of Indonesia's 27 provinces, in which public sector user fees were varied experimentally. Within the two provinces, fees for outpatient services were varied in a staggered fashion (as opposed to being increased uniformly) in order to provide sufficient variation to estimate demand elasticities. Fees were increased in some districts, and not others, and in different types of health facilities.

The study found, among other things, that the price elasticity of demand for services at rural health facilities (health subcenters) was lower than that at more urban "health centers," mainly because of the larger variety of alternative sources of medical care in cities. This observation makes it clear that when interpreting own-price elasticities, it is important to have information on changes in the utilization of other forms of medical care that may accompany price increases for a particular form of delivery. If the price of a specific type of care, or care provided through a particular institution (such as public hospitals), is increased, the demand for other substitutive forms of medical care will likely increase. The price response in the alternative markets determines the overall impact of the particular price increase on total medical care utilization. Also, the study found that the price elasticity of demand for care was greater for children's care than for that of adults.

Summary of Empirical Results

This final subsection provides a partial review of demand elasticity studies, based on the work of Gertler and Hammer (1997). The overwhelming evidence appears to suggest that higher prices do reduce the demand for medical care, but, on average, significantly less than proportionately. In addition, the size of the demand reduction effect varies considerably according to income, age, gender, and so forth on the demand side, and type of health care facility on the supply side. In studying the potential impact of user fees on revenue, utilization, and welfare, Gertler and Hammer (1997) have recently provided a useful summary of these studies, reproduced in table 4.3.

Specific indications from these studies are that the poor tend to have more price-elastic demand than the rich, and that children's utilization suffers relatively more in response to a price rise than does that of adults. Gertler and

Hammer caution against using studies that estimate demand elasticities on the basis of relatively small price differences to infer changes in demand that would be likely to result from large price increases, noting that the elasticity of demand may well be a function of the price level. They also note that omitted variable bias may well be problematic in many studies, either because quality is inadequately controlled for, or because of the endogeneity of publicly set prices and locations of health care facilities (as discussed above).

Table 4.3. *Econometric Estimates of Own-Price Elasticities of the Demand for Medical Care in Developing Countries*

Country	Data	Service type	Own-price elasticity			Source
			Overall	Low-income	High-income	
Burkina Faso	1985	Public provider				Sauerborn and others (1994)
	All ages		−0.79	−1.44	−0.12	
	Ages 0–1		−3.64	—	—	
	Ages 1–14		−1.73	—	—	
	Ages 15+		−0.27	—	—	
Côte d'Ivoire	1985	Health clinic	—	−0.61	−0.38	Gertler and van der Gaag (1990)
		Hospital outpatient	—	−0.47	−0.29	
Côte d'Ivoire	1985–87	Health clinic	−0.37	—	—	Dow (1996)
		Hospital outpatient	−0.15	—	—	
Ghana	1987	Hospital inpatient	−1.82	—	—	Lavy and Quigley (1993)
		Hospital outpatient	−0.25	—	—	
		Dispensary	−0.34	—	—	
		Pharmacy	−0.20	—	—	
		Health clinic	−0.22	—	—	
Kenya	1980–81	Government provider	−0.10	—	—	Mwabu and others (1993)
		Mission provider	−1.57	—	—	
		Private provider	−1.94	—	—	

(table continues on following page)

(Table 4.3 continued)

Country	Data	Service type	Own-price elasticity			Source
			Overall	Low-income	High-income	
Indonesia	1991–93					Gertler and Molyneaux (1997)
	Children	Health center	-1.07	—	—	
		Health subcenter	-0.35	—	—	
	Adults	Health center	-1.04	—	—	
		Health subcenter	-0.47	—	—	
	Elderly	Health center	-0.47	—	—	
		Health subcenter	-0.11	—	—	
Mali	1982		-0.98	—	—	Birdsall and others (1983)
Nigeria						Akin and others (1995)
Pakistan	1986					Alderman and Gertler (1997)
	Female	Traditional healer	—	-0.43	-0.24	
	Children	Public clinic	—	-0.43	-0.23	
		Pharmacist	—	-0.44	-0.25	
		Private doctor	—	-0.17	-0.09	
	Male	Traditional healer	—	-0.60	-0.26	
	Children	Public clinic	—	-0.61	-0.27	
		Pharmacist	—	-0.63	-0.27	
		Private doctor	—	-0.25	-0.10	
Peru	1985	Private doctor	—	-0.44	-0.12	Gertler and van der Gaag (1990)
		Hospital outpatient	—	-0.67	-0.33	
		Health clinic	—	-0.76	-0.30	

(table continues on following page)

(Table 4.3 continued)

			Own-price elasticity			
Country	Data	Service type	Overall	Low-income	High-income	Source
Philippines	1981	Public providers	—	-2.26	-1.28	Chin (1995)
		Private providers	—	-3.93	-2.23	
Philippines	1981	Prenatal care	-0.01	—	—	Akin and others (1986)
Philippines	1983–84	Urban maternity	-0.24	—	—	Schwartz and others (1988)
		Rural maternity	-0.05	—	—	

— Not available.
Source: Gertler and Hammer (1997).

References

Cretin, S., N. Duan, A. P. Williams, X. Gu, and Y. Shi. 1988. "Modeling the Effect of Insurance on Health Expenditures in the People's Republic of China." RAND Corporation manuscript. Santa Monica, California.

Cropper, M. L. 1977. "Health, Investment in Health, and Occupational Choice." *Journal of Political Economy* 85(6): 1273–94.

Dunlop, David W., and J. M. Martins. 1995. *An International Assessment of Health Care Financing: Lessons for Developing Countries.* Economic Development Institute (EDI) Seminar Series. Washington, D.C.: World Bank.

Gertler, Paul, and Jeffrey Hammer. 1997. "Strategies for Pricing Publicly Provided Health Services." Policy Research Working Paper 1762. World Bank, Washington, D.C.

Gertler, Paul, and Jack Molyneaux. 1997. "Experimental Evidence on the Effect of Raising User Fees for Publicly Delivered Health Care Services: Utilization Health Outcomes, and Private Provider Response." Santa Monica, California: RAND.

Gertler, Paul, and Jaques van der Gaag. 1990. *The Willingness to Pay for Medical Care: Evidence from Two Developing Countries.* Baltimore, Maryland: The Johns Hopkins University Press.

Grossman, Michael. 1972. "On the Concept of Health Capital and the Demand for Health." *Journal of Political Economy* 80(2): 223–55.

Ikegami, Naoki, and Toshihiko Hasegawa. 1995. "The Japanese Health Care System: A Stepwise Approach to Universal Coverage." In David Dunlop and J. M. Martins, eds., *An International Assessment of Health Care Financing: Lessons for Developing Countries.* Economic Development Institute (EDI) Seminar Series. Washington, D.C.: World Bank.

Manning, Willard G., Joseph P. Newhouse, Naihua Duan, Emmet B. Keeler, Arleen Leibowitz, and Susan M. Marquis. 1987. "Health Insurance and the Demand for Medical Care: Evidence from a Randomized Experiment." *American Economic Review* 77(3): 251–77.

Manski, Charles, and Daniel McFadden, eds. 1981. *Structural Analysis of Discrete Data with Econometric Applications.* Cambridge, Massachusetts: MIT Press.

McFadden, Daniel. 1981. "Econometric Models of Probabilistic Choice. In C. Manski and D. McFadden, eds., *Structural Analysis of Discrete Data with Econometric Applications.* Cambridge, Massachusetts: MIT Press.

Newhouse, Joseph. 1993. *Free for All: Lessons from the RAND Health Insurance Experiment.* Cambridge, Massachusetts: Harvard University Press.

Phelps, Charles E. 1992. *Health Economics.* New York: HarperCollins.

Smith, M. C., and D. D. Garner. 1974. "Effects of a Medicaid Program on Prescription Drug Availability and Acquisition." *Medical Care* 12(7): 571–81.

World Bank. 1993. *World Development Report 1993.* New York: Oxford University Press.

5

Insurance

Health status and health expenditures are inherently uncertain, and individuals respond by trying to reduce the associated financial and nonfinancial risks. To understand the mechanisms of such risk reduction, this chapter examines the factors that underlie the demand for health insurance and the different types of insurance policies that can be observed in a private market. Following Arrow's (1963) seminal contribution, we identify a number of market failures that derive from information asymmetries that, while present in many other insurance markets, are particularly acute in markets for health insurance. This analysis of the performance and possible failures of private insurance markets will form the basis for our discussion in later chapters of the role of government in the provision or regulation of health insurance.

A particular theme of this chapter is that insurance should not be seen solely as a financing mechanism for health care delivery. On the contrary, the primary role of insurance is as a mechanism to reduce individuals' exposure to risk. The point is that, risk reduction aside, insurance contributions that finance a given level of health care spending represent just one of a multitude of financing options, and without considering the effects on risk, such contributions are unlikely to be optimal financing instruments.

Risk Aversion

Uncertain health status imposes a number of risks on individuals. The most obvious is the loss of health itself, as well as the risk of incurring large financial costs associated with medical treatments aimed at maintaining or improving health. In addition, health deterioration can reduce the ability of an individual to work, or her productivity while working, so that the person faces the risk of lost (market and nonmarket) wages. Finally, individuals may be less able to enjoy other forms of consumption (such as participation in sports) because of their health status, or they may suffer the psychological and emotional trauma associated with physical deterioration.

All of these events and consequences are uncertain, both in size and occurrence. Some, such as the loss of health and the loss of the ability to enjoy other consumption, are difficult to quantify, but the others are more easily measured objectively. Faced with such risks, individuals are typically willing to pay to have them reduced. To understand the mechanisms behind this behavior, we need a descriptive theory of how decisions are made under conditions of uncertainty.

Preferences and Expected Utility

The most widely used model of decisionmaking under uncertainty in economic theory and practice is that of expected utility maximization. For a discussion of aspects of decisionmaking under uncertainty that are not easily dealt with in the expected utility framework, see Machina 1987. Analogous to the theory of choice under certainty (as exemplified by the demand analysis of the previous chapter), in which choices are made to maximize the value of a utility function, in the presence of uncertainty it is assumed that choices are made to maximize the expected value of the utility function (see Mas-Colell, Whinston, and Green 1995, chapter 6, for a thorough but accessible treatment of expected utility theory).

As an example, consider the use in the previous chapter of a utility function $u(c,h)$ to describe an individual's preferences for health and consumption. In that discussion, we assumed that health status was measured by the price of health, θ, which defined the individual's budget set as $c + \theta h = m$, where m is income. Defining the indirect utility function as

$$v(\theta, m) = \max_{c, h} u(c, h) \text{ s.t. } c + \theta h = m$$

we see that in each health state θ, the individual's attainable utility is $v(\theta, m)$. Now let us assume that θ can take on n different values, $\theta_1, \theta_2, \ldots, \theta_n$, and that the probability of θ_i occurring is π_i, with $\pi_i \in (0, 1)$, and $\Sigma_i \pi_i = 1$. The individual's expected utility then is given by

$$V(m) = \sum_{i=1}^{n} \pi_i v(\theta i, m).$$

Notice that expected utility depends on income but not on any particular value of θ, because utilities across health states are averaged.

It turns out that this description of expected utility, while consistent with our discussion of preferences in the previous chapter, can be simplified when considering the basic analytics of risk and insurance. It is more common in elementary treatments to analyze risk in terms of a very simple utility function that depends only on income, $u(m)$. The assumption is that income can vary across states of nature (that is, health states), but that prices do not.[1] For example, consider an individual with income m, but facing the prospect of incurring a loss l with probability π. Average income is then $\mu = (1 - \pi) m + \pi(m - l)$. In this case, the individual's expected utility is just

$$V(m) = (1 - \pi)u(m) + \pi u(m - l).$$

Risk Aversion, Insurance, and Risk Pooling

It is common to assume that an individual's marginal utility of income falls as income increases. In this case, the function $u(.)$ is concave, and we say that the individual is risk-averse. It can easily be shown in this case that the utility of the expected value of a risky level of income is greater than the expected utility of the risky income. That is, faced with an uncertain income, the individual prefers to remove the variability and consume the average income.[2] This is shown in figure 5.1, in which the expected utility of the uncertain income is V_u and the utility of the certain average income, μ, is V_c. Notice that the individual would prefer to face a certain income less than μ, but greater than or equal to $\mu - p$, instead of facing the risky income. The term p is referred to as the risk premium, and it represents the cost associated with the risk exposure.

Now suppose that the individual can trade with an insurance company, and that she pays a premium P in return for the promise that if she suffers the loss l, the insurer will pay her a proportion α of the loss. That is, when no accident occurs, her income is $m - P$, and when an accident does occur, her income is $m - P - l + \alpha l$. The question we wish to answer is what level of α will be chosen by the individual? Choosing $\alpha = 0$ would represent no insurance, because the premium would be zero, and so the individual's income in the two states of the world would be unaffected.[3] In contrast, when $\alpha = 1$, the individual's income is $m - P$ in each state of the world. That is, her income is independent of the state, and she thus faces no risk. We say that in

---

1. In the example above, it is the price, θ, that varies across states of health.

2. This is just another application of Jensen's inequality, already encountered in a somewhat different setting in chapter 3.

3. We refer to the different situations that an individual can find herself in—that is, no accident or accident—as different "states of the world," or "states of nature."

Figure 5.1.   *Risk Aversion and the Risk Premium*

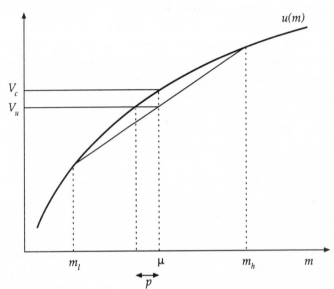

Note: When income can be high, m_h, or low, m_l, each with probability 0.5, the expected income is μ. If received with certainty, this would yield utility V_c. The expected utility of the uncertain income is $V_u < V_c$, and the risk premium p satisfies $0.5u(m_l) + 0.5u(m_h) = u(\mu - p)$.
Source: Author.

this case, the individual has full coverage. When α is between zero and one, we say that the individual has incomplete insurance, or partial coverage.

Suppose the insurance industry is competitive, so that profits are zero, and that insurers are risk-neutral. In this case, the premium charged must be equal to the expected value of payments made by the insurer to the individual in the case of an accident. That is, $P = \pi \alpha l$, in which case the individual's expected utility is

$$V(m, \alpha) = (1 - \pi)u(m - \pi \alpha l) + \pi u(m - \pi \alpha l - l + \alpha l)$$
$$= (1 - \pi)u(m - \pi \alpha l) + \pi u(m - l + \alpha(1 - \pi)l).$$

The first-order condition for expected utility maximization with respect to α is thus

$$\frac{\partial V}{\partial \alpha} = -(1 - \pi)\pi l u'(m - \pi \alpha l) + \pi(1 - \pi)l u'(m - l + \alpha(1 - \pi)l) = 0$$

or

$$u'(m - \pi \alpha l) = u'(m - l + \alpha(1 - \pi)l).$$

Because u is concave, this can only be satisfied if $\alpha = 1$, so that the individual will choose to be fully insured.

This simple model may appear to be of little use, because risk is merely transferred from one individual to another (the insurance company), who was assumed to be risk-neutral. This is a valid criticism when there is only one person on the demand side of the insurance market, but the real role of insurers is not so much to act as holders of risks but as spreaders of risks. Thus, when there are many individuals seeking insurance, they can effectively pool their risks through the insurance company. The only service the insurance company offers is the administrative task of facilitating this pooling of risks.

Risks can only be pooled like this when there is a large number of individuals seeking insurance, and when the risk of any one individual suffering the loss is statistically independent of that of any other. This is illustrated by the difficulty of buying insurance for certain natural disasters (such as earthquakes). If an earthquake occurs, it will likely affect many policyholders simultaneously. In such a case, the insurance company may not be able to pay all claims. When losses are statistically independent, however, the insurer will know with a high degree of certainty the actual number of claims expected each year and will not face any risk. In health insurance, this analysis suggests that insurance against epidemic diseases, which can easily affect entire villages and districts, may best be provided at the national level (either by the national government or by a private insurer with a national client base).

Choosing the pool within which risks are spread can have large effects on the efficacy of risk exposure management. Of particular interest in this regard is the extent of risk sharing across generations—that is, do the elderly (who typically have larger health care costs than the young) insure themselves, or do they spread their risks across other generations? The argument, based on equity that all individuals should share in the burden of insurance, is not particularly strong, but such intergenerational risk sharing can be supported on efficiency grounds as a means of implementing lifetime insurance coverage (see Jack 1998). These issues of who should be in the risk pool are important when we consider the design of public insurance mechanisms.

Three Problems with the Standard Insurance Model

We often find insurance policies that offer less than complete coverage. This is especially true in the context of health insurance, where policies that pay a given proportion of medical costs are far more common, at least in the private sector, than policies that reimburse all medical costs. Also, expenses associated with some kinds of services, such as hospital stays, may be more fully covered than those associated with others, such as drugs. Such incomplete insurance often derives from information asymmetries between insured individuals and insurance companies.

We will examine three kinds of information asymmetry in this chapter that can lead to incomplete insurance and market failure. The first, known as adverse selection, occurs when individuals do not all have the same probability of suffering a loss (that is, of getting sick), and when the insurance company cannot distinguish the good risks from the bad risks. The second, which we will call hidden information moral hazard, occurs when it is difficult for the insurer to know whether or not the individual has suffered a loss or, more generally, when it is difficult to observe the size of the loss. The third, hidden action moral hazard, occurs when individuals can take precautionary actions that alter their probabilities of suffering the loss or that alter the size of the loss when it occurs.[4]

Adverse Selection

When individuals have varying probabilities of suffering a loss, they impose different costs on insurance companies. For example, individuals from families with a history of heart disease might be expected to have a higher than average chance of suffering from heart disease themselves, while those working in dangerous occupations may be expected to suffer accidents more often. If these people are pooled with low-risk individuals—such as white collar workers with no family history of heart disease—and if members of each group are required to pay the same premiums, the latter group will effectively subsidize the insurance coverage of the former. Given this subsidy, individuals with low risks will tend to leave the market, pushing up the proportion of high-risk individuals in the pool, which will increase the premium required. This, in turn, will cause more of the low-risks to leave, and a vicious cycle of market unraveling will ensue, possibly until no one is left purchasing insurance.

---

4. Some authors, including Zweifel and Breyer (1997, chapter 6), refer to hidden action moral hazard as *ex ante* moral hazard, because the unobservable actions are taken before the state of the world is realized. Similarly, hidden information moral hazard is sometimes referred to as *ex post* moral hazard, because the consumption choices that characterize the moral hazard occur after the state of the world is realized.

This kind of a problem will arise whenever a single insurance policy is offered to individuals, and prices cannot (or are not allowed to) vary according to the risk characteristics of the individuals covered. Of course, there are some ethical arguments in favor of charging all individuals the same amount for insurance, independent of their risk; the problem of adverse selection simply means that such a policy will be difficult to implement through the private sector.

There is sometimes confusion over the extent of the market unraveling that will occur. The appendix to this chapter presents a formal model, originally developed by Akerlof (1970), that enables us to identify the factors that determine the degree of equilibrium coverage.[5] If the average medical care costs across the population of potential purchasers is low, there will be no unraveling, and everyone will be insured. In this case, the premium (equal to average medical costs) is not too high, and even the lowest-risk individuals value the reduction in risk and are willing to subsidize those with higher risks. But, if population-average costs are too high—that is, if there are too many high-risk individuals—at least some unraveling is likely, and only a segment of the potentially insured population will be covered in equilibrium.

One way to get around the problem of adverse selection might be for insurers to offer a menu of policies to individuals and to allow them to choose the one most suited to their needs and preferences. Even when prices cannot vary among individuals according to their risks, the insurer will be able to charge different prices for the policies. Thus, the premium charged for a policy that covers 90 percent of medical costs would be higher than that for a policy that covers only 50 percent of costs. The outcome of this strategy may be that individuals with higher risks purchase the higher-coverage option, while those of lower risks purchase the lower-coverage option. In this way, the individuals effectively sort themselves into two groups, although the insurer cannot observe ex ante to which group each belongs.

Although the availability of multiple policies allows the insurer to remove the cross-subsidy between individuals, and thus the incentive for the low-risks to quit the insurance pool, there are two remaining problems with the strategy. First, as shown by Rothschild and Stiglitz (1976) and

---

5. Akerlof's model examined the market for used cars, or "lemons" as they are referred to in the North American vernacular. The discussion here also draws on the exposition of the model in Mas-Colell, Whinston, and Green (1995, chapter 13), which is applied to the labor market.

Wilson (1977), the low-risk individuals will be underinsured—that is, the low-risk individuals will wish to purchase more insurance than is offered, but they will be constrained from doing so because the insurer will not offer more to them. The essential reason behind this is that to stop the high-risks purchasing the insurance contract that is meant for the low-risks (and has an appropriately lower premium reflecting the lower expected costs), the low-risk policy must be made to look suitably unattractive to the high-risks. But this is achieved by making the insurance incomplete. A formal model of this is presented in the appendix.

Second, there may not be a competitive equilibrium in the model, suggesting that the insurance market may "break down" in a fundamental sense. This is a potentially much more worrisome problem than the incompleteness of insurance suggested above. It says, effectively, that attempts at controlling the unraveling market of Akerlof by allowing multiple policies could backfire. Instead of partial unraveling, and hence the incomplete coverage of the lemons model (with a single policy), with some individuals insured and others not, we might observe an unstable insurance market, in which no steady pattern of coverage emerges.

This analysis, which has been only glossed over here, is central to some of the arguments regarding the desirability of public versus private insurance schemes, and for compulsory insurance. We shall return to these issues in greater depth in subsequent chapters.

Hidden Information Moral Hazard

Probably the most common market failure discussed in health insurance economics is that relating to hidden information moral hazard, although many discussions do not distinguish it from the hidden action variety and refer to it simply as moral hazard. Hidden information moral hazard is reflected in excessive consumption of medical services by insured individuals.[6] This statement clearly requires a precise definition of what it means for the demand for services to be excessive.

Let us ignore the issue of risk for now and examine the behavior of an individual who is fully insured against the financial costs of medical care. In a given health state, this individual will have a demand curve for health care

---

6. For early contributions to this literature, see Pauly (1968) and Zeckhauser (1970). In addition, Pauly (1986) and Weisbrod (1991) provide surveys of related literature.

services that is downward-sloping, as in figure 5.2(a). Suppose the marginal cost of producing health services is fixed, and equal to one. If the price faced by the consumer for these services is zero, then the individual's demand will be s_0, where the demand curve cuts the horizontal axis.[7] From elementary microeconomics we know that the benefits received by the consumer from consuming the amount s_0 can be estimated by the consumer surplus, equal to area $A + B + C$.

Of course, the individual must pay a premium that covers the expected costs of medical care consumed. If the individual's health state is known with certainty, this cost is equal to area $B + C + D$, and the individual's net surplus from paying up-front for medical care is equal to $A - D = (A + B + C) - (B + C + D)$.

If instead, the individual were not insured and paid for medical care at its marginal cost (equal to one in this case), the gross consumer surplus would be $A + B$, the costs would be B, and the net surplus would be A. The area D, which is the difference between the individual's net surplus with

Figure 5.2.   *The Tradeoff between Risk Reduction and Distortionary Costs*

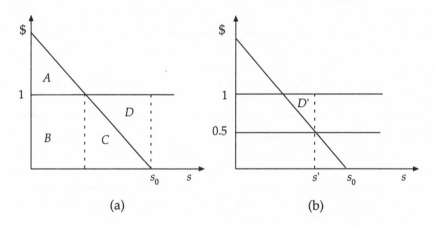

Note: (a) Full coverage of incurred expenses leads to a dead-weight loss equal to area D; (b) Partial coverage reduces demand from s_0 to s', and reduces the dead-weight loss to D'.
Source: Author.

7. For many standard descriptions of preferences, the demand curve will not cross the horizontal axis, and demand at a zero price will be infinite. We assume in this example that even at a zero price, demand is finite.

8. This cost is entirely equivalent to the dead-weight loss associated with commodity taxes and subsidies that may be familiar from standard public finance

and without insurance, represents a dead-weight loss to the consumer.[8]

Alternatively, suppose the individual must pay 50 percent of the medical bills—that is, the individual receives a subsidy at a rate of 50 percent. Demand falls to s', and the dead-weight loss associated with this policy is reduced to D', as shown in figure 5.2(b). Clearly, the higher the level of insurance—that is, the greater the subsidy to medical care—the greater the dead-weight loss incurred.

Now suppose that the individual faces the risk of being in one of two alternative health states, labeled as L (for low health needs) and H (for high health needs). In this case, she can face two different demand curves for health care services, and if she has no insurance (paying a price of one per unit of health care in each state), there is no dead-weight loss. However, her risk premium, p, which measures the benefits of removing all risk, is positive, so some insurance would be desirable.

If the individual had full insurance, she would incur dead-weight losses of D_L and D_H in each state, respectively. Assuming that the probability of the bad health state occurring is π, the expected value of the dead-weight loss is equal to $\overline{D} = (1 - \pi) D_L + \pi D_H$. This loss is balanced against the reduction in risk that the full insurance policy provides, captured by her risk premium, p. If $p < \overline{D}$, it is preferable to have no insurance than to have full insurance. However, the individual could choose an intermediate level of insurance—for example, a policy that obliges her to pay a fraction κ of her medical costs. The expected dead-weight loss then falls to $\overline{D}_\kappa < \overline{D}$. At the same time, the individual is exposed to a positive level of risk, so her risk premium (the value of the reduction in risk from having no insurance) falls to $p_\kappa < p$. If there is a coinsurance rate κ that results in $p_\kappa > \overline{D}_\kappa$, the individual will choose that policy.[9]

This suggestive analysis indicates that the elasticity of demand for health care services will play a crucial role in determining the optimal insurance policy chosen by risk-averse individuals. The dead-weight

---

literature. In those cases, price is distorted away from marginal cost (either above, in the case of a tax, or below, in the case of a subsidy), and individuals are compensated with a lump-sum transfer (which is positive or negative, respectively). In the health insurance example, price is distorted below marginal cost, and the individual is required to pay a lump-sum premium.

9. One can argue that, starting from a situation of no insurance (in which case the coinsurance rate is $\kappa = 1$), it is very likely that a small amount of insurance is desirable (with κ close to, but less than, one). The argument rests on the distortionary dead-weight loss being of second order in the subsidy rate (equal to $1 - \kappa$), so for κ close to one, this cost is small. However, a small reduction in risk has a value that is first order in the subsidy rate, outweighing the cost of the distortion.

losses in each health state, D_L and D_H above, depend on the slopes of the demand curves. When demand is not very elastic (the demand curves are nearly vertical), the dead-weight losses are small, and relatively high levels of insurance (that is, low coinsurance rates) will be desirable. However, when the demand curves are elastic (that is, flat), the dead-weight losses will be large, and the appropriate insurance coverage is much lower, that is, the coinsurance rate is higher.[10]

The dependence of insurance rates on the elasticity of demand helps us understand the observed pattern of insurance of different medical services. For example, the elasticity of demand for hospital care is relatively low compared with that of the demand for physician visits. The dead-weight loss associated with insurance will be correspondingly smaller for hospital services than for physician visits, and the optimal rate of coverage will be higher for the former. Similarly, dental insurance tends to be less extensive than other forms of insurance, because it is more price sensitive.[11]

One might ask how the problem of moral hazard could be corrected. The full description—hidden information moral hazard—gives us a clue. Insurance is incomplete because individuals are given a price subsidy, and making that subsidy excessively high increases dead-weight losses too much. The price subsidy means that the more health care is consumed, the larger is the financial transfer received from the insurer. Suppose, however, that the insurance company could identify the state of health of the individual. In this case, the insurer could give the individual a prespecified income transfer that was independent of the amount of health care expenditures, while allowing the individual to pay the full price of health care services. This would remove the incentives to overspend, while maintaining the desirable reduction in risk. The inability of the insurer to observe the state of health perfectly—that is, the hidden information—thus constrains the efficiency of the contract.[12]

---

10. Jack and Sheiner (1997) show that the optimal coinsurance rate, κ, is determined by the equation $cov(\alpha, q) = -\bar{\alpha}(1 - \kappa) \, d\bar{q}/d\kappa$, where α is the marginal utility of income, q is spending on health care, and bars denote averages across states of health. When demand is inelastic, $d\bar{q}/d\kappa$ is small, and for a given covariance rate, the optimal κ is closer to zero—that is, the optimal level of insurance is higher.

11. The demand elasticities reported in the RAND health insurance study were –0.15 for hospital, –0.3 for outpatient physician visits, and –0.4 for dental services (Phelps 1992, table 10.1, p. 293).

12. The analogy with lump-sum taxation should be apparent from this discussion. Ideally, a government will use lump-sum taxes to redistribute income so as not to distort consumption and labor supply decisions. But when individual

Hidden Action Moral Hazard

Suppose an individual is fully insured against the financial costs of ill health. It is unlikely that this person will be indifferent between suffering bad health and keeping well, because there are certain nonpecuniary costs associated with medical care, including inconvenience, time, pain, and stress, that cannot usually be covered by an insurance contract. Even so, in some circumstances, the removal of all financial risks may induce the individual to be somewhat less careful in preventing illness or bad health than she would be in an uninsured state. If the insurer could observe the precautionary actions taken by the individual, the insurance contract could specify that coverage would be offered only when suitable precautions were taken (such as not smoking, wearing a seatbelt while driving, attending a prenatal clinic, and so on).[13] However, under most circumstances, insurance companies do not have access to this kind of information and cannot put such requirements of prudence into the contracts they offer. Indeed, this is the reason the associated market failure is referred to as "hidden action" moral hazard, indicating that the precautionary actions of individuals are not observable.

When precautionary actions are not observable, or contractible, the premium required by an insurance company offering a full-coverage policy would be proportionately larger than that required of a policy with incomplete coverage. The exposure of the individual to some risk is then desirable, because she saves (proportionately more) on the premium reduction than she suffers through risk exposure.

This intuition can be formalized by modifying the simple model of insurance presented earlier, in which an individual faced the prospect of having an accident that reduced her income by an amount l. In that model, the probability of the accident, π, was assumed to be exogenously fixed. Let us modify the model now by introducing an effort variable e, which can be thought of

---

characteristics are unobservable, optimal lump-sum taxes are not feasible, and distortionary taxes must be used.

13. When actions (or even circumstances, like membership of an exposed group) affect the probability of illness, the arithmetic increase in risk due to a particular action is referred to as the attributable risk associated with the action (see Gordis 1988, p. 53–4.) Similarly, one plus the proportional increase in risk due to the action is referred to as the relative risk. That is, if the probability of contracting an illness given an action is r times the probability in the absence of the action, the relative risk is r, which is usually greater than one (see Selvin 1991, p. 75–7).

as representing actions taken by the individual to reduce the probability of the accident (Laffont 1989 presents a similar model, p. 125–28). Thus, the probability becomes endogenous, and it is denoted $\pi(e)$. We assume that effort must be nonnegative, and that $e = 0$ corresponds to "no effort," at which point the probability of the accident occurring is $\pi_0 \in (0, 1)$. We also assume for convenience that a small amount of effort above zero is productive in reducing the probability of an accident below π_0—that is, $\pi'(0) = -\infty$. The probability function is shown in figure 5.3.

Effort is costly to the individual, and we incorporate this by assuming that her utility function can be written

$$v(m, e) = u(m) - e$$

where $u(.)$ is the original utility of income function.

The individual can purchase insurance by paying a premium P, after which she decides on her effort level. Suppose she has purchased a policy that covers a proportion α of the loss, so her incomes in the two states are $m - P$ and $m - P - (1 - \alpha)l$, respectively. She now chooses effort to maximize her expected utility:

Figure 5.3. *The Impact of Effort on the Probability that an Accident Will Occur*

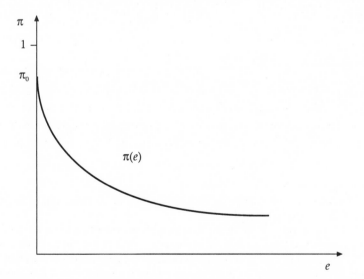

Note: At $e = 0$, the marginal impact of effort is very large, but as effort grows, the marginal impact falls off.

Source: Author.

$$V(m, \alpha, e) = (1 - \pi(e))u(m - P) + \pi(e)u(m - P - (1 - \alpha)l) - e.$$

The first-order condition for effort choice is thus

$$- \pi'(e)u(m - P) + \pi'(e)u(m - P - (1 - \alpha)l) - 1 \leq 0$$

with equality whenever e is strictly positive. If $\alpha = 1$ (full insurance), then the optimal effort choice is zero, and when $\alpha < 1$, the optimal effort choice solves

(5.1) $$\pi'(e) = - \frac{1}{[u(m - P) - u(m - P - (1 - \alpha)l)]}$$

where the denominator is positive. For future reference, this first-order condition can be totally differentiated to yield

(5.2) $$\frac{\partial e^*}{\partial \alpha} = - \frac{u'(m - P - (1 - \alpha)l)l}{\pi''(e)[u(m - P) - u(m - P - (1 - \alpha)l)]^2} < 0.$$

(When $\alpha = 1$, $\partial e^*/\partial \alpha = - \infty$.)

Equation 5.1 defines the optimal effort choice given the level of insurance and the premium, $e^*(\alpha, P)$, and, in turn, the endogenous probability of accident as $\pi^*(\alpha, P) = \pi(e^*(\alpha, P))$. That the premium must be set to cover expected losses, $P = \pi^*(\alpha, P)\alpha l$, means we can implicitly define a function $P(\alpha)$ that relates the level of coverage to the premium.

The individual's expected utility can then be written as a function of the coverage rate, α, as

$$V(\alpha) = [1 - \pi(e^*(P(\alpha), \alpha))]u(m - P(\alpha))$$

$$+ \pi(e^*(P(\alpha), \alpha))u(m - P(\alpha) - (1 - \alpha)l)$$

$$- e^*(P(\alpha), \alpha).$$

The first-order condition for the optimal choice of α is then

$$\frac{\partial V}{\partial \alpha} = - (1 - \pi)\, u'(m - P)P'(\alpha) - \pi u'(m - P - (1 - \alpha)l)P'(\alpha)$$

$$+ \pi u'\,(m - P - (1 - \alpha)l)l$$

$$- \pi'(e^*)\left(\frac{\partial e^*}{\partial P}\frac{\partial P}{\partial \alpha} + \frac{\partial e^*}{\partial \alpha} \right)[u(m - P(\alpha)) - u(m - P(\alpha) - (1 - \alpha)l)]$$

$$- \left(\frac{\partial e^*}{\partial P}\frac{\partial P}{\partial \alpha} + \frac{\partial e^*}{\partial \alpha} \right).$$

Let us calculate the value of this expression when $\alpha = 1$. In this case, the term in square brackets on the third line above is zero. We know that with $\alpha = 1$, the optimal choice of effort is zero, whatever P is, so

$$\left.\frac{\partial e^*}{\partial P}\right|_{\alpha = 1} = 0.$$

Simplifying, we get

$$\left.\frac{\partial V}{\partial \alpha}\right|_{\alpha = 1} = -u'(m - P).P'(\alpha) + \pi u'(m - P).l - \frac{\partial e^*}{\partial \alpha}$$

$$= u'(m - P)(\pi.l - P'(\alpha)) - \frac{\partial e^*}{\partial \alpha}$$

$$= u'(m - P)\left(\pi.l - \pi.l - l.\pi'(e^*)\frac{\partial e^*}{\partial \alpha}\right) - \frac{\partial e^*}{\partial \alpha}$$

$$= -\frac{\partial e^*}{\partial \alpha}(1 + l.\pi'(0).u'(m - P))$$

because $e^*(P(1), 1) = 0$. From equation 5.2 and $\pi'(0) = -\infty$, $\left.\partial V/\partial \alpha\right|_{\alpha = 1} < 0$, so it is optimal to reduce α below one.[14]

Group Insurance and Administrative Costs

Running an insurance plan is costly. Not only does the insurance company have to pay out claims, but it might have to administer and organize the plan, check on the performance of medical providers, screen new members of the plans, advertise and sell the plans, and so forth. To cover these additional costs, insurance companies will charge a "loading fee," usually equal to some percentage of the expected value of claims. The premium thus includes an amount that covers the expected value of claims, plus an amount to pay for the insurance services provided.

The additional costs of running an insurance company tend to be largely independent of the number of members of the insurance pool. This means that large plans have much smaller loading fees than small plans, and that

---

14. When the assumption $\pi'(0) = -\infty$ is not satisfied, it can be shown that the effect of a marginal reduction in the coverage rate below 1 has no effect on welfare, but that a large enough reduction does increase the individual's expected utility. That is, as a function of α, expected utility is flat near $\alpha = 1$, but falls for some α below some critical level $\alpha^c < 1$. Thus, the same qualitative result obtains.

they are thus cheaper for individuals. In addition, if large groups of individuals—a group of employees at a particular firm or the members of a union, for example—purchase insurance together, the insurer will be able to make a good estimate of the expected claims from the group without incurring the costs of examining the behavior and medical history of each new member. Phelps (1992, p. 296, table 10.2) reports that loading fees for group insurance ranged from 15 to 30 percent in the United States, while those for nongroup insurance were as high as 100 percent.

That loading fees fall with increases in the size of insured groups means that adverse selection problems will be mitigated to some degree. For example, consider a group insurance plan that covers the employees of a large firm. Some of these employees will be relatively low risk, while others will be high risk. Because they all pay the same premium for their coverage, the high-risk individuals will, on average, get a better deal than the low-risks, who will thus wish to quit the pool and purchase insurance at a price that more closely reflects their lower risks. However, if a low-risk employee quits the group and purchases insurance individually, that individual will face a much larger loading fee, which could offset the reduction in premium tied to her lower risk. This will constrain the incentive to quit the group and lead to more stable coverage for the group as a whole.

It is important to realize that even when employment-based insurance is purchased by the employer for the group as a whole, the individual workers are effectively paying for the coverage in lower wages. In the example above, we argued that each worker paid the same premium for insurance, which, when the employer pays, reduces to the conjecture that each worker has her wage reduced by the same amount. This may not be exactly true—for example, if wages are determined by collective bargaining—but on average it will be about right. It is certainly unlikely that the employer will bear the real costs of purchasing the insurance.

Responses to Moral Hazard

We saw above that the existence of hidden information moral hazard leads to incomplete insurance and excessive consumption of medical services by the insured. Not only will insured individuals generally purchase too much health care when it is subsidized, but they may also purchase the wrong kind of care, by going to an expensive hospital when a visit to a clinic might have been adequate, for example. To control these cost-increasing practices, a number of alterations to fee-for-service insurance have been implemented, both in the public and private sectors.

Health Maintenance Organizations

Perhaps the most well-known alternative to fee-for-service insurance plans is the health maintenance organization (HMO), which can be thought of conceptually as an insurance company run by doctors. By combining the roles of provider of both medical services and insurance, HMOs can remove at least part of the hidden information problem. Recall that the underlying mechanism by which fee-for-service insurance led to increased consumption of medical care relied on the assumption that the insurance company could not accurately observe the health status of the individual. If the insurance company is run by doctors, however, there is a much better chance that it will be able to observe health needs and rely on nondistortionary insurance mechanisms.

The particular insurance scheme that we suggested earlier to combat moral hazard involved the observation of health status by the insurer, coupled with a lump-sum income transfer. The individual was then free to purchase any amount of health care desired at the unsubsidized market price. While HMOs attempt to improve their knowledge of the individual's health status, they do not offer lump-sum cash payments to those with high health needs. Instead, the HMO will provide the medical care services at essentially a zero price, but it will determine the quantity and not allow the individual to choose an unconstrained level of care. As long as the HMO acts in the interests of the consumer, the outcome of this process is identical to that in which a lump-sum payment is made. One potential problem with HMOs is that, once an individual is covered by the plan, it may be difficult to obtain the quantity or quality of services desired. Because an individual's health status is often observable as much (or more) by a doctor as by the individual, it is difficult for an insured person to argue that the HMO has withheld benefits in a way that contravenes the contract.

Other Organizational Forms

Instead of running the insurance company, doctors might find it more efficient to join loosely integrated groups that contract with insurers and agree on certain medical practices and charges in advance. Such organizations, which include Preferred Provider Organizations (PPOs) and Independent Practice Associations (IPAs), give medical care providers incentives to reduce the cost of care. Again, this cost reduction can be achieved either through a reduction in "unnecessary" care or through a reduction in quality, so the net impact on the value of the insurance may be questionable. Nevertheless, the dead-weight losses associated with overconsumption may be reduced, but the incentive to cut costs might lead to underprovision of quality.

Other mechanisms used by insurers include second-opinion clauses and gatekeeper models. Under the first scheme, individuals who are told by one doctor that a given (expensive) treatment is necessary are required to seek the opinion of a second doctor. If the opinions differ widely, a third opinion may be sought to establish the appropriate course of action. This type of mechanism can reduce the number of medically unwarranted expensive treatments, because while the first doctor may have a financial incentive to suggest treatments with high monetary payoffs, a second (or third) doctor is more likely to consider the desirability of the treatment only on medical grounds. This argument breaks down, of course, when the doctors form collusive alliances and agree to recommend treatments for one another's patients.

Gatekeeper models can be seen as providing "first" opinions. In such systems, individuals do not have immediate access to specialists, whose time is very costly (because of their higher than average wages), but they must first consult a general practitioner or primary care doctor. If that doctor agrees that specialist treatment is required, a referral to the specialist is given, and the insurance company will cover the specialist's charges. These schemes are useful if the additional cost to the insurer of the first consultation is more than offset by the reduction in costs from the smaller number of unwarranted specialist visits. Some versions of the gatekeeper model require that primary care physicians shoulder some of the cost of their referrals, so as to constrain their incentives to refer too many patients. Of course, this has the undesirable consequence of transferring risk from the individuals to the primary care physicians, and such schemes may not be sustainable (Moore, Martin, and Richardson 1983).

Informal Insurance Mechanisms

Private insurance contracts differ from other commodities in that they require a degree of literacy and sophistication on the part of consumers, as well as institutional mechanisms to enforce them. These requirements may mean that poor countries, and poor people in rich countries, will not have the necessary infrastructure and skills to take full advantage of formal insurance markets. When governments do not fill the gap, underinsurance is likely to prevail. While we have identified the inefficiencies associated with excessive insurance, the economic and social costs of underinsurance can be equally important in poor countries.

In response to the absence of formal risk-spreading markets, informal arrangements may evolve that replicate, possibly imperfectly, the functions of a formal market.[15] Let us recall that the function of insurance is to transfer income between uncertain states of the world. That is, if an individual is risk-averse, she would like to be able to transfer income from states in which she is healthy to those in which she is ill, so that she is better able to afford medical care in the latter situations. She can do this as long as there are other individuals who face similar but independent risks, so that a dollar she gives up in a healthy state is transferred to someone who is ill. She is willing to do this under the assumption that, should she fall ill, other members of the group will finance transfers to her.

These kinds of transfers can be implemented in two ways. The first, characteristic of formal insurance markets, is that all members of the group pay a premium before their health needs become known. These funds are used to make payments to individuals in need. Alternatively, the members of the group make no initial contributions, but they agree that if and when a member falls ill, the medical care costs will be financed by all group members (in the form of equal contributions or some other sharing mechanism). At the village level, the second method tends to prevail, because it is easier to deal with the collection of funds only when the need arises.

The singular aspect of such informal institutions is that they rely on self-enforcement—that is, there is no outside actor, such as the government or the legal system, that can compel healthy members of the group to contribute to the medical care needs of the unfortunate ill. In a static view of the world, it would be difficult to explain such cooperative behavior without an outside enforcement agency. However, using models of repeated games, some authors, including Coate and Ravallion (1993) and Kimball (1988), have shown that effectively cooperative informal risk-sharing arrangements can be sustained as a noncooperative equilibrium. In such models, economic agents find it individually optimal to honor group agreements, even if it means that they suffer a loss in the short run. This is because of the repeated nature of the interaction, because they know that with high probability they will face poor health in the future and will need to call on the generosity of other group members.

Typically these models require that individuals live a long time, and that the one-shot games are repeated infinitely often. Such assumptions

---

15. Ravallion and Dearden (1988) examine the empirical evidence for the existence of similar informal mechanisms that facilitate income insurance.

are rationalized by the idea that, in traditional villages at least, the appropriate notion of an agent or player in the game is a dynasty—that is, although a member might not expect to play the game many more times before his death, he may care about the welfare of his offspring enough to act on their behalf by playing cooperatively (Coate and Ravallion 1993). An important implication of this assumption is that if it is foreseen that future members are likely to leave the group, cooperative strategies may not be sustainable. More generally, if the net costs of leaving the group are low, cooperation will typically be more difficult to sustain. Thus, as outside opportunities emerge, and rural-urban migration is facilitated, we might expect to see traditional informal insurance mechanisms begin to break down.

Appendix

In this appendix we present more detailed models of market failure caused by adverse selection.

The Lemons Model—Market Unraveling

First we present Akerlof's (1970) lemons model in relation to the health insurance market, in which adverse selection leads to market unraveling. Suppose there is a single insurance policy to be sold, that removes all medical care risks—for example, there is no moral hazard (of either variety) and all medical expenses are fully reimbursed. Individuals are identical in all respects (for example, they have the same incomes), but they differ only in their risks of falling ill. Those with high risks have high expected medical costs, and those with low risks have low expected costs. Denote the expected value of medical costs for an individual by γ, and assume that $\gamma \in [\underline{\gamma}, \overline{\gamma}]$. That is, an individual selected at random from the population will have expected medical care costs in the interval $[\underline{\gamma}, \overline{\gamma}]$; higher-risk individuals have higher γs. We assume that individuals are distributed on this interval according to the density function $f(.)$.

Individuals value the removal of risk—after all, this is the reason they want to buy insurance. We denote the value to an individual of type γ of the removal of this risk by $v(\gamma)$, and assume that $v(\gamma) \geq \gamma$ for all γ, and that $v(.)$ is increasing in γ. $v(\gamma)$ can be identified with the sum of the risk premium and the expected costs that a γ-type individual is willing to pay to remove the risk associated with uncertain medical care expenses. It is reasonable to assume that this is larger for individuals with higher risks.

Because an insurance company cannot observe each individual's risk type separately, it must charge the same premium to all types. Suppose then that it offers insurance at a premium P: all individuals for whom $v(\gamma)$ $\geq P$ will buy the policy (because it is worth more to them than the price), and all for whom $v(\gamma) < P$ will not buy. Thus the set of individuals who purchase insurance is a function of the premium, and is defined by

$$\Gamma(P) = \{\gamma : v(\gamma) \geq P\}.$$

We assume that competition in the insurance market drives the insurance company's profit to zero, so that in an equilibrium, the premium charged is equal to the average medical costs of all individuals who purchase insurance. That is:

(5.3)
$$P^* = E[\gamma \,|\, \gamma \in \Gamma(P^*)]$$
$$= E[\gamma \,|\, v(\gamma) \geq P^*]$$

where E is the expectation operator. All this condition says is that profits are zero in equilibrium. If the premium is larger (smaller) than the average value of the medical costs of individuals who purchase insurance, the insurance company makes a positive (negative) profit, neither of which are sustainable in equilibrium. If the equilibrium premium is such that $\Gamma(P^*)$ does not coincide with the whole set $[\underline{\gamma}, \bar{\gamma}]$, then there is market unraveling.

We can now examine the extent of market unraveling using a relatively simple graphic approach. In figure 5.4 the horizontal axis measures the premium, P, charged by the insurer. The horizontal axis also measures γ, the expected medical care costs of the different individuals. We can think of the expression $E[\gamma \,|\, v(\gamma) \geq P]$ as a function $g(.)$ of P—that is, $g(P) = E[\gamma \,|\, v(\gamma) \geq P]$. Our intention is to draw this function and see where it crosses the 45 degree line. This crossing point will define the equilibrium premium P^* (according to equation 5.3), *and* the degree of market unraveling—that is, the set of individuals who purchase insurance in equilibrium, $\Gamma(P^*)$.

To construct the graph of $g(P)$, first note that when the premium is equal to the highest possible valuation, $P = v(\bar{\gamma})$, only those with the highest expected medical costs will be willing to purchase. That is, $\Gamma(P) = \{\bar{\gamma}\}$. In this case, the expected value of medical costs of those who purchase is just $\bar{\gamma}$. As the premium is reduced, lower-risk individuals are persuaded to purchase insurance, so the average costs (across those who buy) necessarily falls. That is, $g(P)$ decreases as P falls below $v(\bar{\gamma})$.

Now consider the value of g when the premium is set equal to the lowest possible valuation, $P = v(\underline{\gamma})$. In this case, all individuals, including those with the lowest risk, will wish to purchase insurance—that is, $\Gamma(P) = [\underline{\gamma}, \bar{\gamma}]$, and $g(P) = E[\gamma]$, the unconditional population average of expected medical costs. For all P less than $v(\underline{\gamma})$, the set of individuals who purchase insurance continues to be equal to the entire population, and $g(P)$ is constant.

Figure 5.4.   *Market Unraveling*

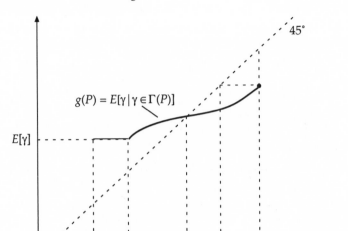

Note: The equilibrium premium is P^*, and only those individuals who value insurance more than P^* purchase in equilibrium.
Source: Adapted from Mas-Colell, Whinston, and Green (1995).

Figure 5.4 is drawn under the assumption that $E[\gamma] > v(\underline{\gamma})$, and the graph of $g(P)$ crosses the 45 degree line at least once. As shown, the equilibrium premium is P^*, and all those with $v(\gamma) \geq P^*$ purchase insurance. If we define the critical level of expected costs, γ^*, by $v(\gamma^*) = P^*$, individuals with expected costs less than γ^* leave the market.

Two extreme examples are when $\gamma^* = \underline{\gamma}$, in which case there is no market unraveling and everyone is insured, and when $\gamma^* = \bar{\gamma}$, in which case the market completely unravels, and only the very worst risks are insured. The first case is shown in panel (a) of figure 5.5. Here $v(\underline{\gamma}) > E[\gamma]$, and the equilibrium premium is low enough that the highest-risks are willing to purchase. In panel (b) we have assumed that $v(\bar{\gamma}) = \bar{\gamma}$ and that $v(\gamma) > \gamma$ for all $\gamma < \bar{\gamma}$. In this case the graph of $g(.)$ does not cross the 45 degree line for any $\gamma < \bar{\gamma}$, and the equilibrium premium is $P = v(\bar{\gamma})$, with virtually all individuals uninsured.

Contrary to some popular understanding of adverse selection in health insurance markets, the case of complete market unraveling appears unlikely to occur. For it to be an equilibrium, we needed to assume that the gross valuation of risk removal by the highest-risk person was equal to her expected

Figure 5.5. *The Extent of Unraveling in the Lemons Market*

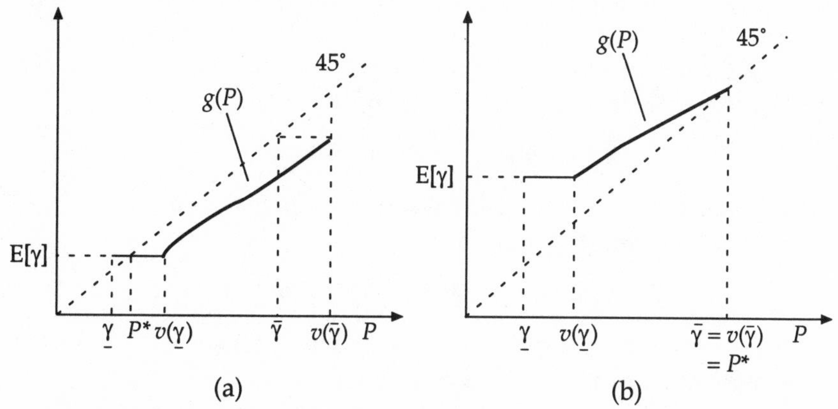

(a)   (b)

Note: (a) when $v(\underline{\gamma}) > E[\gamma]$, there is no unraveling; (b) but when $v(\bar{\gamma}) = \bar{\gamma}$ and $v(\gamma) > \gamma$ for all $\gamma < \bar{\gamma}$, there is complete unraveling.
Source: Adapted from Mas-Colell, Whinston, and Green (1995).

medical cost. This assumption is equivalent to assuming that the highest-risk individual has a risk premium equal to zero, or equivalently that she is risk-neutral. This seems unlikely. However, it is still plausible that $v(\bar{\gamma})$ is only slightly greater than $\bar{\gamma}$, in which case we would expect only a small group of the higher-risk individuals to purchase insurance in equilibrium.

Equilibrium with Multiple Insurance Policies

Here we give a brief geometric review of the model of Rothschild and Stiglitz (1976) and Wilson (1977) of a competitive insurance market with adverse selection. To make things simple, we assume that each individual faces an exogenous shock to income, so that income is either $m_g^0 = m$ in the good state or $m_b^0 = m - l$ in the bad state. There are two types of individual, high-risk and low-risk. The probability of the bad state is π_h for the high-risks, and $\pi_l < \pi_h$ for the low-risks.

Insurance has the effect of redistributing income from the bad state of the world to the good state, and we can describe a contract in terms of the net income received by the individual in each state. Thus, the pair of incomes (m_g, m_b) represents a contract in which the individual has income m_g in the good state and m_b in the bad state. This would be implemented by agreeing with an insurance company that in the good state the individual is paid $m_g - m_g^0$ (which is likely to be negative) by the insurer, and in the bad state is paid $m_b - m_b^0$.

For any contract represented by the pair of incomes (m_g, m_b), the expected utility of an individual of risk type i is

$$V_i(m_g, m_b) = (1 - \pi_i)u(m_g) + \pi_i u(m_b).$$

Similarly, an insurance company that agrees to implement the income pair (m_g, m_b) earns an expected profit of

$$(5.4) \qquad \Pi_i(m_g, m_b) = (1 - \pi_i)(m_g^0 - m_g) + \pi_i(m_b^0 - m_b).$$

When the individual's risk type is observable, the insurer can be certain that it does not make a loss by offering contracts to individuals of risk type i that satisfy $\Pi_i(m_g, m_b) \geq 0$. Competition in the insurance market will force insurers to offer the contract satisfying $\Pi_i(m_g, m_b) = 0$ that maximizes the individual's expected utility. That is, with full information, the equilibrium contract for individuals of risk type i solves

$$\max_{(m_g, m_b)} V_i(m_g, m_b) \text{ s.t. } \Pi_i(m_g, m_b) = 0.$$

The equilibrium contracts under full information—C_h^* for the high-risks and C_l^* for the low-risks—are shown in figure 5.6. Each contract lies on the appropriate zero profit line, *EL* for low-risks and *EH* for high-risks. Also shown in the figure is the average zero profit line, *EA*, along which a contract would yield zero profits if accepted by both risk types.

Now suppose that the insurer cannot observe each individual's risk type but still offers the two contracts, C_h^* and C_l^*. From the figure it is easy to see that low-risk individuals will continue to choose contract C_l^*. But high-risk individuals will also choose this contract, because it provides them with higher expected utility than C_h^*. (Note that in the full information case, high-risk individuals could be prohibited from choosing C_l^* because the insurer could observe their type.) If all individuals choose the single contract C_l^*, the insurance company will make negative profits.

What kind of equilibrium might arise in this case of asymmetric information? There are two potential types of equilibrium: a pooling equilibrium, in which both types of individuals receive the same contract, and a separating equilibrium, in which each type purchases a different contract.[16]

---

16. In the lemons model, the equilibrium is constrained to be quasi-pooling in that all individuals who purchase insurance have the same contract. Here we allow

Figure 5.6. *Equilibrium Contracts under Full Information,* (C_h^*, C_l^*), *and under Asymmetric Information,* (C_h^*, C_l')

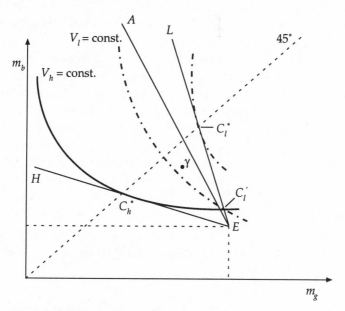

Source: Adapted from Rothschild and Stiglitz (1976).

It is straightforward to show that a pooling equilibrium cannot exist, because the indifference curves of high-risk individuals cut those of low-risk individuals from below. (This is the famous Spence-Mirrlees single-crossing property, characteristic of virtually all models of adverse selection.)

So a potential equilibrium will have two contracts, but these cannot be the full information contracts (C_h^*, C_l^*). To make it unattractive for high-risk individuals to choose the contract proposed for low-risks, that contract must be altered. Now, any contract for low-risks that is part of an equilibrium must be such that it earns zero profits when consumed by the low-risks, so it must lie on the zero profit line for low-risks, *EL*. The contract that provides low-risk individuals with maximal utility, subject to the constraint that high-risks do not choose the contract, is C_l'. This shows that, at a potential equilibrium, while the high-risks are optimally insured, the low-risks are less than fully insured (their income pair is not on the 45 degree line).

---

two contracts to be offered: in the full information case the equilibrium was separating, because two contracts were offered.

In addition, the pair of contracts (C_h^*, C_l') may not constitute an equilibrium. To see this, notice that if there is a sufficient number of low-risk individuals, the average zero profit line, EA, is close to the low-risk zero profit line, EL. In this case, an insurance company could offer the contract γ as marked in figure 5.6. This contract would be accepted by both high- and low-risks (because it lies above the indifference curves through C_h^* and C_l', respectively) and would earn positive profits. However, as a pooling contract, it cannot be an equilibrium. Thus we have a situation in which the potential separating equilibrium cannot be sustained, and the market breaks down completely. When the proportion of low-risks is small, however, a contract that makes positive profits like γ will not exist, and the pair (C_h^*, C_l') will constitute a separating equilibrium.

References

Akerlof, George. 1970. "The Market for Lemons: Qualitative Uncertainty and the Market Mechanism." *Quarterly Journal of Economics* 84: 488–500.

Arrow, Kenneth J. 1963. "Uncertainty and the Welfare Economics of Medical Care." *American Economic Review* 53: 941–73.

Coate, Stephen, and Martin Ravallion. 1993. "Reciprocity without Commitment: Characterization and Performance of Informal Insurance Arrangements." *Journal of Development Economics* 40: 1–24.

Gordis, Leon. 1988. *Epidemiology and Health Risk Assessment*. Oxford, U.K.: Oxford University Press.

Jack, William. 1998. "Intergenerational Risk Sharing and Health Insurance Financing." *Economic Record* 74(225): 153–61.

Jack, William, and Louise Sheiner. 1997. "Welfare Improving Health Expenditure Subsidies." *American Economic Review* 87(1): 206–21.

Kimball, Miles. 1988. "Farmers' Cooperatives as Behavior Toward Risk." *American Economic Review* 78: 224–32.

Laffont, Jean-Jaques. 1989. *The Economics of Uncertainty and Information*. Cambridge, Massachusetts: MIT Press.

Machina, Mark J. 1987. "Choice under Uncertainty: Problems Solved and Unsolved." *Journal of Economic Perspectives* 1(1): 121–54.

Mas-Colell, Andrew, Michael Whinston, and Jerry Green. 1995. *Microeconomic Theory*. New York: Oxford University Press.

Moore, S. H., D. P. Martin, and W. C. Richardson. 1983. "Does the Primary-Care Gatekeeper Control the Costs of Health Care? Lessons from the SAFECO Experience." *New England Journal of Medicine* 309(22): 1400–04.

Pauly, Mark V. 1968. "The Economics of Moral Hazard: Comment." *American Economic Review* 58: 531–37.

_____. 1986. "Taxation, Health Insurance, and Market Failure." *Journal of Economic Literature* 24:629–75.

Phelps, Charles E. 1992. *Health Economics*. New York: HarperCollins.

Ravallion, Martin, and Lorraine Dearden. 1988. "Social Security in a Moral Economy: An Empirical Analysis for Java." *The Review of Economics and Statistics* 70(1): 36–44.

Rothschild, Michael, and Joseph Stiglitz. 1976. "Equilibrium in Competitive Insurance Markets: An Essay on the Economics of Imperfect Information." *Quarterly Journal of Economics*: 629–49.

Selvin, Steve. 1991. *Statistical Analysis of Epidemiological Data*. Oxford, U.K.: Oxford University Press.

Weisbrod, Burton A. 1991. "The Health Care Quadrilemma: An Essay on Technological Change, Quality of Care, and Cost Containment." *Journal of Economic Literature* 29: 523–52.

Wilson, Charles. 1977. "A Model of Insurance Markets with Incomplete Information." *Journal of Economic Theory* 16: 167–207.

Zeckhauser, Richard J. 1970. "Medical Insurance: A Case Study of the Trade-off between Risk Spreading and Appropriate Incentives." *Journal of Economic Theory* 2: 10–26.

Zweifel, Peter, and Friedrich Breyer. 1997. *Health Economics*. Oxford, U.K.: Oxford University Press.

6

The Supply of Physician Services and Other Medical Services

In the previous two chapters we have studied the determinants of demand for medical services, and, given the uncertainty surrounding health needs, the associated demand for insurance. An implicit assumption that permeated the whole of the analysis was that individuals had well-defined and well-informed preferences for health and health care, and that they made their consumption and risk-reduction decisions rationally. When we consider the supply of medical services, this assumption, which is basic to most economic analysis, must be tempered to some degree, because it becomes clear that as well as providing operational services (that is, injections, surgery, and the like), one of the primary roles of a medical care worker is the provision of information that affects the demand for services. The implications of this connection for the level and quality of care can be significant and lead us to question the likely efficiency of a market-determined allocation of resources in the health sector.

This chapter considers the motivation and behavior of physicians and other health sector workers, the institutions within which they operate, and the resource allocation outcomes that alternative financial structures and other incentives might yield. Of particular concern is the efficiency of health service production, the appropriateness of the services, and the allocation of physician and other labor to rural and urban areas. We will also examine the use of other inputs into the production of health, including prescription drugs and capital equipment.

The final part of the chapter examines the behavior of physicians in the market. The analysis is essentially one of the equilibrium between supply and demand, and it might be better addressed in a separate chapter linking both sides of the market. However, the special position of medical care providers in relation to their patients means that demand may be in some sense a function of the behavior of suppliers, so it is natural to include such an analysis here. We are particularly interested in the extent to which physicians can induce consumers to purchase more medical care than they would if they were fully informed about its effects, and the impact such strategies might have on market responses to supply shocks and the effectiveness of government price interventions.

Inputs into the Production of Health Care

This section describes the individual actors and physical inputs in the health production process and the institutional and cultural settings in which they are organized. The purpose is to examine the combinations of inputs and the subsequent outputs in the health care sector, which, in a formal sense, is akin to determining the health production function, albeit at a very general level of abstraction. We do not include inputs that traditionally fall outside the health care sector—for example, sanitation, infrastructure, education, and so on—but concentrate solely on health care delivery. In the following section we shall examine the incentives medical care providers face and the likely resource allocations that result when these incentives are coupled with the generic production function.

Physicians

A defining characteristic of the demand side of the health care market is the lack of information that individuals have about the cause, nature, and treatment of disease. Unlike the demand for food, clothing, and other standard consumption commodities, individuals often have poorly defined preferences over health care services. Of course, there may be little reason to think that they have poorly defined preferences over health (as described in chapter 3), but if their knowledge of the way in which health care services can be used to improve health is limited, they will have little basis for making decisions about appropriate methods of care.

Given this essential feature of demand, physicians of all kinds and specialties play two distinct roles as health care providers. First, they provide information and advice to patients on the nature of their conditions; the likely impacts of particular treatments, both positive and negative; and their recommended course of action. In addition to these services, physicians engage in the physical delivery of services, including surgery, administering of injections, writing of drug prescriptions, and so forth. If individuals were fully aware of the effects of various treatments in improving their health, they would not require the first kind of service—the provision of information—and physicians would be just like bakers and barbers.

Of course, there are many other producers in the economy that have similar dual functions, including car mechanics, accountants, and teachers. In these situations, economists find it useful to think of the service provider as the "agent" of the consumer. Of particular relevance is that the agent—the physician or other health care provider in our case—has more extensive information about the consequences and costs of his or her actions than does the patient (who is known in the literature as the "principal").

It is necessary to note two important points regarding this description of the roles of physicians. The first is that it is possible, at least in principle, to imagine some physicians providing just advisory services, and other physicians providing the executive or operational services, in which case the dual roles would be separated to some degree.[1] This could have important effects on the pattern and cost of services delivered.

The second point to note is that, while they are usually better informed than their patients, physicians are unlikely to have full information about the consequences of their actions either. Evidence for such uncertainty is found in the large range of treatments and drug use exhibited among physicians with similar training and backgrounds, and while there are recommended responses to many conditions, the physician must often make decisions based on partial and incomplete information.

Other Medical Personnel

Physicians, who have typically undertaken extensive training, make up only a fraction of the personnel resources used in the health care sector. Also included are nurses, administrators, clerks, receptionists, traditional healers, and general staff. Some of the labor services provided by such individuals are substitutes for each other and for the work of physicians. For example, trained nurses can administer injections and oral drugs, monitor patients, and so forth. Receptionists could probably manage the taking of a temperature, but their productivity in doing so would likely be much less than that of a nurse, because they may make mistakes.

Of course, it is not the absolute level of productivity in performing a task that should determine the allocation of tasks among individuals, but

---

1. The separation is unlikely to be complete, because advising physicians will often need to engage in operational actions—performing examinations, ordering diagnostic tests, and the like.

the relative productivity, or comparative advantage. Thus, even though the physician may be a better typist than the receptionist, it is economically efficient for the receptionist to type up prescriptions and let the physician concentrate on diagnosing and treating patients.

One potentially important substitute for physician services is lower-level medical services (provided by nurses or other clinicians, for example) delivered at the appropriate time. It may be possible to substitute the use of a doctor's labor at a time when a patient has developed a severe illness for the use of a clinician's time at a much earlier stage in the patient's life, for example. This is essentially an argument about the possibility of preventive care reducing the need for future curative care. Notice that the desirability of this substitution depends on the relative costs of the two types of care, the costs imposed on the patient (in ill health and the like) and other social costs. Most analysts argue that the returns from such a substitution are substantial in Sub-Saharan Africa, but some studies in more advanced economies suggest that intensive preventive care, such as screening for certain types of cancer, may or may not be desirable (or "cost effective"—see chapter 9).

Nonlabor Inputs

Medical supplies, particularly drugs, instruments, and capital equipment, are essential inputs into the production of health services. There may be some degree of substitutability between labor and nonlabor inputs, such as consultations with other physicians that might reduce the quantity of drugs required for a given patient, or the use of additional secretarial services in place of office equipment. But many drugs do not have close non-drug substitutes and represent complements to physician care rather than substitutes. Absence of these inputs can constrain the productive capacity of the medical services significantly, just as the absence of left shoes would constrain the production of pairs of shoes.[2]

It is of concern in some developing countries that the quality of inputs is sometimes very difficult to discern. This is particularly the case with drugs, which often have a nondescript appearance in tablet form. If labeling can be altered at low cost, the scope for fraud is wide, and high-quality

---

2. More specifically, the absence of left shoes would constrain the production of "miles walked"—an output that requires both left and right shoes.

drugs may be unavailable, except on the black market. This can have two effects: first, treatments may not be provided, and second, treatments with poor-quality drugs may lead to serious unintended effects. In addition, drugs are most effective when prescribed in the correct dosages and in conjunction with suitable complementary treatments and actions (such as abstinence from drinking alcohol). If physicians are unaware of the recommended uses, and patients do not follow instructions, the effectiveness of drugs can be severely limited.

While capital goods are important inputs in hospitals, they tend to make up a much smaller share of costs in lower-level outlets, such as clinics. As well as the financial costs involved in procurement of the equipment, resources must be spent to keep them in good working order. These costs are essentially depreciation costs and are incurred with all machines that do not last forever. The problem is that the rate of depreciation can be a function of the uses of the equipment, and inappropriate use can increase the rate at which the stock of physical capital becomes ineffective. This, coupled with the possibility that local workers might be untrained in the maintenance of the machines, can impose additional real resource costs on health care service organizations.

Incentives and the Allocation of Resources

Given the technical relationships between inputs and outputs described in rather general terms in the preceding section, what patterns of resource allocation are we likely to see in the health care sector? Such resource allocations can be effected either through direct administrative procedures (for example, by governments) or as a consequence of decisions made by private economic agents in the economy. Although governments play a large role in the delivery and management of health care services, they still rely on the choices and behavior of physicians and other providers of labor and physical inputs within institutional settings to implement their preferred resource allocations. We examine here the incentives of agents on the supply side of the health sector, and the implications of different financial and other structures in the determination of resource use.

It is useful to identify two margins on which the allocation of resources may be inefficient. First, incentives may induce agents on the supply side to produce too much or too little care of a particular kind, and second, a given level of care or output may be produced inefficiently—with the wrong mix of inputs, for example. Deviations from efficiency on the first of these margins represent allocative inefficiencies, while those on the second represent so-called X-inefficiencies.[3]

Physicians' Objectives and Behavior

It is common in economics to describe resource allocations as the outcome of optimizing behavior of economic agents who have explicit objectives and capacities and who face given financial (and other) reward structures. Within this general framework, physicians can be thought of both as supplying orthodox labor services and, primarily because of their privileged possession of information about the health production process and the needs of their patients, acting as entrepreneurs. As the suppliers of labor, their behavior can be analyzed in a similar fashion to that of other workers as resulting from a tradeoff between consumption of goods purchased in the market (financed by earned income) and leisure. As medical entrepreneurs, the objectives that determine their behavior must be expanded to include such dimensions as effort on the job, prestige and reputation, the well-being of their patients (both generally and specifically with regard to their health), and other ethical considerations.

INVESTING IN HUMAN CAPITAL—THE DECISION TO BECOME A DOCTOR. Faced with market- or government-determined compensation (that is, wage) rates, individuals make decisions on whether to become doctors, the type of speciality (if any) to undertake, and their hours of work. Like any investment decision, the decision to undertake a typically long-term commitment to study must be made with the opportunity costs in mind. These include forgone current income and any direct financial costs. Of potentially more significance, however, is that, unlike many other investment choices, investment in human capital may be difficult to finance through capital markets. That is, when ownership of individuals is not permitted, a person who invests in human capital through education has no associated physical capital to offer a lender as collateral. Faced with such capital market imperfections, only those with existing assets (that is, the well-off) will be able to attain costly

---

3. At a conceptual level, it is not always easy to separate these two notions of efficiency. Given a production function, allocative efficiency requires that the right quantity be produced, as defined in some way on the basis of the estimated social benefits and costs. However, if production is not undertaken efficiently, the "right" level of output may change, and allocative efficiency would be defined in some constrained second-best fashion.

education. On the assumption that the potential returns to human capital investment are independent of an individual's existing social status, such an allocation of investment resources is likely to be inefficient.

At the same time, much of higher education in developing countries is provided free by the state, so the direct financial costs incurred by individuals are low. This would suggest that opportunity costs would be relatively more important in determining education decisions. Under the assumption that individuals from wealthier backgrounds have higher opportunity costs than others, we might expect them to have a lower demand for eduction than others. Two factors oppose this conclusion, however. First, to the extent that individuals from better-off backgrounds have access to family financing (financial support from their families during their studies), they suffer relatively small opportunity costs. Second, and unfortunately, in many countries it is not just the failure of the capital market that directs education resources to the better-off. Because access to higher education is often as much a function of previous education opportunities and political connections as current resources, it is the elite who dominate.

We should note that while financial returns are likely to be of central concern to individuals in deciding on investments in human capital, other factors will also influence their choices. In some societies, being a member of the medical profession avails an individual of a certain degree of prestige and social status superior to that enjoyed by others with similar incomes. Somewhat more altruistically, many individuals choose to enter the medical profession based on an explicit concern for the health of others or because of their interest in scientific pursuits. A final influence on many young students may be the wishes of their parents, who may themselves belong to the medical profession.

LABOR SUPPLY. Having received their training, physicians must make decisions about the amount of work they intend to do and where they will do it. The hours decision, although empirically difficult to estimate, is captured conceptually through the standard income-leisure tradeoff as a function of net wages. As net wage rates increase, the price of leisure effectively increases, and the *substitution effect* induces individuals to supply more labor. In opposition to this, higher wages effectively increase each individual's wealth, and the *income effect* induces the individual to consume more leisure (that is, to reduce the labor supply). It is usually assumed that the first effect dominates, at least over the relevant range, and that the labor supply curve slopes up. Thus, one way to encourage doctors to supply more services (or at least more hours) is to pay them more.

The location decision presents policymakers with perhaps one of the more challenging dilemmas in health care provision. Because of the greater availability of both private and public goods and services in urban areas, compensation payments to physicians must usually be correspondingly greater in rural areas to persuade them to locate outside major cities. Although money prices of some goods are likely to be greater in cities, the effective prices of others may well be extremely high in rural areas, where the particular item is unavailable (such as opera tickets). In addition, if incomes are lower in rural areas, the supportable prices that physicians can charge will be lower, so some form of public subsidy is likely to be necessary. Of course, when the required subsidy is sufficiently high, it is likely to be much cheaper for the government to encourage nonphysician health workers to practice in rural areas, although there will be a tradeoff between lower costs and lower medical skills. To the extent that many required health care services in rural communities can be provided easily by clinicians and nurses, the impact of lower-skilled health providers on the quality of care may be relatively small.

In addition to the rural-urban decision, physicians might have the option of locating outside their home country, moving to neighboring countries where their incomes could be higher. Of course, this incentive can work in the opposite direction, with doctors trained in Western countries willingly sacrificing large salaries to work in developing countries with international agencies. In the presence of significant net out-migration of state-trained physicians, the government might be advised to examine the net social return to publicly funded medical education.

MANAGERIAL ACTIONS. Even within the strictures that a salaried government appointment might impose, physicians often have sufficient discretion over choices of techniques and practices to suggest that they be considered as filling managerial or entrepreneurial roles. This discretion arises from the physician's private information regarding the effects and costs of various treatment strategies, and it means that the way the physician is paid can affect her supply decisions. In this section, we will think of the physician as a firm that makes production decisions to maximize some generalized objective function. Faced with various payment mechanisms—all of which are observed in some guise in health care systems around the world—we examine the incentives physicians have to efficiently supply medical care, both in the allocative and X-efficiency dimensions.

Consider a physician as a producer of the final good health, h. As we have mentioned on numerous occasions, the measurement of h is likely to be problematic—this is one of the sources of inefficiency below—but we ignore this for now. The physician can choose from a variety of inputs in treating patients, including drugs, diagnostic tests, days in hospital, the physician's own effort, the length and frequency of visits, and so forth. Given the particular health status of an individual—the disease she suffers from, her symptoms, and the like—certain combinations of these inputs can improve the health of the individual by varying degrees. Let us model this process formally by labeling the individual's health status, as before, by θ, and letting $z = (z_1, \ldots, z_i, \ldots, z_n)$ be a vector of n health care inputs. Suppose for now that these inputs can be purchased by the physician in competitive markets at a price vector $w = (w_1, \ldots, w_i, \ldots, w_n)$. We suppose that the improvement in the individual's health is given by the production function:

$$h = f(z, \theta).$$

Corresponding to this production function is the cost function, $c(h, \theta, w)$, which is the minimum cost of producing h units of health improvement for an individual with health status θ, and is given by

$$c(h, \theta; w) = \min_z w.z \text{ s.t. } f(z, \theta) = h.$$

This description of the available choices open to the physician is identical to the neoclassical theory of a competitive firm, where h is output (the number of widgets) produced.

Now suppose that there are $j = 1, \ldots, J$ possible health statuses, and the physician must treat n_j individuals with health status θ_j. The health improvement of each θ_j-type individual is given by $h = f(z_j, \theta_j)$, and the cost function for each is $c(h_j, \theta_j, w) = \min_{z_j} w.z_j \text{ s.t. } f(z_j, \theta_j) = h_j$, where $z_j = (z_{1j}, \ldots, z_{ij}, \ldots, z_{nj})$ is the vector of inputs used in treating a type-θ_j individual. The vector of health outputs is $h = (h_1, \ldots, h_j, \ldots, h_J)$, and total costs are $C(n, h, \theta; w) = \sum_{j=1}^{J} n_j c(h_j, \theta_j; w)$, where $n = (n_1, \ldots, n_j, \ldots, n_J)$ and $\theta = (\theta_1, \ldots, \theta_j, \ldots, \theta_J)$.

Recall from neoclassical economic theory that, under certain convexity assumptions, the first and second fundamental theorems of welfare economics tell us that market allocations will be Pareto-efficient (see chapter 7 for a definition of Pareto efficiency) and that any particular Pareto-efficient allocation can be implemented as a market equilibrium with suitable lump-sum transfers. The abstract description of the production of health by physicians here is meant to be as consistent with the standard theory of the firm as possible to allow us to focus on the ways in which inefficiencies may arise without letting the different nature of health confuse the issue.

Given the description of production possibilities, to determine likely allocative outcomes we must also define the objectives of physicians.

Extending the analogy of the market for widgets, suppose (implausibly) that physicians are paid on the basis of the health improvement of their patients, h_j, at a rate p_j per unit. These prices can vary according to the health status of the patient. A physician's profit is then $\Sigma_j n_j p_j h_j - C(n, h, \theta; w) = \Sigma_j [n_j p_j h_j - w.z_j(p_j, \theta_j, w)]$, where $z_j(p_j, \theta_j, w)$ is the input bundle chosen for treating patients of type θ_j, given the price received for treating them, and the input prices. Because we have included elements such as physician effort in the vector of inputs, z_j, we do not need to account for them separately.

This objective function—profits—can be further altered in many ways. For example, an additional motivating force affecting physicians' behavior might be the health of their patients, not just because of any potential monetary rewards it might bring, but also as a primitive element of physicians' preferences. Physicians may also have preferences for the health of some individuals above that of others—on the basis of income, for example, as in a preference for serving the indigent. The effects of these alterations are discussed later.

To fix ideas further, let us now assume that there is a given population of individuals with a distribution of health statuses, and a single institution—perhaps the government or a large insurance company—wishes to purchase health care services on their behalf from physicians. For each j, the institution decides on a value h_j^*, which is the level of health improvement it requires for an individual in state θ_j. The term h_j^* could be interpreted as the improvement in health that restores the individual to *full* or *normal* health. If both health status and health improvements were observable by the purchasing agent, it could agree to pay the physician an amount $pj = c_j^* \equiv c(h_j^*, \theta_j; w)$ for each individual of status θ_j whose health the physician improves by h_j^*. The physician will then treat all individuals using an efficient mix of inputs, because if she uses an inefficient mix, she will make a loss. Note that we can think of the health improvements of individuals with different needs as representing different goods, with different costs of production. Thus, the physician is like a multiproduct firm, producing more than one output.

Now suppose that health outcomes are observable, but health needs, or status, are not. If the physician is paid the average of each of the c_j^*—that is, $p_j = \bar{p} = (\Sigma n_j c_j^*)/(\Sigma n_j)$—then she will have an incentive only to treat patients with relatively minor health needs. From those individuals, she makes positive profits; patients with more extensive needs create a loss. Because a uniform price is charged for different goods, we should expect the firm (the physician) to direct production to goods with the highest markup.

If health outcomes are not observable, but health status is (based on diagnosis), physicians could be paid c_j^* for each individual with status θ_j. Whatever services are rendered will efficiently produce a given level of health improvement, but this level (which is not observable by the purchaser) cannot be specified in the contract, and there is little reason to expect that it will equal the desired level, h_j^*. When physicians do not care about the health outcomes of their patients, they will provide only enough services to convince the purchaser that the patient was treated. Of course, physicians do tend to place a positive value on the health of their patients, and some treatment is to be expected, but the level of treatment may not be as high as would be required.

Because of the limited capacity to observe health status and the unpredictability of the effects of health care interventions, it is difficult to make payments contingent on either health status or health outcomes. It is therefore common for physicians to be paid in other ways, either related to incurred costs, on the basis of fixed salaries, or some combination of these.

Suppose physicians are paid on the basis of reimbursement of incurred costs. It should be noted that not many productive firms are paid on this basis (although in equilibrium it might turn out that price equals average cost). Cost reimbursement is equivalent to the firm receiving a 100 percent subsidy for the costs of its inputs, but receiving nothing for its outputs. In this case, the level of production is indeterminate, because any level of output will result in zero profit. If costs are reimbursed subject to some output target (for example, treatment of all individuals who want attention), we might expect the target to be met, but there is no particular guarantee that the output will be produced efficiently. Because resource costs do not depend on input choices, physicians will—at best—choose the inputs somewhat arbitrarily. Worse, however, they may choose unnecessarily expensive methods of treatment, such as the use of costly new capital equipment that they enjoy using but that is of little help to patients.[4]

It is very rare for all costs to be reimbursed; generally, only financial costs, such as the costs of purchases of inputs from other parties, are reimbursable. It is unusual for physicians' costs of effort to be explicitly reimbursed, for example, because such costs are difficult to observe. This means that cost reimbursement typically results in a large subsidy to some kinds

---

4. A similar incentive is faced by the economic theorist, who might be tempted to ask for the latest computer technology when a pencil and paper will suffice.

of inputs, but not to others, which distorts input choices toward the subsidized set. In the case where drug costs are reimbursed but physician time is not, we might thus expect to see greater reliance on drug therapy than on consultations. This is an example of the payment mechanism resulting in X-inefficiency—that is, the production of a given level of output (health improvement) is effected with an inefficient mix of inputs.

Examples of distorted input choices abound in the health financing literature. For example, suppose hospital physicians are reimbursed for the number of days individuals stay in hospital, which is meant to proxy for their health needs. The subsidized input is bed-days, and there will clearly be incentives for patients to be kept in hospital longer than if the physicians were paid a lump sum. If the opportunity costs incurred by physicians in keeping individuals in hospital are small enough, lengths of stay may well increase significantly.

Another easily observable input is the number of visits by a patient to a physician. If doctors are paid on the basis of the number of visits and not the services provided, excessive checkups and referrals may occur. An alternative payment system would pay the physician on the basis of the number of patients seen, independent of the number of times they see the physician. This arrangement would clearly be biased against individuals with chronic diseases that require recurrent treatment—individuals with "bad" θs—and against those unlucky enough to suffer more than one health impairment—against those with multiple θs. Again, if payments could be based on these (unobserved) health statuses, the problem would be mitigated.

A final alternative is that physicians are paid a salary, like many workers in long-term contractual arrangements, with nonlabor-input costs reimbursed. The pattern of input use will be shifted toward nonlabor inputs, with care being produced inefficiently. In addition, because at least some physician time is required for each patient, it may be expected that the quantity of services will be suboptimal. A variant on this mechanism is one in which physicians are paid a salary and allowance, and they must finance purchases of inputs other than their own labor from the allowance. Efficient use of nonlabor inputs is likely, although the scale of service provision might be reduced and the physician would face potentially large financial risks if a greater than average number of relatively sick individuals need care. This is the *fundholder* model of the United Kingdom, to be discussed at greater length in later chapters.

MOONLIGHTING. A final aspect of physician labor supply that deserves attention, particularly in the context of developing countries, is moonlighting.

This is the practice of workers (not necessarily physicians) taking on a second job in addition to their primary employment. Typically the second job will be in the informal sector of the economy, characterized by a lack of formal administrative structure (labor laws, unions, and so on) and incomplete tax coverage. There are positive and normative issues that may be of concern to a policy analyst with respect to moonlighting. On the one hand, it is useful to understand the forces that lead to multiple job holdings; on the other hand, it is important to know the welfare implications of such activities. Should they be controlled, and if so, how?

To understand why physicians might engage in both formal and informal sector labor supply, we can begin by describing a scenario in which such multiple job holdings would not be desirable to the individual. Suppose that wages in both sectors are fixed, that the worker can work as much as he wishes at the going wage (that is, the labor market is competitive), and that the disutility of work is the same in both sectors. In this case, the optimal labor supply choice is to work in the sector with the highest net wage, and moonlighting would not be observed. However, the conditions imposed in this example suggest situations in which multiple job holdings would be desirable. [5,6]

First, if the worker cannot choose hours of work freely, then he may face a constraint in one job that makes the second job attractive. For example, suppose the formal sector wage is higher than that in the informal sector, but that no overtime work is permitted (or at least remunerated) in the formal sector. The worker will optimally work as much as possible in the higher-paid job but may choose to work additional hours in the lower-paid informal sector.

Second, the worker may be concerned about the stability of his income, as well as its average value. If wages in the informal sector are higher but more volatile than those in the formal sector, he may wish to provide himself with some insurance by working in both sectors. Note that full insurance could be obtained by working only in the low-paid formal sector, but that this may not be optimal if average wages in the informal sector are high enough, or if the individual is not too risk-averse.

---

5. Note that differential tax enforcement does not constitute a reason for multiple job holdings. If effective tax rates differ across sectors, then, other things being equal, the worker should work solely in the sector with the lower rate.

6. One empirical study that addresses moonlighting explicitly in the developing country context is van der Gaag, Stelcner, and Vijverberg (1989).

Of course, if there is a well-functioning insurance market, the individual would work only in the informal sector and would purchase insurance against volatile wages. Such formal insurance markets are imperfect in industrial countries, however, and often nonexistent in developing countries, and multiple job holdings can be an effective substitute.

A third reason to have jobs in both sectors is that there might be private economies of scope in labor supply. That is, working in one sector may increase the individual's productivity in the other sector. The most likely cases are when formal sector employment increases informal sector returns. For example, some kind of training may be provided in the formal sector job that increases both formal and informal sector productivity. Alternatively, attributes of the formal sector job could be used as inputs in the informal sector, such as office equipment and stationery, professional status and reputation, and access to patients (who are subsequently treated outside of office hours). Some of these attributes, such as status, human capital, and reputation, have a public good aspect, and their use in the informal sector represents a social economy of scope. Others, however, such as use of formal sector inputs, permit the worker to achieve private economies of scope without any social equivalent. That is, these second activities tend to reduce productivity in the formal sector, but they may not reduce the individual's formal sector wage (the private return).

The issue of private and social returns to moonlighting suggests that as well as identifying the determinants of this aspect of labor supply, it is important to understand its normative implications. Should all forms of moonlighting be discouraged, and should this be achieved by increasing formal sector wages or increasing penalties on informal sector activities? Should formal sector employment arrangements be made more flexible—either by allowing more discretion in decisions about formal sector labor supply or by allowing outside work—in order to improve the efficiency of labor allocation?

Some recent literature (see Bardhan 1997 for a review and also Bigsten and Moene 1996 and Mauro 1995) has begun to address the question of the impact of corruption in general on economic growth and well-being. The standard view is that corruption represents rent-seeking activities undertaken by agents that do not increase output or social welfare but detract from the available resource base of the economy. An alternative thesis is that corruption is an attempt by rational economic agents to circumvent obstructive rules and regulations that are imposed by inefficient and politically motivated bureaucracies. As long as all parties that are affected by corruption agree to the actions (there is a Pareto improvement), such behavior should not have a negative effect on welfare.

The trouble is, of course, that both of these effects will likely coexist, and the net impact is difficult to measure. Indeed, it is quite a job simply to measure corruption, let alone its impact on economic performance. Very little empirical work has been done on this subject in the medical care market.

Drugs

Despite the scope for substitution among inputs, modern drug therapies play an essential role in the treatment of many diseases, and they are second only to personnel costs in their share of recurrent costs in African economies (World Bank 1994, p. 67). They represent complementary inputs to physicians' visits in health production as is evidenced by large positive correlations between the supply of drugs and the demand for health facility visits.

By far the greatest component of the cost of production of most drugs is incurred at the research and development stage, and the marginal costs of production are often close to zero, except when transportation and storage costs are significant. This characteristic of the production process has at least two important implications. First, to give drug companies incentives to incur the large investment costs required, new drugs can be patented, allowing the producer to exercise monopoly power. These patents typically last for a limited amount of time, and when they expire, the drugs can be produced (at low marginal cost) and sold by other companies. Competition then forces prices down, and the drugs become much less profitable. At this stage, drugs with expired patents become known as "generic" drugs. They may have similar properties to other patented (and more expensive) drugs in their effectiveness in combating disease, but they are usually much cheaper. The existence of products that appear to be different, but are actually similar, means that information problems at the consumer level that are significant in the market for drugs might be exacerbated. While one might expect that in such situations uninformed individuals could choose cheap but inappropriate drugs, it is also possible that they will infer that there are additional benefits associated with the more expensive varieties. Some accounts (World Bank 1994, chapter 5) suggest that the predilection of consumers for specialty drugs over their generic equivalents can be extremely costly.

The second implication of the heavily investment-intensive nature of drug production is that, because many developing countries have very low absolute levels of savings and generally suffer shortages of many forms of capital (such as public infrastructure), they are at a distinct comparative (and absolute) disadvantage in the development of new drugs.

Thus it is rational for most developing countries to import a large share of their prescription drugs. Sometimes it is economical for countries with low labor costs to import the drugs in some easily transported form (such as powder) and to process these raw materials locally into tablet form. In any case, the large, and possibly complete, component of imported inputs allows the government to exert more control over the procurement and distribution of drugs than might otherwise be the case, because of the administrative economies associated with a small number of ports of entry. This, however, can be either a blessing or a curse. In its role as a benevolent planner, the government can regulate the quality and price of drugs to protect and promote consumer well-being. However, to the extent that border control personnel and governments can engage in corrupt activities, it increases the rents available to corrupt officials.

On the positive side, a single importer may be able to exercise some level of monopsony power in purchasing large quantities of drugs on behalf of the country. The possibility of such action is increased in the market for drugs in comparison with other imported commodities to the extent that the relative size of fixed costs is much higher for drugs. This means that if suppliers can price discriminate among countries—charging some countries more than others—the countries that are willing and able to pay more might be induced to pay a larger fraction of the fixed costs than poorer countries. If a large number of small purchasers in a country were to bargain individually with a large international drug company, they would be unlikely to achieve such discounts.[7]

Bulk purchases are not only economic at the import stage, but also at the stage of distribution within a country. Economies of scale in transportation and storage mean that it is preferable for regional health centers, and even clinics, to receive supplies that can last a reasonable length of time. In such cases, if health facilities are required to purchase the drugs in advance, they will require either an existing source of capital or access to reasonably well-functioning capital markets. In the absence of these resources, facilities will find it difficult to take advantage of the economies associated with bulk purchases, even if they are able to charge consumers sufficiently high prices at the time of use to cover the costs. Solutions to this problem have included

---

7. This process is taken one step further in practice, with groups of developing countries banding together to purchase bulk supplies from international drug companies. This strategy is implemented through the United Nations Children's Fund (UNICEF), which purchases large quantities of cheap drugs to distribute to developing nations.

the institution of so-called "revolving drug funds," which essentially amount to policies directed at capital market failures.[8] Under such schemes, the government (or a donor) provides the financial resources for the purchase of an initial quantity of drugs that are then sold to consumers. The revenues are available for subsequent purchases, and the cycle continues. The optimal size of the fund depends on, among other things, the economies of scale in bulk purchasing (the greater the discount for bulk purchases, the larger the fund), the storability of the drugs (longer life implies a larger fund), and the inflation rate (the higher the inflation rate, the smaller the fund).[9]

Once drugs reach health facilities and physicians, they must be used effectively. There are two reasons that drugs are inefficiently used in practice. First, medical care workers with inappropriate or insufficient training may not prescribe drugs in the correct dosages or regimens. When they are available, multiple drugs are sometimes prescribed, either because the health worker lacks knowledge of the patient's medical condition or does not understand the effects of the drugs. A shotgun strategy, whereby the undefined target is "sprayed" with potential solutions, is then adopted. This is costly with regard to the resources used, and also to the extent that it may lead over time to some drugs (especially antibiotics) becoming ineffective, even when used appropriately.

The second reason that drugs might be used inefficiently is that they are often administered by the patients themselves (particularly in oral form). Individuals may forget to take the prescribed drugs, take them in the wrong dosages, or fail to complete a course. Such behavior may severely curtail the effectiveness of the drugs in alleviating or curing the disease. The effectiveness with which individuals use their prescribed drugs is often a function of their level of education; illiteracy is associated with particularly negative outcomes (see Frack and others 1997 for a related study).

Hospitals

Hospitals combine a large number of inputs and treat a wide variety of conditions, ranging from the mundane to the exotic. To be able to make sensible policy decisions regarding the allocation of resources to and

---

8. Such funds have been introduced in many Sub-Saharan African nations (World Bank 1994, p. 79).

9. A higher inflation rate means that revenues collected from sales early in the cycle are not worth much, and therefore they do not contribute enough to the financing of future bulk purchases.

within hospitals, it is necessary to have a model (explicit or otherwise) of how these institutions function and means of explicitly measuring their performance. The standard theory of the firm is not much use to us here. On the one hand, the goals and decisionmaking processes of hospitals are not necessarily well described by the neoclassical model, because describing the organization of a hospital in economic terms can be difficult when orthodox notions of ownership and control are ill-defined, and the objectives of those in control are only vaguely characterized. On the other hand, measuring a hospital's performance—in productivity terms, for example—is notoriously difficult, given the myriad services they offer. We address the positive theory of hospital organization and "behavior" in the next subsection, followed by a discussion of issues surrounding the objective measurement of performance. The reader is referred to Phelps (1992, chapter 8) for a brief survey, and Barnum and Kutzin (1993) for a discussion of the production and organization of hospital services in developing countries.

Hospital Motives and Behavior

A striking feature of many nongovernment hospitals in some countries is that they deem themselves "not for profit" organizations. Exactly what such status means for the behavior of decisionmakers within these hospitals is not always clear. One would hope, for example, that such a status did not mean that resources were wasted, so that any potential profit would be removed by inefficiencies. This hardly seems a reasonable goal for any organization to espouse, nor for a government to foster.

The best way to understand the nature of a not-for-profit hospital is, first, to consider its alternative—a profit-maximizing hospital. As with any other productive firm, the profits from such an enterprise measure the economic surplus from production (the value of outputs sold over inputs used) that typically accrue to the owners of the firm—the shareholders. Under the assumption that the owners of the hospital control decisions regarding its business activities (including the kind of doctors to hire, the suppliers from whom to purchase inputs, the potential patients to target in advertising campaigns, and so on), the surplus represents a return to their capital investment and entrepreneurial actions.[10]

---

10. In practice, of course, boards of directors and chief executive officers (CEOs) make such business decisions. When shares in the enterprise are widely held, the link between ownership and control is severed, and the returns to shareholders may not be maximized (see Tirole 1988).

The profits are typically distributed to the shareholders on a regular basis, such as at the end of each year.

Now suppose that for some reason a particular group of individuals involved in the activities of the hospital happen to be the owners. For example, the resident physicians and attending specialists might be the sole shareholders, or the administrators could be in this position. Alternatively, the patients who are served by the hospital might own it. In each case, the distribution of profits could be effected through an explicit financial transfer, as in the case of the previous paragraph. A similar transfer could be implemented by altering the prices at which the owning group trades with the hospital. For example, physicians' salaries might be increased by an amount that compensates them both for their labor services as physicians and for the capital (if any) they have invested in the hospital plus their entrepreneurial services. Alternatively, the transfer could be made in kind, with physicians acquiring various perks (such as membership in a hospital-funded social club) that do not show up as earned income. In either case, the hospital would show no accounting profit, but all the surplus would accrue to the physicians. A similar situation could easily be imagined in the case of a hospital owned by an administrator.

When the surplus is to be distributed to the consumers of hospital services, the transfer can be implemented by charging prices below cost or by offering nonmedical services in conjunction with the primary product. For example, such hospitals might provide care of a higher quality than is necessary, or ancillary services such as meals and entertainment. One problem that arises in this case (and in the previous two, but to a lesser extent) is that although the surplus is meant to be distributed implicitly to consumers, the design of mechanisms for achieving this distribution is usually delegated to a manager. If this manager has his or her own idea about what is valued by consumers—color televisions more than better medical equipment, for example—the distribution of the surplus is likely to be inefficient.

The question that naturally arises in cases like these is why would shareholders wish to receive transfers of surplus by these indirect means, rather than directly as owners? A simple answer in many countries is the tax system. Not-for-profit hospitals receive favorable tax treatment, not only on their economic profit, but also in their use of otherwise taxable inputs.[11]

---

11. Note that in most countries with advanced tax systems, if firms attempt to distribute profits indirectly, the tax authorities have ways of levying taxes on these distributions in lieu of the corporate profits tax.

Thus, the inefficiencies that can arise from indirect allocation of profits might be offset by the tax advantages.

Weisbrod (1975) has provided an alternative explanation for the emergence of not-for-profit hospitals (and other organizations) based on the theory of public goods. Suppose that the level of a publicly provided public good in a community is determined on the basis of the preferences of the median voter. In general, the level determined in this manner will be too large for those who do not greatly value the good, and too low for those with greater valuations. The latter group may cooperatively decide to provide themselves with additional services to better satisfy their personal objectives. To the extent that the economic surplus from such activities accrues indirectly to members of the group, as consumers of medical care, for example, the enterprise will appear to be operating on a not-for-profit basis.

There are alternative theories of the forces that motivate hospital decisions. Newhouse (1970) suggested that hospitals of any variety should be seen as maximizing some utility function defined over the quality and quantity of services provided. Unfortunately, it is difficult to explain any incentives for X-efficiency in such a model, unless one supposes that the hospital in question has a fixed budget (so internal efficiency is necessary to maximize output). But firms (apart from public hospitals, perhaps), unlike consumers, do not really have budget constraints in an economic sense, so to support internal cost control, hospitals must place some weight on minimizing costs.[12]

Pauly and Redisch's (1973) theory of hospitals as physicians' cooperatives bridged this gap and is consistent with the discussion above regarding the distribution of surplus to physician "shareholders." It is important to note that physicians may come to be effective shareholders in a hospital without making any kind of capital investment of their own. Because of their privileged possession of health-care-related information, they

---

12. That is to say, a utility-maximizing consumer's problem can be written in general as max $u(x)$ subject to a budget constraint $p.x \leq m$, where $u(.)$ is the utility function, x the vector of goods, p the vector of prices, and m income. A profit-maximizing firm's optimization problem is to max $p.y$ subject to a feasibility constraint $y \in Y$, where y is the vector of net outputs, and Y is the production set. The consumer's constraint fixes the available quantity of resources, while the firm's constraint fixes the feasible combinations of resources, but not necessarily the scale of production (see, for example, Mas-Collel, Whinston, and Green 1995, chapter 5).

may be in a position to dictate the transfer of surplus to themselves without the knowledge of hospital administrators. For example, they may claim that the hospital should fund expensive new technologies when such investments serve mainly to increase the physicians' prestige and outside employment options, or that attendance at overseas conferences (particularly to the other hemisphere during the winter) is vital for them to keep up with the latest surgical techniques.

Finally, Harris (1977) models hospitals as noncooperative organizations of physicians and administrators who bargain over the surplus they jointly create. (In Pauly's model, the physicians effectively have all the bargaining power.) This interpretation helps explain why the various inputs into a hospital's production tend not to be internally traded at "market-determined" prices, but that negotiations and rules of thumb govern the allocation of resources (this issue was first observed by Coase 1937 in discussing the nature of the firm). A significant difference between hospitals in many developing countries and those in more advanced economies is that explicit internal markets tend to be more prevalent in the former than in the latter. Patients are often required to supply their own food (and sometimes medicines), and doctors might pay their colleagues for medical supplies.

Measuring the Performance of Hospitals

A description of a hospital's costs and productivity requires output to be measured quantitatively. At a conceptual level, hospitals produce health, and the amount they produce depends on the number of patients they admit, the health status of the patients, and the inputs they use and how they use them. As noted above, if we assume there are J possible health statuses, we can think of the hospital as producing quantities of J different goods, the quantity of good j being equal to $n_j h_j$, where n_j is the number of individuals with health status θ_j, and h_j the amount of health improvement for each, or, alternatively, the health status of each individual upon discharge from the hospital. We might calibrate the model by assuming, for example, that an individual who fully recovers has health status at discharge equal to 1, and one who dies has health status at discharge equal to zero. In practice, the output of each good is often measured simply by the number of admissions of each condition.

When estimating total output of a hospital, we need to aggregate the goods that the hospital produces—the treatments of different types of illnesses and conditions—in a meaningful fashion. The usual way to do this is by weighting the outputs of each good by its average or, preferably, marginal cost. With this one-dimensional measure of output, we can ask questions about the existence of increasing, decreasing, or constant returns to scale. Hospitals are usually assumed to have increasing returns over some range, because they require certain capital equipment and buildings. As Phelps (1992) has pointed out, however, one necessary input into a hospital's production process is the patient, and if patients must travel a long distance to reach the hospital, total marginal costs may start to increase at some level. This may be particularly important in developing countries with poor transportation infrastructure. In addition, the unidimensional output measure, in principle, allows the estimation of improvements over time in productivity, while accounting for possible changes in the mix of patient conditions (the "case mix").

A substantial impediment to accurate cost and productivity estimation arises from the difficulties of measuring the quality of health care. Health status upon discharge can vary continuously from zero to one, so that the number of discharged patients is a very poor measure of the actual amount of health improvement generated by the hospital. A second dimension of quality is associated with the costs born by consumers in using the hospital facilities. Transport costs were mentioned above, but these costs also include waiting times, the pleasantness of the surroundings, the friendliness or compassion of medical staff, and the like (the last two are negative costs to the consumer). If these costs are not included in the estimation of hospital costs, measures of productivity will be biased.

In addition to admission rates, other practical measures of the outputs of hospitals include number of bed-days, costs of inputs used, and other input measures. The implicit assumption behind all of these measures is that there is a stable and monotonically increasing relationship between inputs and output, and if the first increases, so does the second. But increases in input levels coupled with inefficient use or poor management can easily lead to less than proportional output increases, or even to reductions in output. Thus, a hospital that increases the length of stay of patients may be providing more comprehensive treatment, and thus better-quality health care, in which case an inference of higher output would be valid. But longer hospital stays may also be the result of poor organization and staffing, and patients may spend most of their time waiting for physicians and supplies to turn up. Certainly, if input costs are used as a proxy for output, then productivity, as measured by the ratio of this output proxy to costs, will remain fixed at unity, independent of changes in the resource costs used in producing health improvements.

Medical Care Suppliers in the Market

A recurring question in health economics regards the ability of physicians to induce consumers to purchase more medical care than they otherwise would. If such forces exist, it is natural to hope that restricting the supply of doctors might reduce consumption. However, economists usually expect reductions in supply to increase prices. To fully understand these possibilities, it is necessary to examine the interaction of supply and demand.

Interactions of Demand and Supply—Standard Analysis

So far we have examined the nature of the production processes of medical care and the incentives suppliers face in determining the type and quantity of care provided and the inputs used. In particular, the influence of prices and other financial variables on supplier behavior was addressed. Abstracting from issues regarding the choice of inputs (that is, production techniques), it seems reasonable to suggest, as we did, that higher prices for physicians' services will lead to an increase in the quantity that physicians desire to supply. Although there will be offsetting income and substitution effects, we usually assume that the labor supply curve S_0 (measuring, for example, hours worked) is upward-sloping. In a free, competitive market, the observed equilibrium price, p_0, of medical services (or the hourly wage rate of physicians) is then determined by the intersection of the supply curve and the demand curve D_0, as in figure 6.1. Note that the supply curve here measures total hours of work by all physicians, and it can be thought of as the horizontal sum of individual supply curves for each physician. Thus, total services provided are $Q_0 = n_0 q_0$, where n_0 is the number of physicians and q_0 is the number of hours (or services) supplied by each. The income of each physician is $y_0 = p_0 q_0$.

While the relationship between the price received by physicians and the quantity they desire to provide, as described by the supply curve, is likely to be upward-sloping, we usually expect the relationship between the quantity actually supplied and the *equilibrium* price to be negative for a given demand curve. For example, suppose that the number of physicians in the marketplace increases (for example, because the government increases the number of places available at a public medical school or relaxes immigration controls for foreign doctors). There is no effect on the individual supply curves of physicians who were initially active in the market. However, the total supply curve is now the horizontal sum of a larger number of individual

Figure 6.1.   *Effects of an Increase in the Number of Physicians on Prices and Physician Incomes, Assuming Orthodox Demand and Supply Dynamics*

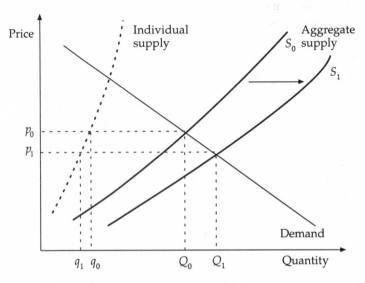

Source: Author.

supply curves because of the new entrants, and it shifts out to S_1, as shown in figure 6.1. The equilibrium price of health services has fallen to p_1.

What does this change imply about individual physicians' incomes? Assuming that each physician has the same individual supply curve, we see that the hourly rate has fallen (from p_0 to p_1), and the hours supplied by each physician have fallen from q_0 to q_1. Thus, individual incomes are reduced to $y_1 = p_1 q_1 < y_0$. Under the assumption that demand is relatively elastic, however, the total amount of health care expenditure increases from $e_0 = n_0 y_0$ to $e_1 = n_1 y_1$. The combined effects of the increase in supply are then reductions in the unit price ($p_0 \downarrow p_1$), the number of hours each physician supplies ($q_0 \downarrow q_1$), and physicians' personal incomes ($y_0 \downarrow y_1$); however, total services provided ($Q_0 \uparrow Q_1$) and total expenditure on physician services ($e_0 \uparrow e_1$) increase.

In practice, this kind of negative relationship between equilibrium prices and quantities does not always obtain in medical care markets. One example is the relative supply of physician services in urban and rural areas. As discussed earlier, there may be many reasons that physicians prefer to practice in cities rather than rural areas, including better facilities, greater access to consumption goods, and so forth. Suppose that over time the rural and urban populations remain more or less constant, but that the supply of physicians steadily increases. If all the physicians locate in the cities, the analysis above suggests that average physician incomes will fall in cities (as the supply curve shifts out) relative to those in rural areas. At some point, we expect that the real incomes that can be earned in rural areas would become sufficiently higher than those in urban areas that physicians would begin to migrate to the countryside. In practice, however, such equilibrating movements are seldom seen, and physician incomes appear, if anything, to *increase* in urban areas.

This raises at least two interesting issues. First, what economic mechanisms are at work that allow such a counterintuitive relationship between equilibrium prices and quantities to be sustained? And second, what does such a phenomenon imply for the effectiveness of prices in reallocating supply (to rural areas, for example)?

Supplier-Induced Demand

The market analysis above assumed that the demand curve did not change when the supply curve shifted. This is a very orthodox assumption in microeconomic theory, the demand curve being the derived relationship between price and desired consumption, taking preferences (including health status), prices, and incomes as fixed. The behavior of suppliers, in particular, influences the *equilibrium* price and quantity consumed but not the demand curve. As we saw earlier in the chapter, in the case of health care, consumers rely on physicians for at least two qualitatively different kinds of service: the provision of information and the execution of care. The information provided can relate to the effects of certain treatments, their likelihood of success, possible side effects and other risks associated with them, and the effect of having no treatment. Given this information, individuals make better-informed choices about the type and quantity of care they desire.

The trouble is, of course, that individuals have little opportunity to verify the information provided, and when the providers of the information stand to gain from providing misleading information, it is unlikely that correct information will be forthcoming. Thus, if the provider of information is the same person as the provider of medical services (which is often the case), individuals may be induced to consume more than they would if they had access to purely objective information. The position of the demand curve might thus be affected by the supplier of services.

This possibility does not answer our question about the way in which a positive relationship between equilibrium prices and supply may arise. Indeed, if physicians can influence demand, why do they not push the demand curve out indefinitely and earn higher and higher incomes? There must be some force that restrains suppliers from acting in such a fashion. One possibility is that physicians feel guilt from effectively "fooling" patients into having more treatment than is necessary, and this disutility acts as a constraint on the extent of induced demand (see McQuire and Pauly 1991).

An alternative, and perhaps more natural, constraint on the ability of physicians to induce demand is competition. Overservicing imposes some costs on individuals (even if they are fully insured against the financial costs of care), and if one physician is found to continually overservice, that individual will lose patients to other physicians. In a perfectly competitive market, this mechanism would restrain the ability of physicians to overservice completely, and they would provide correct information. It is generally acknowledged, however, that the market for physician services is better described as monopolistically competitive (see Hart 1985) because of consumer search and switching costs. Thus, each supplier exercises a degree of monopoly power over his or her own patients, who incur additional costs if they switch to other doctors. These costs include the time it takes to find a new doctor with whom the patient feels comfortable, the uncertainty about the quality of a new doctor, and the additional visits, if any, that are required for the new doctor to establish the patient's medical history and condition.[13]

Given such local monopoly power, physicians will be able to exercise a degree of demand inducement. The observed positive relationship between equilibrium price and quantity can then be rationalized by assuming that when faced with an increase in the number of physicians, and thus an outward shift in the supply curve, each physician increases the amount of demand inducement he or she exercises. The effect is to shift the demand curve out to D_1 in figure 6.2. At the new equilibrium—the intersection of D_1 and S_1—the price is p_2 and the total quantity is Q_2. Personal income of each physician is $y_2 = p_2 q_2 > y_1 = p_1 q_1$.

---

13. For an application in the context of physician supply, see Satterthwaite (1985). Other models of partial market power along these lines are spatial models of product differentiation (Salop 1979). In such models, suppliers are located at regular intervals on, and consumers are distributed uniformly around, a circle. Consumers

Figure 6.2.   *Supplier-Induced Demand*

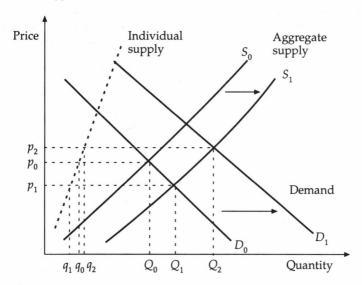

For this story to hold water, there must be some reason that the increase in supply has made it either more profitable or, alternatively, less costly for each physician to induce additional demand. One hypothesis is that physicians have a "target income," and that when they see their income fall to y_1 with the initial increase in supply, they try to retain their previous income level of y_0 by inducing demand. This is not particularly compelling, however, because the question immediately arises as to why the physician would have been satisfied with an income y_0 at the initial equilibrium. It would also imply that, faced with an increase in income following a fall in aggregate supply, physicians would reduce overservicing in order to reattain the lower income level.[14, 15]

---

incur travel costs that increase with the distance from their supplier. These costs, which can be interpreted as generalized switching costs, give each supplier a limited amount of market power over consumers that are "close" to it. See Tirole (1988) for a full treatment of this subject.

14. It is important to remember that we are discussing the relationship between *equilibrium* prices and quantities.

15. A somewhat more sophisticated version of the target income hypothesis might argue that the medical profession, as a relatively close-knit community with

Two more plausible explanations for the posited change in the level of inducement when the supply curve shifts out relate to possible changes in the level of competition and changes in opportunity costs. First, suppose that one of the switching costs that individuals incur in changing physicians is that they are uncertain about the quality of their new physician. They must gather information about each potential choice and make a decision based on this information. Suppose also that as the number of physicians increases so does the variance of their quality. In this case, individuals will have to consider relatively more physicians before they are confident a "good one" has been found. These higher search costs increase the monopoly power that each physician can exercise over patients, and the physician may be able to induce a higher level of demand. While the number of patients will fall in proportion to the increase in the number of physicians, this may be at least partially offset by an increase in the intensity of the treatment of the remaining patients.

The second mechanism that might increase demand inducement following an increase in supply relates to the extent of the loss a physician experiences when a patient leaves the practice because of overservicing. The initial increase in supply leads to a fall in unit price. Under our assumption of relatively inelastic demand, this will lead to an increase in the demand by each patient, but to a *reduction* in the amount of the expenditures. Therefore, the revenue that the physician earns from each patient falls, and the opportunity cost of losing a patient because of overservicing also falls. That is, the "price" of overservicing falls, so we expect more of it. Of course, such a partial equilibrium argument only holds if incomes and other variables are fixed, and we know that the physician's income has fallen because of the reduction in the number of patients, as well as the reduction in revenue per patient. However, the price or substitution effect points in the direction of increased inducement following an outward shift in the supply curve (see Dranove 1988 for a model).

From the equivocal discussion above, it should not be a surprise that health economists are divided regarding the existence of, and underlying mechanisms behind, induced demand. There are many studies that attempt to empirically document the existence of the phenomenon, with mixed success.[16]

---

various associations and networks, may have considerable political power, which it can use to maintain the incomes of its members. Again, this begs the question of how the particular targets are chosen, but within a political economy framework it is possible that such targets are more defensible.

16. Fuchs (1978) is the most widely cited empirical paper supporting the supplier-induced demand hypothesis. Also see Richardson (1998) for a review,

Some Policy Issues

What does the preceding discussion imply about the use of prices and quantities in allocating resources? Suppose the government wishes to attract physicians to rural areas, and it does so by paying rural doctors sufficiently more than those in urban areas. One way to do this might be to put a tax on urban doctors. This price reduction has a similar effect to an increase in the supply of physicians, and it could lead to demand inducement that increases incomes enough to make the initial tax ineffective in motivating physicians to move to the countryside. To effect a net migration, the government may have to increase rural physician wages by a much larger amount, which could be costly for the budget and politically untenable. Direct regulation of the supply of physicians—by mandating that all new graduates spend a certain number of years in rural communities, for example—might have some advantages, although this may well affect the number and quality of medical students.[17]

Alternatively, the government may wish to control the level of medical expenditure, especially if much of this is financed from its budget. From a normative point of view, such a desire must be based on the assumption that at the margin, the value of the services provided (measured by the consumer price) is less than their social opportunity cost. Suppose that the government can set physician wages independently of the price consumers pay for physician visits, and that to control public expenditures, it lowers such wages. In the standard model of market dynamics, this will lead to a reduction in supply, and in the case of fixed consumer prices, excess demand. Public expenditure will fall, as will the level of consumption (consistent with the normative objective).

Suppose, however, that physicians are paid by the visit, and (for illustrative purposes) that the price initially paid by consumers is equal to that paid to physicians. In this case, demand and supply curves are functions of the number of physician consultations, and the equilibrium is at price p_0 and quantity q_0, as shown in figure 6.3. Physicians' income is equal to the rectangular area $A + B + D$. If the government reduces the fee paid to physicians for

and Ramsey and Wassow (1986). Phelps (1992, footnote 12, p. 211) contains a long list of references.

17. It is arguable that the effect on the type of medical student might be positive, because those who enter the profession only for financial reward will be deterred relative to those who have more altruistic and noble aspirations. As always, these arguments are difficult to quantify economically.

Figure 6.3.   *Supply and Demand Responses to Change in the Fee Paid to Physicians Per Consultation*

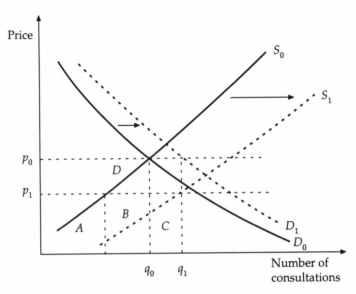

Source: Author.

each visit to p_1, one possible response is that they will reduce the length of time of each visit (or some other input, such as effort). Under the assumption that the original supply curve, representing physicians' supply of hours worked, does not move, the supply of patient consultations will shift out to S_1, as in figure 6.3. That is, if the horizontal axis measures the number of patient visits, then by reducing the input of time or effort for each consultation, the physician lowers the (marginal) cost of each visit, and thus is willing to supply more visits at any given price.

This strategy offsets some of the income loss that would otherwise occur, assuming that the demand for physician services does not fall, assuming the consumer price is held fixed at p_0, so demand continues to be q_0, and income is equal to area $A + B$, instead of area A, as it would be if there were no supply response. Such an assumption about demand not responding to the length of visit (or more generally, the quality of care) requires that physicians are able to exercise some inducement. But they can do even better: by engaging in still further inducement, not only can they stop the demand curve from moving in, but they can also shift it out from its initial position, to D_1, increasing their income to area $A + B + C$.

Notice that the effect of the policy to reduce physicians' fees has been to increase the number of visits and to have an indeterminate impact on total government expenditures (that is, physicians' pay). Public expenditures may actually increase, and they are certainly unlikely to fall in proportion to the fee reduction. The welfare impact of the increase in visits is also unclear. The objective was to reduce the use of medical services, suggesting that the welfare impact of the increase is negative. However, adjusted for quality, real resources per visit have fallen, so total resources dedicated to medical care may have fallen as well.

This brief discussion suggests that the effects of price interventions in medical care markets may differ from those cited in textbook models of supply and demand. An underlying problem is that actions of physicians and other providers are difficult to regulate, because quality and on-the-job effort (including just showing up for work) may be difficult to monitor. This is a theme we shall return to in further discussions of market intervention and the organization of medical care systems, and derives from the notorious difficulty of measuring output, the improvement in the health of patients. Because output cannot easily be measured and specified in a contract, payments are made on the basis of inputs, and this introduces myriad opportunities for suppliers of services, given their privileged access to information, to distort the allocation of resources.

Manpower Planning

The policy issues addressed in the previous subsection represent issues in what has become known in the health economics literature as the area of *manpower planning*. Such a label is suggestive of a central planning approach to the allocation of resources in the health sector and derives from the tendency of governments to be big players in health delivery markets. We will have more to say about government intervention in the following chapters, but it is natural to address some topics in medical labor markets here.

The central concern of manpower planning is the allocation of human resources (labor) in the health sector. Questions include the correct number of doctors, the optimal mix of doctors and nurses, and the relationships these variables should have to the size and demographic structure of the population. When the allocations of labor resources are not at their desired levels, shortages or excess supply will be observed and corrected using either price or quantity instruments, as described above. It is useful to first review some standard administrative measures of labor allocations, and then to compare these with economic measures of shortages and their alleviation.

Conventional Measures of Labor Allocations

Because the output of medical care is difficult to measure, the adequacy of physicians and other labor supplies are measured directly. The most common measure is the physician-population ratio. The assumption that underlies the use of this measure is that a certain number of physicians is required to deliver appropriate medical care and, more specifically, that the number is proportional to the size of the population. We expect the number of physicians required to deliver a given standard of care to increase with the population, but strict proportionality is only necessary when the production of care (or improved health) exhibits constant returns to scale. To the extent that physicians provide advice to other health care providers, there may well be decreasing returns to scale. For example, if a physician's main function is to provide information to nurses and other practitioners, this output is a public good, and having two physicians produce the good does not increase total output proportionately. We may then expect to observe an increasing but concave relationship between the size of the population and the number of physicians required to deliver a given quantity of care, as shown in figure 6.4. Such a relationship would imply that the optimal physician-population ratio falls as population size increases.

Conversely, on the demand side, as population size increases, it is possible that the health needs of each person increase—because of crowding in urban areas, for example. To attain a given quality of health outcomes, the quantity of medical care inputs may need to increase more than proportionately with population, implying a convex relationship and an increasing physician-population ratio.

Even with a population of fixed size, the appropriate number of physicians may vary according to their productivity. Again, it is necessary to recall that we are interested in the output of medical care—improved health—and that some populations may require larger medical care inputs, including physician services, to achieve a given output level. The obvious example is an aging population: as populations age, their health needs tend to become more acute, and the medical care inputs required to attain a given level of health increase. Again, aiming for a fixed proportion of physicians to population size is unlikely to be optimal, unless the population is adjusted for its demographic composition.

A more detailed approach to manpower planning would integrate other factors of production, such as nonphysician labor, material inputs, drugs,

Figure 6.4. *Nonlinear Relationships between Population Size and the Number of Physicians Required to Deliver a Given Level of Care*

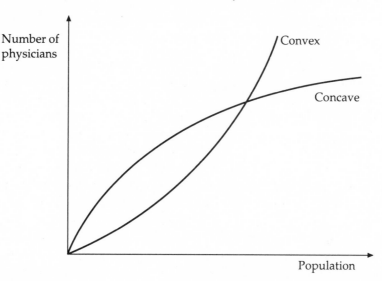

Source: Author.

and the like. From the above example, however, it is clear that assigning inputs on the basis of fixed proportions, independent of population size and structure, is unlikely to be optimal.[18]

Economic Measures of Shortages

Using administrative measures such as the physician-population ratio above, it is possible to identify "shortages" in factor markets. One way an economist would measure a shortage is in the excess of demand over supply. Such shortages can only arise when prices do not adjust to equilibrate the market. The most common example of such disequilibrium in the labor market, however, is one of excess supply—that is, unemployment—that arises when wages do not fall low enough. In some cases, however, if governments control physician wages at low levels, the market will exhibit excess demand. These two possibilities are shown in figure 6.5.

It is important to note that equality of demand and supply—that is, the absence of shortages or excess supplies—does not necessarily mean that

---

18. Such an approach implicitly assumes a Leontief health production function—that is, one in which there is no substitutability among the factors.

Figure 6.5.　*Shortages and Oversupply*

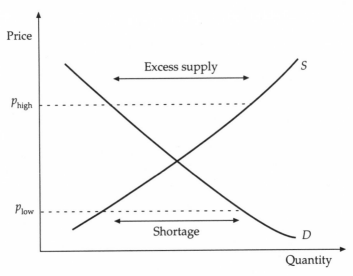

Note: Shortages exist when prices are low and there is excess demand for physican services. Excess supply is characterized by prices that are too high.
　　Source: Author.

the quantity of services or physicians is socially optimal. For example, if the prices paid by consumers are lower than those paid to providers, it is possible that demand equals supply, but that the quantity of services is above its optimal level. Such a situation is shown in figure 6.6, and it may occur as a result of the subsidization of medical training (which increases the effective wage) and the existence of insurance (which reduces the consumer's price of care). If the market is competitive, the optimal allocation of physicians is q^*. A complete analysis of the appropriate quantity of physician services would require a thorough treatment of failures of other markets, including capital and insurance markets, that lead to the subsidies implicit in figure 6.6.

Note that the natural response to a shortage like that in figure 6.5 is to expand the supply of physicians, shifting out the supply curve. Under the assumption that demand is independent of supply, this expansion will remove the shortage at the given price. In the presence of supplier-induced demand, however, such an expansion of supply may lead to an outward shift in the demand curve of the same magnitude, and the observed shortage would not be affected. Increasing the price paid to providers would

Figure 6.6.   *The Inefficiency of Excess Supply*

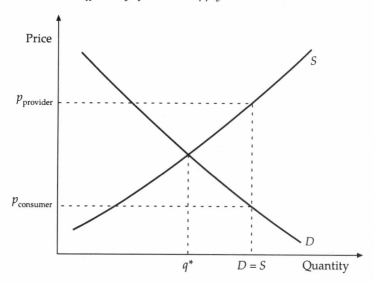

Note: Even when demand is equal to supply, if demand and supply prices are not equal, it is unlikely that the observed quantity of services is optimal.
Source: Author.

not have such a demand-inducement effect, and indeed, could lead to negative demand inducement, or a contraction of demand. This suggests that if demand inducement is significant, prices may be more effective in ameliorating shortages than quantity instruments.

References

Bardhan, Pranab. 1997. "Corruption and Development: A Review of Issues." *Journal of Economic Literature* 35(3): 1320–46.

Barnum and Kutzin. 1993. *Public Hospitals in Developing Countries.* Washington, D.C.: World Bank.

Basmann, R., and G. Rhodes. 1986. *Advances in Econometrics,* 5. Greenwich, Connecticut: JAI Press.

Bigsten, Arne, and Karl-Ove Moene. 1996. "Growth and Rent Dissipation: The Case of Kenya." *Journal of African Economies* 5(2): 177–98.

Coase, Ronald. 1937. "The Nature of the Firm." *Economica* 4: 386–405.

Dranove, David. 1988. "Demand Inducement and the Physician/Patient Relationship." *Economic Inquiry* 26(2): 281–98.

Frack, S. A., S. I. Woodruff, J. Candelaria, and J. P. Elder. 1997. "Correlates of Compliance with Measurement Protocols in a Latino Nutrition Intervention Study." *American Journal of Preventive Medicine* 13(2): 131–36.

Fuchs, Victor R. 1978. "The Supply of Surgeons and the Demand for Operations." *Journal of Human Resources* 13(Suppl): 35–56.

Harris, Jeffrey E. 1977. "The Internal Organization of Hospitals: Some Economic Implications." *Bell Journal of Economics* 8: 467–82.

Hart, Oliver. 1985. "Monopolistic Competition in the Spirit of Chamberlin: A General Model." *Review of Economic Studies* 52: 529–46.

Inman, R. P., ed. 1985. *Managing the Service Economy.* Cambridge, U.K.: Cambridge University Press.

Mas-Collel, Andrew, Michael Whinston, and Jerry Green. 1995. *Microeconomic Theory.* New York: Oxford University Press.

Mauro, Paolo. 1995. "Corruption and Growth." *Quarterly Journal of Economics* 110(3): 681–712.

McQuire, Thomas G., and Mark V. Pauly. 1991. "Physician Response to Fee Changes with Multiple Payers." *Journal of Health Economics* 10(4): 385–410.

Newhouse, Joseph. 1970. "Towards a Theory of Nonprofit Institutions: An Economic Model of a Hospital." *American Economic Review* 60: 64–74.

Pauly, Mark, and Michael Redisch. 1973. "The Not-for-Profit Hospital as a Physician's Cooperative." *American Economic Review* 63: 87–100.

Phelps, Edmund S., ed. 1975. *Altruism, Morality, and Economic Theory.* New York: Russell Sage Foundation.

Phelps, Charles E. 1992. *Health Economics.* New York: HarperCollins.

Ramsey, J. B., and B. Wassow. 1986. "Supplier Induced Demand for Physician Services: Theoretical Anomaly or Statistical Artifact? An Econometric Evaluation of Some Important Models in Physician Services Markets." In R. Basmann and G. Rhodes, eds., *Advances in Econometrics.* Greenwich, Connecticut: JAI Press.

Richardson, Jeff. 1998. "Supplier Induced Demand Reconsidered." Paper presented to the 20th Annual Conference of the Health Economics Society of Australia, Sydney, July.

Salop, Steven. 1979. "Monopolistic Competition with Outside Goods." *Bell Journal of Economics* 10: 141–56.

Satterthwaite, Mark A. 1985. "Competition and Equilibrium as a Driving Force in the Health Services Sector." In R. P. Inman, ed., *Managing the Service Economy.* Cambridge, U.K.: Cambridge University Press.

Tirole, Jean. 1988. *The Theory of Industrial Organization.* Cambridge, Massachusetts: MIT Press.

van der Gaag, Jacques, Morton Stelcner, and William Vijverberg. 1989. "Wage Differentials and Moonlighting by Civil Servants: Evidence from Côte d'Ivoire and Peru." *World Bank Economic Review* 3(1): 67–95.

Weisbrod, Burton. 1975. "Towards a Theory of the Voluntary Non-Profit Sector in a Three Sector Economy." In Edmund Phelps, ed., *Altruism, Morality, and Economic Theory.* New York: Russell Sage Foundation.

World Bank. 1994. *Better Health in Africa.* Development in Practice Series. Washington, D.C.

Part III

Normative Analysis for Health Policy and Projects

7

Market Failure and Public Intervention

In this chapter we examine the role of government in the health care sector. Based on the analysis of the preceding chapters, we can identify resource allocations that are likely to be suboptimal, in a social sense, and whose distribution might be improved by government intervention. One underlying and important assumption of the chapter is that the government behaves in a responsible fashion—that is, it does not waste resources and it allocates them in a socially desirable way. This assumption is often not met in many countries where institutional capacity is weak or corruption rife. Such issues of government failure, particularly as they impact on the health sector, will be touched upon in subsequent chapters, although a comprehensive analysis of political economy is beyond the scope of this text.

An important theme of the chapter is that government intervention should be used to correct observed inadequacies of the private market and not to replicate private sector actions where these are satisfactory. Government intervention may be viewed as taking two forms. The first and somewhat indirect intervention can be described as serving an "enabling function," in which the government adjusts the environment in which private economic agents make decisions. This may occur through the introduction of taxes and subsidies that alter private incentives or through other forms of regulation of individual activity. The second and more direct kind of intervention is characterized by public provision of resources that are not provided at correct levels by the private sector.

Before we can properly examine the alternative instruments available to the government, it is necessary to establish normative guidelines that help us measure the goodness of different resource allocations. This is done briefly in the next section (for a more complete discussion, see chapter 8).

Social Objectives

It is common to judge the desirability of alternative resource allocations by their efficiency and equity. We will discuss in much greater depth the meaning of these concepts and their operationalization in chapter 8, but for now it is sufficient to give relatively informal definitions. In simple terms, we will say that resources are used and allocated efficiently if there is no waste. Efficiency would appear to be a reasonably uncontroversial social objective, because if a particular pattern of resource use were inefficient, the wasted resources could be used to make at least some people better-off.

Two types of efficiency are sometimes identified, depending on the economic activity under consideration. If we are examining the use of a fixed quantity of resources in producing a collection of outputs, we say that the production process is technically efficient if it is not possible to rearrange the way the in which the inputs are combined in order to produce more of some of the outputs, and not less of the others. When just one output is being produced, it is not possible to use the inputs in a different way that increases the level of output. Equivalently, the use of resources is efficient if reducing the quantities of any of the inputs reduces the amount of output. For example, we considered in chapter 6 the production of medical services using physician time, nursing staff, drugs, and other inputs. Some allocations of these inputs can be used to produce given levels of health improvement more efficiently than others.

The second type of efficiency incorporates not only the production of goods (and services), but also their distribution among individuals. We say that a resource allocation is allocatively efficient if it is not possible to redistribute the available resources in a way that makes at least some people better-off without making others worse-off. Notice that a change from an allocatively inefficient use of resources to an allocatively efficient use may make some individuals worse-off. The requirement is that from the new arrangement of resource use, it should be possible, in principle, to compensate those who were made worse-off, while maintaining the winners at a level of well-being greater than their initial level.

The simplest illustration of the concept of allocative efficiency is the division of a fixed quantity of a good between two individuals, labeled $i = 1, 2$. Suppose there is an amount Q of the good available, and individual i's consumption is q_i, with $\Sigma q_i = Q$. The marginal benefit schedule of individual i is denoted MB_i, and it is assumed to be downward-sloping. These schedules are shown in figure 7.1, with q_1 measured from the left-hand side, and q_2 from the right. The allocatively efficient distribution (q_1, q_2) is the one that

Figure 7.1. *Allocative Efficiency When a Fixed Quantity of a Good Is to Be Divided between Two Individuals*

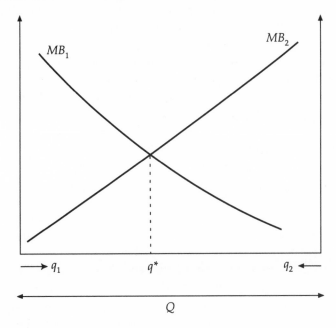

Source: Author.

maximizes total benefits, which in turn is characterized by the point where the marginal benefit curves cross. Any move away from this allocation would increase the benefit of one individual less than it would decrease that of the other, and there is no possible redistribution that will leave both individuals at least as well-off as they were before the move.

We will examine examples of resource use in the health sector that exhibit productive and allocative inefficiencies. Thus, there is likely to be a role for some government intervention at both the production stage (in the organization of hospitals, the accreditation of physicians, and the like) and at the consumption stage (use of preventive care, smoking habits, and so forth).

In addition to the objectives of technical and allocative efficiency, societies usually have preferences regarding the equity of the distribution of resources. An inequitable but efficient distribution of resources may not be desirable or politically sustainable. A particular manifestation of a preference for equitable resource allocation in the health sector is the often-expressed view that health care should be available to all. In practice it may be difficult to determine what constitutes equal availability of health resources if individuals' needs differ (because of different living environments, occupations, and so on), if the quality of services differ (for example, because of differences in physician training), and if access costs differ (for rural versus urban dwellers, for example). In addition, if the general distribution of income is very uneven, an equal distribution of health care may not be the most effective way of improving the well-being of the poor. For example, equal provision of high-quality medical equipment may be valued much less by poor urban laborers than general income transfers. Nonetheless, equal access to health care and health insurance has been a stated goal of governments in both past and current reform strategies.

Market Failures

In this section we examine three situations in which resource allocations produced in private markets are likely to be inefficient.[1] Such situations are routinely referred to as market failures, in the sense that the existing markets do not deliver socially desirable outcomes. In fact, the inefficiencies can be attributed to the absence of certain markets, suggesting the importance of these complementary markets. Given the market failure, an interventionist approach might be to rely on public action in the actual production and delivery of the good or service in question—that is, to replace the existing market—while a more market-friendly approach may be to facilitate the creation and improvement of the missing complementary markets. Which of these interventions is more suitable depends on the nature of the market failure and the institutional capacity of the government.

Externalities

Sometimes the production or consumption activities of an individual directly affect the well-being of others. The classic example of a production externality is that of a factory discharging an effluent into a river as a by-product, which subsequently reduces the quality of water used by a downstream producer (such as a fisherman). One of the effects of the factory's

---

1. One market imperfection that we do not address in detail is that of uncompetitive behavior on the part of firms. We touched on issues of monopoly power in discussing incentives for research and innovation in drug markets, and we dealt with imperfect competition in the market for physician services in chapter 6.

actions—the reduction in the profitability of the fisherman—is external to it. This negative effect is not taken into account when the factory owners choose how much to produce, and thus how much to pollute, and the factory is likely to pollute too much. By too much, we mean that the total value of the joint output of the factory and the fisherman could be increased if the factory produced less, enabling the fisherman to produce relatively more.

Note that this argument does not suggest that the efficient level of pollution by the upstream factory is zero. Indeed, this is unlikely to be the case, because the marginal cost of the first small amount of pollution in reduced output of the fisherman is likely to be small, while the marginal benefit from associated factory production may be large. The optimal level of discharge is shown at point y_0 in figure 7.2, where effluent discharge is measured along the horizontal axis. The marginal benefits to the factory of increased discharge (in greater profits) are shown as declining, *MB*, while the marginal cost to the fisherman is shown as an increasing function, *MC*. When the factory is allowed to pollute as much as it wishes, the outcome is a discharge level of y_1. Reducing effluent levels by an amount dy below this level will

Figure 7.2.   *Optimal Effluent Discharges Trade Off the Benefits of Production and the Costs of Pollution*

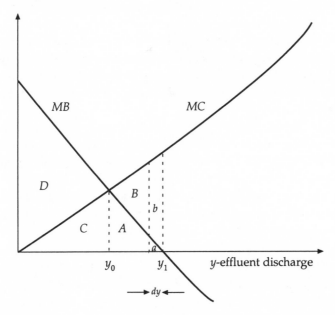

Source: Author.

reduce profits by an amount equal to the area a. However, such a reduction will reduce the costs imposed on the downstream fisherman by an amount equal to the area $a + b$, so that the net benefit is positive. Further reductions in effluent discharge continue to have net positive effects until the level y_0 is reached. Additional reductions beyond this point would hurt the profits of the factory more than they would increase the benefits to the fisherman.

The allocation y_0 is allocatively efficient; it maximizes the sum of the profits of the factory and the fisherman. Compared with a position of excessive pollution y_1, the fisherman gains an amount $A + B$, and the factory suffers a loss equal to the area A, so the net gain from reducing the discharge to y_0 is B. Alternatively, compared with the position of zero effluent, the factory makes profits equal to the area $C + D$, while the fisherman suffers a loss equal to the area C, and the net gain from increasing emissions is equal to D.

The size of the gain and the distribution of the gains and losses depend on the initial starting point, particularly on the initial distribution of property rights. If the factory owns the right to discharge effluents, the initial discharge is y_1, and reduction to y_0 hurts the factory and benefits the fisherman. It is more convenient to think of the factory owning the rights to clean water, and it uses these rights by discharging effluents into the river. If, instead, the initial rights to clean water are owned by the fisherman, the efficient amount of pollution leads him to suffer a loss, and the factory owners are made better-off.

Note that above we assumed that the government could implement the desired emission level, y_0, and was then only concerned about the distribution of gains and losses. In the next subsection we will address the instruments that the government might use to induce economic agents to choose efficient allocations.

It should be noted at this point that some important assumptions underlie the simple argument above. First, it has been implicitly assumed that a schilling of profits earned by the factory owners is worth as much (in terms of social value) as a schilling earned by the fisherman. When this is the case, we can easily add positive benefits and negative costs to arrive at net social benefits, which are maximized at y_0. But what if the owners of the factory are rich, and the fisherman is poor? Should we still weight the factory profits equally with the fisherman's? Or what if the factory is owned by a multinational corporation? Should a government take such issues into consideration when deciding on the optimal level of effluent?

The answer to these questions depends on whether the government can easily redistribute income. For example, if redistribution is costless (in administrative and other costs), the optimal level of discharge is y_0, independent of how the welfare of factory owners and fishermen is weighted. The reason is simply that when the level of discharge is y_0, the "size of the pie" (aggregate resources) is maximized, and under the assumption of costless redistribution, these resources can be used as the government wishes. For example, starting from a position of zero emissions, the government may wish to implement the optimal level, y_0, but to compensate the fisherman for his loss by transferring an amount C from the factory to him, leaving the factory owner better-off by the amount D.

When redistribution is costly, however, y_0 may no longer be the socially most desirable discharge level. Suppose the government has an ineffective and costly tax system, so that taxing the profits of firms (in particular the factory) produces little revenue and distorts the decisions of factory owners and other economic agents. As an extreme example, suppose that it is impossible to transfer income from the factory owners to the fisherman (because all revenue collected in taxes ends up in the hands of corrupt officials, for example). In this case, allowing emissions of y_0 and taxing the factory an amount C results in net benefits of D to the factory, but none of the cost to the fisherman is offset, and he still suffers a loss equal to area C. The government may well choose to ban emissions entirely in this case, if it reasons that the increase in profits of the factory is not large enough to offset the reduction in well-being of the fisherman.

This example is extremely important, because it illustrates how constraints on the instruments and policies available to a government can influence normative choices. Here, if a pie cannot be divided costlessly, it is no longer necessarily true that the government should aim to maximize its size. The example illustrates, albeit informally and incompletely, the tradeoff between efficiency (the size of the pie) and equity (its distribution).

Externalities in Health and Health Care

The example above is illustrative of the general nature of externalities, which lead to situations in which the level of resource use is inefficient. We will now examine four examples of externalities more closely related to health and health care. The first deals with the potential negative effects of smoking by some on the health of others and is qualitatively similar to the example of a polluting factory. The second relates more directly to the use of health care and examines possible failures in the market for immunizations. In this example, it is the *lack* of action (not being immunized) rather than the action itself that imposes a cost on other individuals. The third example is of preventive care and its possible underconsumption, and the last example relates to the possible overconsumption of antibiotics.

SMOKING. Secondhand smoke (that produced by smokers) can cause discomfort and more serious long-term health problems for individuals, both those who do not smoke and those who do. One way to model the effects of smoking simply is to assume that the extent of discomfort or damage suffered by a nonsmoker is positively related to the number of individuals who smoke, so that this becomes the variable that corresponds to the "effluent discharge" of the previous model. Now label individuals in the population by $i = 1, ..., I$, and let us assume that individual i places a value v_i on being allowed to smoke. There will be some individuals in the population who gain great satisfaction from smoking, so their values of v_i will be relatively high. Other individuals will enjoy smoking to some degree, but they do not put such a high value on it. Finally, v_i can be negative for those who would choose not to smoke. Now, if we order individuals according to the strength of their preference for smoking, with $v_i > v_j$ if and only if $i < j$, then the graph of v_i follows *MB* in figure 7.3. This graph represents the marginal benefit enjoyed when an additional person smokes. The person located at $i = i_0$ has a zero value of smoking and can be thought of as indifferent between smoking and not smoking.

On the cost side, we assume that everyone—smokers and nonsmokers alike—suffers from secondhand smoke. This assumption is probably qualitatively valid, although it is likely to be inaccurate on a person-by-person level. The extent of discomfort or damage is likely to differ for smokers and nonsmokers, but for now we will leave this issue to one side. In general, we expect that damage to individuals will increase with the amount of secondhand smoke, which is proportional to the number of smokers, and that the marginal impact of increases in the level of secondhand smoke will be increasing. The marginal cost per person, multiplied by the size of the population, gives the marginal social cost, *MC*, of additional smokers, as shown in figure 7.3.

It is clear from the figure that the efficient number of smokers is given by i^*. But efficiency requires not only that this number of people smoke, but that the identities of those who smoke coincide with those of the i^* individuals who value smoking most. The total gross benefits that accrue to smokers are represented by the area $A + B$, and the total cost of smoking suffered by all individuals is equal to area A (and the per capita cost is A/I).

As before, if the government has full control over the distribution of income, it should implement the efficient level of smoking (i^*) and redistribute

Figure 7.3.   *Marginal Benefits and Costs of Cigarette Smoking and the Determination of the Optimal Level of Cigarette Consumption*

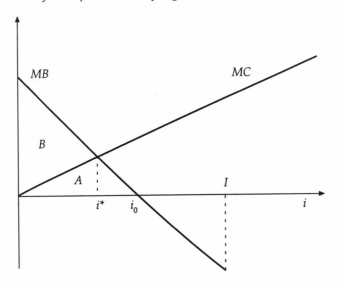

Source: Author.

income *ex post*, if it so desires. This may require, for example, that the government be able to identify (costlessly) individuals who would have smoked but have values of smoking that lie between v_i and zero, or that it identify those who suffer most from positive levels of smoking (although in this model, we have assumed for simplicity that all individuals suffer the same negative effects from secondhand smoke). When such identifications are costly or impossible, it may be second-best optimal for the government either to allow anyone to smoke who wants to or to ban it entirely.

Clearly an aspect of the real world that is missing from this model is that the effects of smoking are relatively location-specific. This suggests that the policy instruments available to the government may be significantly more elaborate, and that restrictions on smoking in certain places and at certain times would be preferred to blanket bans or unregulated consumption.

IMMUNIZATION. There are two types of benefits associated with an individual being immunized. First, the chance of the immunized person contracting the particular disease is reduced, sometimes to zero. This is clearly beneficial to the individual concerned. But if the chance of contracting the disease is related to the number of people carrying it, then by becoming immunized, an individual reduces the chance that other people will become ill. While the individual might care about the well-being of others to some extent, it is usually assumed that she will not consider the benefits that accrue to others because of her actions—the external benefits—when deciding whether to incur the costs associated with immunization (travel to the clinic, pain, side effects, and so on). Because these external benefits are not fully weighted, it is likely that the extent of immunization in the population will be less than optimal. Thus, the "consumption" of immunizations will be inefficiently low. (A full analysis of the allocation of immunization resources is presented in the section "Immunization—An Example of an Externality.")

PREVENTIVE CARE. Individuals may consume too little preventive care if they have to pay for it and if it is impossible for society to withhold expensive curative care from them later, even if they cannot pay for it. In this case, there is an externality associated with the consumption of preventive care, because such consumption lowers the costs that are imposed on those who provide or finance future curative care. If society could credibly commit to withholding curative care from those who had not properly undertaken preventive actions, then the incentive to underconsume preventive care would be removed. In the absence of such credible commitment, however, an externality exists.[2]

ANTIBIOTICS. The discovery of penicillin as an antibacterial agent led to a sudden improvement in the ability of medical science to successfully combat disease. Since then, the development of further antibiotic drugs has widened the variety of diseases that can be treated with such agents, which have become relatively cheap. However, associated with the widespread use of antibiotics is the ability of some organisms through natural mutations to develop resistance to drugs if the drugs are used excessively. When some antibiotics become widely used, their effectiveness in controlling particular diseases can be compromised by the generation of new strains of bacteria, which in turn require suitably adapted drugs for their control. The result of such a process can be either that the new drugs are more

---

2. It should not be understood from this statement that the inability of society to make such a commitment is a bad thing—it helps distinguish humankind from less social creatures.

expensive than the old (and so are not available to as many people), or that it becomes impossible to find effective drugs. In this case, the incidence of infection may increase to levels similar to the prepenicillin days.

Such a situation arises through an externality that is qualitatively similar to that characterizing the market for immunizations. In the immunization example, consumption of the good (an inoculation) confers a benefit on the individual, but it also benefits other individuals in the population by reducing the probability they face of becoming ill. In the case of antibiotic use, there is a similar, private benefit to consumption of the good (the drug). But, if the resistance of a bacterium to a drug is positively related to the ambient concentration of the drug in the population, there is a negative externality imposed on other members of the community, for whom the effectiveness of the drug is reduced. Thus, from a social perspective, overconsumption is likely.[3]

Public Goods

Public goods and services are characterized by the feature that use by one individual does not preclude use by another. Common examples of public goods are defense, police forces, and street lighting. The benefits of these goods can be enjoyed by individuals without reducing their availability to others.[4] It is surprisingly difficult to find examples of pure public goods, because even those mentioned above have limits. For example, if a population becomes large enough, its defense force may not provide as secure a defense as it did when protecting a smaller population.

Some forms of health care are often argued to have public good characteristics. However, many of the benefits of health care accrue directly to the individual and are not public in nature—for example, the main outcome of consumption of curative drugs is the improvement in health of the particular consumer. It is true that healthier individuals may impose fewer costs on the rest of the population and may be more productive, but these attributes do not make health care a public good. For example, if an individual earns wages based on productivity, it is the individual that captures the financial

---

3. Note that if there are other imperfections in the delivery of drugs that restrict their use—such as poor transportation infrastructure, improper storage facilities, or corrupt middlemen—underuse may easily occur.

4. Although defense represents a public good, it can often be overprovided. We discuss briefly below the determinants of the optimal level of public good provision, but initially we are interested only in characterizing goods with public good aspects.

return of improved health; it does not accrue to others. If for some reason the individual were paid less than is commensurate with her productivity, the benefits of improved health would accrue to others (in lower prices of the good she produces or higher profits for the owners of the firm for which she works), but not in the manner of a public good. In this case, there are externalities associated with her consumption of health care.

Some health goods and services, however, do represent public goods. These goods can be categorized into two distinct classes. Goods in the first class are characterized by their impact on the physical or environmental conditions surrounding individuals as they live and work. Those in the second class have no direct physical effect, but they provide information, which is perhaps the purest of public goods.

Of goods in the first class, the more important examples in developing countries include actions that improve the quality of the environment, such as vector control (spraying for mosquitoes) and air quality control (from reduced pollution). Again, the line between public goods and goods with externalities can be somewhat fuzzy: for example, education is sometimes said to have public good aspects, particularly when mothers receive it. There is strong evidence to suggest that children of educated mothers have better prospects, but as above, this is more representative of an externality than a public good.

The second class of public goods includes information provided to allow individuals to make better decisions or to save them the costs of finding the information themselves. Such services include accreditation of physicians, which relieves individual consumers of the task of having to judge the quality of doctors, a job they may not be able to do very well and may not have time to do—for instance, in an emergency. Similarly, control of the quality of drugs by a public authority means that physicians and individuals can be sure of the nature of the medications they prescribe and consume. Of course, the public needs to have some degree of trust in the government to provide correct and accurate information—that is, the quality of the public good must be sufficiently high for it to be valued by consumers.

The problem with public goods is that firms will have little incentive to produce them, because virtually all the benefits accrue to others. If a firm could charge others for the benefits they receive from a public good it provides, this problem would be easily overcome, and the private market would provide adequate levels of public goods. But such a charging mechanism requires, first, that the firm is able to levy charges, and second that it can stop individuals who have not paid from using the good. The second requirement of excludability is often not met, so private providers are unlikely to be able to reap sufficient financial returns to cover the costs of provision. Because private agents left to themselves are not likely to provide sufficient public goods, we say that there is a market failure.

So what determines the appropriate or socially desirable level of provision of a public good? In most of economic analysis, we identify optimal allocations by the condition that the marginal cost of provision is equal to the marginal benefit received by consumers (assuming certain convexity regularities). For public goods, there is nothing specifically different about the nature of marginal costs (although it is likely that there will be large fixed costs and relatively small variable costs). At the same time, as the benefit of an additional unit of the good accrues to many individuals, the marginal social benefit is equal to the sum of the individual marginal benefits from consumption by each individual. This is the basis of Samuelson's rule for optimal public good provision, as illustrated in figure 7.4.

In the figure, the quantity q of the public good is shown on the horizontal axis, and we assume that there is a constant marginal cost of provision, MC. There are I individuals, labeled $i = 1, ..., I$, with marginal benefit curves (demand curves) MB_i. In the figure, $I = 2$. If the good were a normal private good, the efficient output would correspond to the value $\bar{q}$, where the marginal cost curve intersects the aggregate marginal benefit curve, or aggregate demand curve, D_h. This aggregate demand curve is constructed by adding the private demand curves horizontally. For a public good, however, the relevant aggregate marginal benefit curve is the *vertical* sum of the private marginal benefit curves, labeled D_v, and the efficient output is q^*, where D_v and MC cross.

Merit Goods and Information

Sometimes governments impose their own preferences on individual consumption patterns, especially with regard to the consumption of particular goods. When these impositions can be supported by the presence of externalities, it is not so much that the government imposes its own preferences on individuals, as that it weighs the preferences of some against those of others. However, when the intervention is not based on a desire to offset external effects, the motivation for the imposition is based on the presumption that the government "knows best." Such a basis for policy can be quite dangerous if governments use it in an unchecked manner, as in assigning individuals to occupations against their will in the "national interest." In some cases, however, it may well be true that the government knows best, or at least that the government enjoys a cost advantage in the acquisition of relevant knowledge. In this case, it may be efficient for the government to know best and to direct consumption patterns accordingly.

Figure 7.4.   *Optimal Public Good Provision*

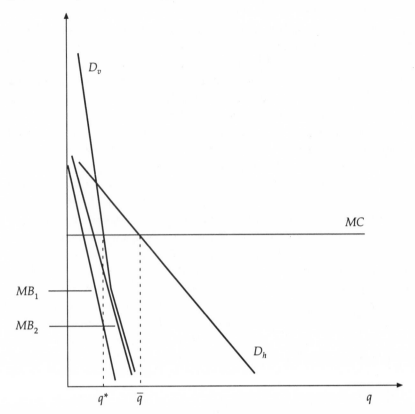

Note: The optimal provision of public goods is q^*, where D_v crosses the marginal cost curve. In contrast, the optimal quantity of private goods is $\bar{q}$, at the intersection of D_h and the marginal cost curve.
Source: Author.

Examples of these so-called "merit goods" (or symmetrically, if the government wishes to reduce consumption, "demerit goods") include preventive medical care, health insurance, and smoking cessation. Individuals may not correctly recognize the benefits of having regular checkups, the size of the financial risks they face, or the negative effects (on themselves) of smoking. While there may be financial or real externalities associated with consumption of these goods, this lack of appreciation of their effects means that even absent such external effects, they may be consumed at incorrect levels. This market failure does not arise because of any coordination problem between producers and consumers (as in the public good case) or between consumers (as in the externality case), but because individuals make their decisions based on erroneous or incomplete information. There might be a role for government intervention in such cases. As pointed out above, however, merit good arguments should be viewed with some skepticism, because they are particularly open to political abuse, especially when the government has monopoly control over selected information sources.

This argument stresses the role of information in the determination of merit goods (such a characterization has been suggested by Sandmo 1983). As we saw in the previous section, information is a classic example of a public good that may not be provided at appropriate levels in the free market. Indeed, one can view information as being a good that is consumed jointly with other goods—for example, an individual, when deciding whether to smoke, would ideally find out about the effects of cigarettes and make his decision based on that information. If information acquisition is costly, however, he will, as with his consumption of all goods, economize and make his smoking decision based on, at best, partial information. Such so-called transaction costs limit the efficiency of private decisions. Now, one might argue that economizing on costly information is not inefficient, and that the resulting resource allocation cannot be said to be inefficient when these costs are included. However, it is not the fact that information is costly that leads to inefficient consumption, but that once attained, it can be used by all individuals at (close to) zero cost (it is a public good) and so will not be provided in sufficient quantities.

If the information is provided by the government (as in the case in the previous section), there is no need for additional government-mandated consumption patterns, because consumers are in a position to properly judge the effects of their actions. But, if it is costly not only to acquire the information, but also to distribute it to individuals in a way that is understandable, it may be preferable for the government to give specific directions regarding consumption. There is some logic to this argument, but note that it has at least two imperfections. First, a strictly benevolent government could be entrusted with this role of assigning consumption patterns, but such governments tend to be thin on the ground. Second, and more fundamental, in order to make the proper assignment of consumption bundles, the government needs not only to know the effects of consumption of certain goods—for example, the increase in risk of cancer from smoking or the reduction in financial risk from being insured—but it also must know individuals' preferences. Thus, while one individual may cease to smoke if the negative effects are made clear, another may continue to engage in the activity if it provides enough pleasure. Although we might be willing to agree that monopoly production of information about the effects of certain behaviors is efficient, it is surely inappropriate to accept that the government can accurately identify individuals' diverse tastes.[5]

Policy Responses to Market Failures—Market-Improving Instruments

The market failures we examined above were characterized by consumption or production of a good that differed from its socially desirable level. We also suggested that in such cases, there may be a role for government intervention in effecting a more efficient outcome. But what instruments might a government use to implement efficiency-improving policies? As we suggested at the beginning of this chapter, the instruments can be divided into those that seek to improve the performance of markets and those that seek to replace markets. Journalists and ideologues may have preferences for one kind of instrument over another as a matter of principle, but it is the job of the serious economist to examine which instrument is best-suited to a given institutional and political environment. We examine each of the three types of market failure—externality, public good, and merit good—in turn.

Externalities

Let us consider again the pollution example. Like figure 7.2, figure 7.5 shows the marginal benefits and costs of effluent emission. Upon reflection, one can interpret the figure as a regular graph of demand and supply for a good. The quantity of the good is measured along the horizontal axis, and its price along the vertical axis. In simple partial equilibrium models, agents trade at the point of intersection of demand and supply, point y_0, which is the efficient amount. It was argued that in an unregulated setting, the equilibrium

---

5. Besley (1988) presents a utilitarian model in which the social planner, when calculating social welfare as a function of utilities, assigns an adjusted weight to consumption of a given good in determining individuals' utility levels. If the adjustment to the weight is positive (negative), the good is a (de)merit good. The adjustments represent paternalistic impositions by the planner on individuals and need not derive from information imperfections at the consumer level. It is not clear, however, what the normative relevance of such adjustments is when they derive from the preferences of a social planner and not from the preferences of individuals (including, potentially, future generations).

Figure 7.5.   *Gains from Trade in the Effluent Discharge Case*

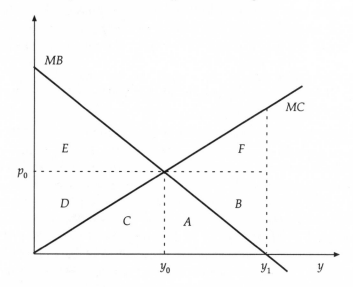

level of emissions would actually correspond to point y_1. What is the explanation for this divergence?

The problem is that the good on the horizontal axis, effluent discharge, is not traded between the factory and the fisherman. Suppose we were to think of the marginal cost curve of the fisherman as being his "supply of emissions curve." Recall that a supply curve represents the amount a producer needs to be paid, at the margin, to increase the availability of a good. The marginal benefit curve of the factory would be their "demand for emissions curve." The purchase of y units of emissions by the factory from the fisherman would then be interpreted as the fisherman granting the factory the right to emit y units of effluent in return for a payment. Assuming that the market worked competitively (which is, of course, unreasonable in the simple example of a single agent on each side of the market), the equilibrium allocation of effluent rights would be y_0, and their price would be p_0. Note that we have implicitly assumed that it is the fisherman who initially holds all the rights to effluent discharge, so that before any trade in emission rights takes place, there would be no pollution. Opening the market for pollution rights results in an increase in welfare for the fisherman equal to area D (because he receives revenue $D + C$, but it costs him C in lost fishing revenue) and an increase in the welfare of the factory owners of E (because they earn $C + D + E$ additional profits, but pay $C + D$ of this to the fisherman). In this case, not only has the market increased the size of the pie, it has also made both parties to the trade better-off, compared with the assumed initial resource allocation.

Suppose now that the factory initially has the rights to pollute, and it thus emits y_1 units of effluent. Now read the diagram from right to left (considering point y_1 to be the new origin). The original marginal benefit curve of the factory is now upward-sloping to the left and can be interpreted as its supply curve for emissions reduction, while the original marginal cost curve of the fisherman now slopes down to the left and can be interpreted as his demand curve for emissions reduction. Again, if the market for emission rights is opened, equilibrium will be established at y_0, with the same price as before, p_0. The fisherman will pay the factory owners an amount $A + B$, so that the owners will reduce emissions to y_0. This will make the fisherman better-off by an amount equal to F and will make the factory owners better-off by an amount equal to B (because they suffer a cost in lost profits equal to A). Again, both parties are made better-off compared with the initial resource allocation.

Notice that the trading mechanisms described above result in efficient resource use and two specific distributions of income, depending on the initial allocation of rights. There is, in principle, nothing to suggest that either income distribution is optimal, and the government may prefer any of a large number of alternative distributions between the fisherman and the factory owners. Without studying the determinants of the optimal distribution of income, it is useful here just to note that the government is able to affect such redistribution that it desires either *ex post*, by making cash transfers between the agents, or *ex ante*, by choosing a particular allocation of emission rights. For example, suppose the government allocated y_0 units to the factory owners, and $y_1 - y_0$ units to the fisherman, and it allowed trade between the two. No trade would take place, and the factory would emit y_0 units of effluent. However, compared with an initial situation of no emissions, the factory owners receive all the efficiency gains, equal to area $C + D + E$, and the fisherman suffers a loss equal to C. Compared with an initial situation in which y_1 units of effluent are emitted, the fisherman receives all the efficiency gains from the reform ($A + B + F$), and the factory loses A.

This discussion suggests that a simple way for government to implement an efficient allocation of resources is to establish a market for the good that implicitly is not traded when an externality exists. Such markets can be observed in some countries (such as the United States) where pollution permits are traded between firms.[6] The role of the government is primarily to establish an initial allocation of property rights, to regulate the ensuing trading environment—for example, by ensuring that agents' actions comply with their holdings of rights (that is, making sure that factories do not pollute more than their holdings of pollution rights allow)—and to facilitate a competitive market (recall that only in a competitive market will the allocation of resources necessarily be efficient).

The natural question that arises from this analysis is why do economic agents affected by externalities (such as the factory and the fisherman) not get together and agree on a reallocation of resources that enables each of them to improve their position relative to the status quo? That is, why is the government needed at all? The general answer to this, given originally by Coase (1960), is that the agents may face transaction costs that impede trade. These may differ from the information-based transaction costs that were identified in the discussion of merit goods, but they generically represent impediments to bargaining that lead to inefficient resource allocations.[7]

The example of smoking-related externalities is one in which the lack of a market (for smoke) is easier to explain. When there is a large number of individuals on one or both sides of a market, it may be difficult to organize trade between them. By establishing a market that reduces the negative effects of smoking, nonsmokers will experience a positive externality among themselves, because any reduction in smoking is of benefit to all nonsmokers, and not just those who organize the market. This type of externality is referred to as the free-rider problem.

When the creation of a market is impossible or economically infeasible, the government may be able to improve the performance of existing markets instead. Consider the effluent discharge example again. In an unregulated environment, the factory chooses to emit y_1 units of effluent, where the net marginal benefit of doing so is zero. The net marginal benefit consists of the gross benefits from higher sales of output, less the costs of inputs required to produce that output. By taxing either the output or the inputs used, the government can effectively alter the position of the net

---

6. See Baumol and Oates (1988). Such tradable permits are usually traded among polluters and not between polluters and pollutees (that is, fishermen). However, U.S. environmental groups such as the Sierra Club often enter the market and purchase permits that they leave inactive, reducing the total level of emissions.

7. Some have argued (Hurwicz 1997; Pitchford and Snyder 1998) that the celebrated Coase Theorem is not much of a theorem, because it does not in fact explain the endogenous existence of transaction costs.

marginal benefit curve. By choosing the tax rates carefully, the net marginal benefit curve can be shifted down, so that it crosses the horizontal axis at the point y_0. Faced with such a constraint, the factory owners will choose the efficient level of effluent discharge. Note that the fisherman is not directly involved in the process—he does not engage in any trade with the factory owners. The government effectively replaces the fisherman by "selling" the right to pollute at a price determined by the taxes on output and inputs. The revenue from these sales goes to the government, and it could in principle be distributed either to the fisherman, the factory owner, or both, or to some other agents in the economy.

This use of taxes to implement an efficient resource allocation, originally suggested by Pigou (1947), allows the government to intervene in the market without interfering directly in production and consumption decisions. It is important to note that the taxes used should, as far as possible, be levied on outputs and not inputs. The reason for this is that output taxes will tend to affect the level of output (and thus emissions) directly, but input taxes will affect both output (and emissions) and the mix of inputs used. The second effect tends to reduce the productive efficiency of resource allocation, without necessarily improving its allocative efficiency, and should be avoided. Strictly speaking, this argument is valid only when a full set of taxes on outputs is available (Diamond and Mirrlees 1971), and this is often not the case. Despite the adjustments that would be required in the more realistic situation of a constrained tax system, however, the general principle that distortionary input taxes should be avoided remains relevant.

Now consider again the example of smoking. A simple way to reduce the number of smokers is to levy a tax on cigarettes, assuming that there is some non-zero elasticity of demand.[8] The previous paragraph suggests that it is better to tax cigarette consumption directly than to tax the inputs used in the production of cigarettes because of the distortionary effects of the latter policy. But one may be concerned about the distributional impact of a tax on cigarettes, particularly if it is found that cigarettes are predominantly consumed by the poor. Again, in this case we would be faced with the tradeoff between efficiency and equity, which may influence our choice of instrument.

A final example is that of preventive care, which is associated with a positive externality if society cannot commit to withholding future curative care.

---

8. Indeed, one can easily show that if the elasticity of demand is zero, there is no need for government intervention based on externality arguments.

If preventive care is underconsumed, there might be an argument for subsidizing it, either on the demand side (by lowering the market price paid by the consumer) or at the physician level on the supply side (by increasing the price received). The important lesson to learn from the general discussion on the use of input and output taxes is that the subsidies should be designed to minimize the distortion in the production techniques employed in the delivery of preventive care.

Public Goods

The scope for market improvement to correct the underprovision of public goods is more limited than in the case of externalities. One approach is for the government to first allocate property rights to some (possibly one) individuals or firms, and second to facilitate a pricing mechanism for the compensation of the selected provider. Recall that because one characteristic of a public good is the difficulty of excluding nonpayers from using the good, facilitation of a pricing arrangement is important. An example of this approach is that of parks and recreation facilities, for which the government might grant a license and the ability to charge an entry fee to a private provider.

In the case of a pure public good, the costs of providing the good do not depend on the number of users. This means that the marginal cost arising from use by an extra individual is zero, and that allocative efficiency requires that the marginal price to the individual of additional use will also be zero. In the example of a national park, such a pricing rule would mean that individuals would be charged an annual fee, for example, but they could have free access to the park whenever they wanted at no additional charge. (If the park became sufficiently crowded in the summer months, an additional charge could be levied, because the marginal cost imposed on other users would be positive.)

Both the exclusion from use and the pricing of public good services provided by vector control appear to be sufficiently impractical that market-improving solutions are unlikely to be effective. An important difference in the national park example is that individuals benefit from mosquito control when they live in a sprayed area. Visiting a sprayed area now and then will offer them essentially no benefit (they will be exposed to the disease at all other times), so exclusion would require the government to be willing to forcibly relocate nonpaying individuals from a sprayed area (as opposed to keeping them out of a park that they may only wish to visit periodically). Given the potentially large areas affected by spraying, this would require implausibly large migrations for little improvement in allocative efficiency. Of course, the negative equity impact—one only has to imagine forced repatriation of the poor into unsprayed slums—would clearly make such a policy socially unpalatable and politically untenable.

A health-related public good whose allocation has been regulated with market-improving policies is medical research, particularly drug discovery and development. As we saw earlier, much of the cost of producing drugs is incurred at the research stage during scientific investigations. It is useful to think of the output of the research stage as "knowledge"—information regarding the medical effects of certain combinations of chemicals. This knowledge has the property of a public good, because its use by other firms does not reduce its availability to the originating firm. Thus, after the research has been performed, allocative efficiency requires free dissemination of the information to all who wish to use it. If such dissemination results in a large number of firms producing the new drug, the market price is likely to equal the marginal cost of production. The firm that incurred the research and development expenses will not be able to charge enough to cover those investment costs and will thus incur a loss. Faced with such a prospect, it will not engage in the research. From an *ex ante* point of view, an allocatively inefficient level of research will be performed, and the public good—knowledge or information—will be underproduced.

A kind of second-best market-improving response to this market failure is for the government to grant firms that engage in scientific research monopoly rights to produce and market their discoveries for a fixed period. During this patent period, other firms are excluded from using the information, and the firm is in a position to earn sufficient profits to cover their research costs. Although the restriction on use of information during the patent period involves some temporary allocative inefficiency (because the monopoly price is set above marginal cost), this social cost is traded off against the alternative dynamic inefficiency that would occur if, when faced with negative returns to investment in scientific research, firms desisted from engaging in research and development activities (see Arrow 1969 for a formal model of optimal patent life).

Merit Goods

We argued above that merit (demerit) goods are under- (over-) consumed, because individuals do not appreciate or know of the full effects associated with their use. On the face of it, the simple solution to this problem is for the government to provide them with the information. But if individuals do not possess the relevant information because it is too costly, a more direct market intervention may be to improve the information-dissemination environment rather than to provide the information directly. At the same time, it may be impractical to improve the dissemination of information—which we saw has the attributes of a pure public good—through the market sufficient to ensure that correct quantities of merit (demerit) goods are consumed, and direct provision of information, in the form of public campaigns, can be employed instead. Examples include campaigns encouraging people to give up smoking, to exercise more, to drink less, and to wear sunscreen. Note, however, that while these approaches are characterized by public provision of information, they do not require the public provision of the merit good itself. For example, the government may inform the public about the likelihood of developing skin cancer if individuals are overexposed to the sun without protection, but this does not require that the public sector produce or distribute sunscreen. Similarly, public advice on the negative effects of alcohol need not necessarily be coupled with direct public control of the sale and purchase of alcohol.

Instead of providing information about the effects of selected consumption goods, the government may choose to impose subsidies or taxes to encourage or discourage their use. Thus, the theory would suggest, individuals would continue to act on the basis of uninformed preferences, but they would be induced to act as if they were well informed by the presence of price distortions. This may be preferred to information campaigns if such campaigns are expensive, or if it is believed that some individuals cannot process information on the effects of consumption of certain goods as effectively as they can respond to price signals. In the case of demerit goods, there is an added payoff to the government from imposing taxes in the revenue collected. This is one reason that taxes on cigarettes and alcohol tend to be at much higher rates than on most other commodities.

Immunization—An Example of an Externality

Communicable diseases in human populations can be transferred from one individual to another through various forms of contact and social interaction. The chance of a particular individual contracting the disease is thus a function of exposure to other infected individuals, and the fewer the number of carriers in the population, the smaller is the likelihood that an uninfected individual will become ill. Another factor that influences the chance of individuals contracting the disease is susceptibility to the infection, which can be affected by general health status, behavior, and, in particular, whether they are vaccinated against the disease or not. In practice, the effectiveness of vaccinations can range from below 50 to virtually 100 percent—that is, vaccinated individuals may still be susceptible to the disease, albeit at a reduced rate, although in some cases vaccination may provide virtually complete protection.

As well as conferring benefits on the individual who is vaccinated, immunization reduces the chance that an unvaccinated person will come into contact with an infected individual and contract the disease by reducing the number of infected individuals in the population. This additional benefit, which is not captured by the vaccinated individual, represents an externality, which in general is expected to be only partially incorporated into an individual's decision to be vaccinated. Assuming that all the costs of the vaccination (including travel and time costs, as well as the costs of the vaccines themselves) are borne by the individual, it is reasonable to expect that the number of individuals immunized will be fewer than would be socially desirable.

This line of reasoning is often used to argue in favor of subsidized immunization programs. However, there is sometimes a corollary presumption that complete immunization of the population is a desirable target. But we will see below that such a policy goal is rarely justified on economic grounds, and that good-specific equity concerns, concern for future generations, or the inevitability of nonuniform implementation, may be required to support such an objective.[9]

To formally model externalities in immunization, suppose there is a population of individuals whose number is normalized to unity. Let $n \in [0, 1]$ be the fraction (number) of individuals immunized against a particular disease. Suppose that when no one is immunized, the chance of any given individual contracting the disease is p_0. We argued above that as n increases from zero, this probability falls, so we can say that the chance of contraction is equal to $p(n)$, where $p'(n) < 0$. The shape of the function $p(n)$ is an empirical epidemiological matter, and it can differ among diseases. Some diseases have probability functions that show a uniform decline as n increases (see figure 7.6(a)), while others seem to show no noticeable decline until some threshold coverage is reached (figure 7.6(b)). For illustrative purposes, we

---

9. A number of recent papers address the issue of externalities and immunizations in a more formal fashion. See, for example, Britto, Sheshinski, and Intrilligator (1991), Francis (1997), and Geofford and Philipson (1997). Francis' paper presents a special case of a dynamic model in which there is no net externality. The analysis below, based on Siepert (1997), is static in nature and exhibits the traditional externality.

Figure 7.6.   *Probability of Contracting a Disease as a Function of the Number of Immunized Individuals*

The linear case

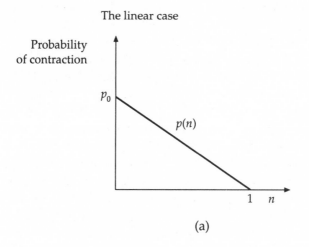

(a)

The threshold case

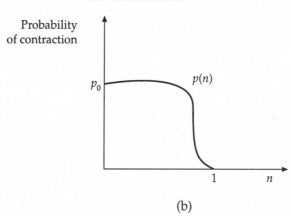

(b)

Source: Author.

will assume that the probability falls linearly with n, so that $p(n) = p_0(1 - n)$. Notice that when the whole population is immunized ($n = 1$), the probability of contraction is zero, and the disease is effectively eliminated. This reflects an initial assumption that the vaccination is 100 percent effective.

We also assume that individuals are identical in all relevant respects, and that the cost imposed by having the illness is the same for all, and normalized to one. In this case, if n individuals are immunized, the expected cost of not being immunized is just equal to $p(n)$ ($= p(n).1 + (1 - p(n)).0$), which is the same as the expected private benefit of immunization of an additional individual, at the margin. The function $p(n)$ can then be interpreted as the aggregate inverse demand curve for vaccinations, under the assumption that individuals make decisions based on the expected costs of disease, and it measures the marginal private benefit of immunization. If the marginal cost of vaccinations, c, is constant, then in market equilibrium n^* individuals will be vaccinated, where $p(n^*) = c$ in figure 7.7

We may now ask, starting from a situation in which n individuals are vaccinated, what is the social benefit of a marginal increase in the number of individuals immunized? If an extra dn individuals are immunized, the benefit to each of them is $p(n)$, as above, and so the total private benefit is $p(n)dn$. Assuming that the vaccination is 100 percent effective, there is no additional benefit to the n individuals who are already vaccinated. For each of the $(1 - n)$ individuals who is not vaccinated, however, the probability of being infected now falls by $dp = p'(n)dn$ (which is negative). Thus, the group of nonvaccinated individuals receives a total benefit of $-(1 - n)p'(n)dn$. The aggregate benefit accruing to all individuals is thus $p(n)dn - (1 - n)p'(n)dn$.

Figure 7.7.   *Equilibrium Immunization Coverage with No Public Intervention, n^**

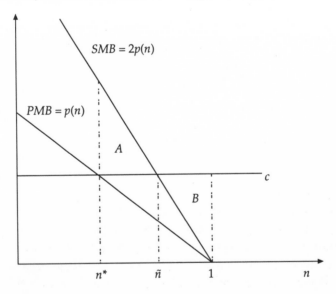

Source: Author.

An alternative interpretation of this condition is as follows. When n individuals are immunized, the aggregate expected cost of disease to the population is $(1 - n) p(n)$ (equal to the expected cost for each of the unimmunized $(p(n))$, times their number $(1 - n)$, plus the expected cost for the immunized (zero), times their number (n)). When the number of immunized individuals increases at the margin by dn, the aggregate expected cost of disease increases by $-p(n) + (1 - n)p'(n) < 0$. Equivalently, the social benefit of the marginal increase is $p(n)dn - (1 - n)p'(n)dn$. In the special case of a linear probability function, $p(n) = p_0(1 - n)$, the social benefit of the marginal increase is just $2p_0(1 - n)dn = 2p(n)dn$. Thus, the social marginal benefit curve is equal to twice the private marginal benefit curve, as shown in figure 7.7.

The socially optimal number of immunized individuals is $\tilde{n}$, at which social marginal benefits and costs are equalized. Notice that $\tilde{n}$ is greater than n^*, as we would expect in the presence of a positive externality, but that $\tilde{n}$ is less than one, midway between n^* and unity. That is, the socially optimal immunization coverage in this model is incomplete. This is not because we have assumed that the costs of immunization become large as larger numbers of individuals are covered—we have assumed constant marginal costs. The incompleteness of optimal coverage stems instead from the fall in the social benefits of immunization as the number of immunized individuals increases, both because the chance of a given nonimmunized individual contracting the disease falls and because fewer people are nonimmunized.

Somewhat more striking is the observation that the welfare loss from the externality—that without government intervention only n^* individuals are covered instead of the socially preferred $\tilde{n}$—is precisely the same as if a policy of full immunization were adopted. To see this, note that the welfare loss from underimmunization is equal to the area A in figure 7.7. This triangle measures the excess of aggregate social benefits over the social costs of immunizing the additional $\tilde{n} - n^*$ individuals. If the whole population is immunized, there is a welfare loss equal to the size of area B, representing the excess of social costs over social benefits when the additional $1 - \tilde{n}$ individuals are immunized. It is easy to see that these two costs are identical.

How can the government implement the socially optimal immunization strategy? One possibility is that it chooses $\tilde{n}$ individuals randomly from the population and provides them with the vaccines. Alternatively, as suggested earlier in this chapter, it can subsidize the private cost of immunization to encourage a larger number of individuals to voluntarily choose to be vaccinated. In the example here, the optimal subsidy rate is 50 percent; this induces an immunization rate of $\tilde{n}$. In practice, of course, the private costs of immunization include more than just the monetary cost (if any) of the vaccine and incorporate travel and time costs, inconvenience, pain, and the like. Suppose, for example, that these non-vaccine costs were about the same as the cost of the vaccine. In this case, providing the vaccine free would amount to a 50 percent subsidy to the total private cost of vaccination. If the non-vaccine costs were greater than the cost of the vaccine, then a monetary (or in-kind) payment may be necessary to induce the optimal number of individuals to become immunized.

RELAXING SOME OF THE ASSUMPTIONS. Three assumptions of this analysis are potentially troubling. The first is that the probability function is linear. Can nonlinearities, which almost certainly exist for real diseases, change the nature of the results? Second, is the assumption of constant marginal costs of immunization realistic, and does it hide some salient features of the optimal policy? And third, what happens if the vaccine is not 100 percent effective, as we have assumed above?

The existence of nonlinearities in the probability function changes the optimal number of immunized individuals, and it is no longer true that the socially preferred coverage rate is midway between the private market equilibrium rate and full coverage. Nevertheless, it remains true that full immunization is not optimal, and, more important, that the welfare loss from the externality continues to be precisely equal to the welfare loss that would obtain under full immunization.

The easiest way to see this last result, which exactly generalizes that of the linear case, is to consider the aggregate costs associated with the laissez faire equilibrium and those associated with full coverage. Consider figure 7.8, which now shows an arbitrary nonlinear probability function $p(n)$, interpreted as the private demand function. At the unsubsidized equilibrium, n^*, individuals are immunized, and pay a total of cn^* in immunization costs, but they suffer no costs of disease. The $(1 - n^*)$ nonimmunized individuals, in contrast, pay no direct immunization costs, but they have expected costs of illness equal to $(1 - n^*) p(n^*)$. Thus, total economic costs associated with the disease, given the observed immunization rate, are $cn^* + (1 - n^*) p(n^*) = cn^* + (1 - n^*) c = c$ (because $c = p(n^*)$).

In contrast, consider the total economic costs associated with complete immunization of the population. Each individual would incur a cost of c to be vaccinated, and the expected cost of illness for each person would be zero. Thus, aggregate costs are $c.1 = c$. The only difference between the two situations is that the costs of illness that are borne by $(1 - n^*)$ individuals in the laissez faire case become direct immunization costs in the complete coverage case.

Figure 7.8. *The Economic Costs of Suboptimal Immunization Are Identical to Those of Full Coverage*

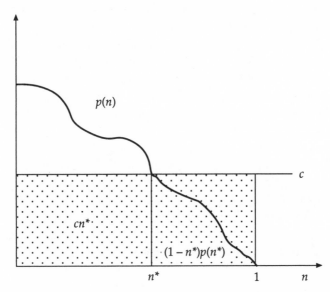

Source: Author.

Note that the optimal immunization level, which continues to fall between n^* and unity, is characterized by the number $\tilde{n}$ that minimizes the total economic (illness plus direct immunization) costs of the disease. As a function of n, these costs are equal to $nc + p(n)(1-n)$. At the optimal immunization level, $\tilde{n}$, total economic costs of the disease are equal to some number c_0, which, because it is minimal, is less than (or equal to) c (being the total costs associated with two particular, and not necessarily optimal, immunization levels, n^* and one). Thus, the welfare loss associated with the externality is equal to the difference between total economic costs under laissez faire and total costs at the optimum—that is, $c - c_0$. This is exactly equal to the welfare loss associated with full immunization.

We have assumed somewhat unrealistically that the marginal cost of immunizing individuals is constant, but they are likely to differ widely as the level of immunization increases and as different kinds of recipients are immunized. It is useful to distinguish between direct and indirect immunization costs here. The direct costs include the costs of the vaccines, the salaries of the medical staff who provide the vaccination services, the costs of traveling to villages to deliver vaccines, and so forth. Indirect costs are essentially those borne by the individual and do not compensate the provider, including travel and time costs, pain, inconvenience, and so on, as discussed above. Some individuals, particularly the highly paid, may have especially high indirect costs, reflecting the high opportunity costs of their time. Others, often the poor, will face high travel costs if they live in remote rural areas without access to health facilities. The split between direct and indirect costs is clearly endogenous to the choice of provision methodology—low direct costs of a small number of immunization posts are likely to be offset by the high indirect costs associated with the large distances individuals must travel to acquire the vaccines.

For a given choice of production technology (such as clinic location, training of medical officers, opening hours, quality of vaccine, and the like), it is possible, in principle, to order individuals according to their private cost of being vaccinated. Those with low costs—the low-paid residing in close proximity to clinics, or those with a high tolerance for the pain and inconvenience associated with the immunization—can be placed at the beginning of the list, and those with high costs—including the high-paid living far from clinics (or the squeamish)—can be placed at the end. Placing this list of individuals along the horizontal axis and plotting the cost of immunization for each, an increasing marginal cost curve is produced. The analysis then proceeds as before, with the qualitative result that, if the number of individuals immunized under laissez faire is the same as in the constant marginal cost case, the socially desirable number with increasing marginal costs is strictly less than that with constant costs.

One complication to this story is that we have continued to assume that the costs of illness are the same for all individuals. But because many of the costs of illness represent opportunity costs associated with foregone labor income, those who have large indirect immunization costs are also likely to have large illness costs. This means that we can no longer use the function $p(n)$ as a demand curve but must weight it according to each individual's illness cost.

Vaccines are seldom fully effective, and they tend to lower, but not necessarily eliminate, the chance of contracting a disease. The main implication of this for our analysis is that the socially optimal immunization program will vaccinate relatively more individuals than when the vaccine is fully effective. This apparently counterintuitive result stems from the benefit of the immunization of additional individuals realized by an immunized person who continues to be susceptible to the disease. That is, an additional immunization not only lowers the probability that a nonimmunized individual will contract the disease, but it also lowers the probability that an immunized individual will, albeit from a lower base.

The result is somewhat counterintuitive, because it appears that when technology is inadequate (that is, when a vaccine is not very effective), we use more of it (we require greater vaccination rates). But this clearly is not equivalent to the proposition that poor vaccines should be used instead of highly effective ones. The essential idea is that we can see immunization as a production process: the inputs are the vaccine and the immunized individuals. These two inputs are, in a sense, substitutes for one another: when we use more of the vaccine per person—that is, when the vaccine is more effective—it is not necessary to use as many individuals. Of course, when more effective vaccines are more costly, and when marginal indirect costs do not increase too rapidly, there is a substantive tradeoff to be made between wide coverage rates with adequate but not fully effective vaccines, and smaller coverage rates using highly effective vaccines.

FOUR REASONS FOR FULL COVERAGE. Given the ubiquity of calls for immunization rates as close to 100 percent as possible, it is useful to examine plausible additional arguments within the framework of the model above in favor of rates higher than $\tilde{n}$. The first relates to risk aversion. At the efficient immunization rate, $\tilde{n}$, the direct cost borne by each immunized person (c) is equal to the expected illness cost $(p(\tilde{n}) = c)$ borne by each nonimmunized person. However, it is clear that the risk exposure of the nonimmunized is greater than that of the immunized, so a somewhat higher rate of coverage is appropriate. Nevertheless, it is still unlikely that the optimal rate will be 100 percent.

Second, while the economic costs borne by the immunized and the nonimmunized are identical at $\tilde{n}$, a society may not feel easy about directly comparing the two. This may stem from a preference for good-specific equity, or from a concern that direct comparison of costs is only justified when the relevant goods are tradable. Because it is difficult to sell one's health (although this often occurs implicitly, as when individuals choose dangerous occupations in return for higher wages), it might be considered inequitable for some individuals to suffer nontradable illness costs, while others incur tradable direct immunization costs.

Third, and perhaps more compelling, the analysis above assumed that individuals in a population are exposed randomly to disease, so that the probability of a nonimmunized person becoming ill was a function of the total number of immunized individuals in the population. But this ignores the plausible possibility that immunizations will be provided nonuniformly across a population—village by village, for example. In such a case, if the $(1 - \tilde{n})$ individuals who are not immunized at "the optimum" all live together, their probability of becoming ill will be much higher than $p(\tilde{n})$. It would be optimal, within the strict framework above, to immunize a proportion $\tilde{n}$ of each village, but given the very low marginal costs of vaccinating the additional individuals in each village, it is no longer implausible that the optimal rate is close to 100 percent.

Finally, the static analysis presented in this section cannot account for intergenerational effects of immunization. Although complete immunization may not be optimal when considering the welfare of the current population, if such a policy is effective in eliminating the disease, then future generations benefit. As long as the social rate of discount is not too high, such an elimination could well be optimal from an intertemporal perspective.

Prevalence Feedbacks and Disease Control

Immunization is one example of an action that an individual can take for protection (full or partial) against disease. Of course, there may be other mechanisms that can affect such protection, including both modification of certain activities and abstinence from others. These mechanisms can be broadly identified with the level of care individuals adopt in order to reduce their exposure to disease. A primary example is the evolution of sexually transmitted diseases such as HIV and AIDS.

In general we would expect individuals to increase the level of care as the prevalence of disease in the population increases. These endogenous reactions to increased risks have implications for the effectiveness of policy interventions and the timing and design of disease control programs. A number of papers by Philipson and his colleagues (see Geoffard and Philipson 1996, 1997; Philipson and Posner 1993, 1995) have explored the impact of modeling the economic behavior of individuals in disease environments and the implications for policy.

SUBSIDIZED PREVENTIVE ACTIONS. The essential feature of much of this strand of the literature is that individuals can and do change their behavior in response to increases in the prevalence of disease, contrary to purely epidemiological models, which effectively assume that risk-related behavior is fixed. Indeed, this effect was the driving force behind the downward-sloping demand curve for immunization in the previous section: when fewer individuals are immunized, the prevalence of the disease is greater, and the demand for protection (immunizations) is higher in consequence.

However, there are other reasons to expect the demand curve for immunizations, or protection more generally, to be downward-sloping, for example, when individuals differ in their incomes, exposure to the disease, or risk aversion. The important implication of allowing behavior to depend on prevalence is that the elasticity of demand for risk-reducing care, be it in the form of immunization, condoms, boiled water, or some other measure, is increased. For example, consider using price and quantity data to estimate individuals' demands for condoms. In an environment with a given prevalence of HIV, P_0, the demand curve may look like $d(p, P_0)$ in figure 7.9, where p is the price of condoms. When the price of condoms is p_0, the initial demand for condoms, given the prevalence of HIV, P_0, is d_0. Now consider a subsidy meant to increase the use of condoms to d_1. Usually it would be argued that a subsidy of s per unit would be required to affect such an increase in demand, where s satisfies

$$d(p_0 - s, P_0) = d_1.$$

Suppose the subsidy does create an increase in demand, and that as a result the incidence of HIV falls. This will mean that over time, the prevalence of the disease also falls, say to P_1.[10] But a reduction in prevalence is likely to reduce the willingness of individuals to pay to reduce the chance of contraction—that is, the demand curve for condoms is likely to shift down, to $d(p, P_1)$ in figure 7.9. At the subsidized price, demand is now only $d_1' = d(p_0 - s, P_1) < d_1$.[11]

The feedback of prevalence on demand for care means that the elasticity of demand for care may be much higher than the estimate if prevalence were fixed. Indeed, the relevant demand curve, for the purposes of estimating the required subsidy rate to increase demand to d_1, is

$$\tilde{d}(p) \equiv d(p, P(p))$$

which accounts for the effects of price on prevalence, and hence demand. It is clear that a much higher subsidy may be required when this feedback effect is incorporated. When, as in most developing countries, public funds are scarce, these high required subsidy rates mean that careful targeting and policy design are necessary to improve the efficiency of interventions subject to tight budget constraints.

---

10. Recall that the incidence is the number of new cases each year, and the prevalence is the stock of infected individuals.

11. This will be an equilibrium demand if, at the subsidized price, the demand for condoms is just enough to ensure a steady-state prevalence of P_1, taking into account deaths.

Figure 7.9.   *Prevalence-Dependent Demand*

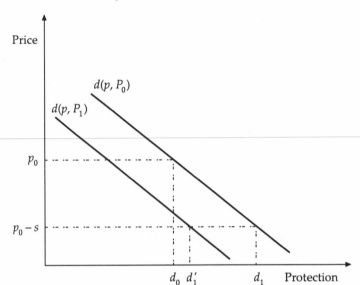

Note: For a given disease prevalence, the demand for protection (condoms) is downward-sloping. Higher prevalence shifts the demand curve up.
Source: Author.

MANDATED VACCINATIONS. A similar effect is at work when we consider the impact of mandatory vaccinations that cover only part of the population. Suppose that in the absence of the mandatory scheme, a proportion $v_0 = 0.5$ of the population would be vaccinated. What is the effect of requiring 50 percent of the population, chosen at random, to be vaccinated? It is tempting to assume that of those in the mandated pool, half would have voluntarily sought vaccination in any case, so the net effect of the program is to achieve a 75 percent coverage rate.

If vaccinating half the population reduces the incentives of others to be covered, however, then fewer than 50 percent of those outside the mandatory pool will choose to be vaccinated. This is a case of a government program effectively crowding out some of the private demand, and the net effect of the program might be to increase coverage from 50 percent to, for instance, only 60 percent of the population. This relationship is shown in figure 7.10 (taken from Geoffard and Philipson 1997). The horizontal axis measures the proportion of the population that is required to be vaccinated, and the vertical axis measures the total number of vaccinated individuals (including both those in the mandatory pool and those

Figure 7.10.   *Prevalence-Dependent Demand and Crowding Out*

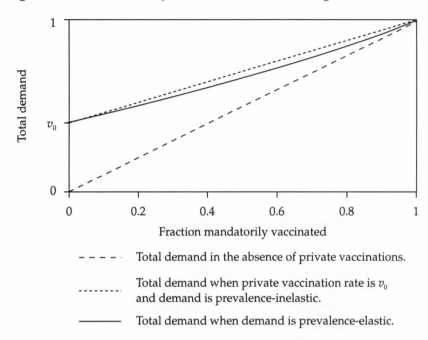

- - - -   Total demand in the absence of private vaccinations.

- - - - -   Total demand when private vaccination rate is v_0 and demand is prevalence-inelastic.

————   Total demand when demand is prevalence-elastic.

Note: A mandatory public vaccination program can crowd out private demand for the vaccine, because of the impact of reduced prevalence on demand.
Source: Adapted from Geoffard and Philipson (1997, figure 1, p. 228).

who choose voluntarily to be covered). When there are no private vaccinations, the relationship is given by the long-dashed 45 degree line. In the
presence of private vaccination, and under the simplistic assumption that
the government program does not affect private demand, the relationship is given by the short-dashed line starting from v_0 and increasing linearly to the full coverage point. When the demand for private vaccination
is prevalence-elastic, however, the relationship is shown by the full curved
line, increasing from v_0 at a slower rate, until full coverage is only attained when a 100 percent mandate is imposed.

TARGETING AND TIMING OF POLICY INTERVENTIONS. The two examples above
highlighted the dependence of the effectiveness of any policy intervention
in reducing the incidence of infectious diseases on the elasticity of care
with respect to the intervention. In addition to price subsidies and mandatory vaccinations (when they exist), other interventions include education

campaigns and attempts to alter social norms that may encourage the spread of disease. In many circumstances the targeting and timing of such campaigns can have a significant influence on their effectiveness, because the underlying elasticities vary across individuals and over time.

For example, Geoffard and Philipson (1996) suggest that in the fight against AIDS, targeting information and education campaigns to uninfected but susceptible groups is likely to have a larger impact than directing such resources toward those who are already infected. The argument is that, aside from altruistic motives (which may, of course, be strong), members of the infected group have little to gain from taking precautions in their sexual activities. Uninfected individuals, in contrast, have much to gain, so they are likely to be more responsive to policies designed to affect their behavior. In addition, in a statistical sense, members of the infected group reveal themselves, on average, to have a relatively higher cost of protection. This issue is particularly relevant in many Sub-Saharan and other developing countries in which female prostitutes are a major source of transmission. The earnings of such individuals often depend greatly on the extent to which they expose others to the disease, and reducing such exposure is costly when alternative earnings possibilities are scarce. Targeting information campaigns to the demand side of the sex industry may be more effective in reducing the rates of transmission.[12]

Because demand may be prevalence-elastic, a given subsidy (or other intervention) is likely to be relatively more effective when the prevalence of a disease is low. As Geoffard and Philipson argue, prevalence and subsidies to protection tend to compete to induce protection (that is, they crowd each other out), so the best time to offer incentives for protection is early on in the development of the disease. Quick, forceful intervention is likely to be the most efficient mechanism, in resources used, for limiting the spread of an infectious disease. The trouble with such a prescription is that it requires a substantial amount of political will and foresight. When new diseases emerge, it is difficult to tell early on the possible extent of the problem and the effectiveness of alternative interventions, leaving aside the issue of demand response.

---

12. A longer-term strategy aimed at improving the lot of prostitutes would require providing them with broad-based education opportunities so that they were better able to access alternative job markets.

Policy Responses to Market Failures—Public Provision

The interventions above were able to alter the market environment of decisionmaking by private economic agents. These interventions typically do not involve the government engaging in any kind of productive activity, at least not with respect to the particular good with a market that is deemed to have failed. By adjusting the decisionmaking environment, the government induces private agents to produce or consume socially desirable quantities of goods and services. An alternative strategy is for the government to more actively intervene in the allocation process, either by imposing specific requirements regarding resource allocation or by explicitly producing or delivering the resources in question. The health sector is one in which governments in both developing and industrial countries have often been, and continue to be, heavily and directly involved.[13]

There are a number of well-established arguments that favor the production and delivery of some kinds of medical and insurance services in a regulated environment. For example, possible scale economies in the delivery of hospital services suggest that a small number of large hospitals may be more efficient than a large number of smaller establishments. Similarly, if the government has a health-specific equity objective, such as equality of service for all, unfettered competition in the health delivery or health insurance markets may not produce socially desirable outcomes. This might be the result of so-called cream-skimming actions by producers, for example, in which they attempt to serve only low-cost and low-risk individuals, while dumping higher-cost and higher-risk individuals.

The question of public provision then turns on the extent to which direct public provision outperforms regulated private provision. That is, while it might be reasonable to assume that unrestricted private competition may be inappropriate, the choice between regulated private provision and public production may be much more acute. In practice, a mixed approach is often taken—coupling publicly provided insurance with private provision

---

13. To provide a satisfactory analysis of the appropriate division of public and private production—that is, the appropriate extent of public provision of goods and services—we would need to examine the theory of ownership and privatization. This would require the study of resource allocation mechanisms in the context of asymmetric information and incomplete contracts, a topic that is well outside the scope of this text. The interested reader is referred to Hart, Shleifer, and Vishny (1997), and the references therein.

of physician services, for example. One rationale for such a system might be that the government wishes to ensure equal treatment for all, independent of risk and income, and that the private sector cannot be relied upon to provide uniform insurance coverage. Once individuals have insurance, however, there will be less of a reason for medical care providers to discriminate on the basis of risk type or income, and the incentives for cost control and efficient production that characterize private provision of services may be harnessed effectively (see chapter 10 for more details).

The choice between public production and regulated private provision also depends on the regulatory instruments available to the government. For example, Weitzman (1974) examined the relative merits of using prices and quantities as regulatory instruments and found that in some cases quantity rules were preferred. In a regulatory setting, a price instrument may correspond to a tax or subsidy imposed on the provider, that is meant to induce a certain output response, while a quantity instrument corresponds more closely to direct delegation of production requirements. For example, to ensure full immunization through private provision, the government may choose either to subsidize the cost (to correct the externality) or simply to instruct a private firm to immunize all individuals. Implicitly this instruction carries with it a large penalty if the target of full immunization is not reached. Thus, the quantity instrument as a means of regulation can only be preferred to the price instrument if the threat of sanctions is credible. If this is not the case, direct provision by the government may be preferred to either kind of regulation.

The role of corruption may also influence the choice of regulation or direct provision. Suppose a price instrument were to be used to offset some market failure—say preventive care visits are to be subsidized. If it is difficult to validate the provision of preventive care services and their quality, the subsidy may create an opportunity for fraud that is difficult to control. It should be noted that there are varying degrees in the operation of such fraud. Relatively mild fraud might be characterized by provision of services that are not very useful, but nonetheless valued by consumers. More significant fraudulent behavior would involve claims for services rendered when no care was provided.

Of course, public sector employees must also be motivated to act in the public interest, and the relevant issue is whether a worker within the institutional setting of the public sector can be motivated more effectively than one in the regulated private sector. If public sector employees are not paid highly enough, their incentives to perform well and keep their jobs will certainly be weak, and moonlighting and fraud may be endemic. The security of tenure and other in-kind or deferred compensation, such as subsidized meals and pensions, may act as sufficiently strong incentives to induce at least partial compliance with the prescribed goals of the government.

Financing Public Expenditures

In the preceding sections we identified cases in which the government might intervene in the markets for medical care, or health-related goods and services in general. Some of these interventions involve the government giving instructions to private economic agents—for example, "individuals should not smoke on public transport," or "all insurance companies should provide certain basic coverage to individuals," and the like. Such instructions or regulations have no direct impact on the government budget, although there might be an indirect effect.[14]

Other interventions, including tax and subsidy instruments and public provision of goods and services, have direct effects on government revenue. Although some interventions, such as taxes on alcohol, result in higher revenues, many health care interventions reduce public revenues. The resources required to pay for these revenue-decreasing and expenditure-increasing interventions must be raised from some source. Optimal financing arrangements must specify (1) what revenue sources will be tapped, (2) what tax instruments will be used to extract revenue from these sources, (3) the administrative organization of the system of collection, and (4) the allocation of funds to alternative bureaucratic institutions.

The orthodox theory of optimal taxation usually concentrates on the first two issues, exploring optimal tax rates on various revenue sources. This approach implicitly assumes zero or low administrative costs, and it excludes any active role for tax collectors and administrators. Some revenue sources, however, are more costly to administer than others, and tax collectors must be motivated to act in the public interest and to desist from corrupt or arbitrary enforcement of tax laws. The orthodox approach also assumes that all revenues are funneled into a central budget, from which expenditure allocations are optimally made. In such an environment there is no substantive role for health-specific budgeting, and no normative reason for requiring cost-recovery on a service-by-service basis. We will argue below that in designing financing mechanisms for health

---

14. For example, if there is an existing tax on cigarettes, then upon the introduction of regulations that reduce the demand for smoking, public revenue may fall.

sector interventions, the principles of optimal taxation should indeed be followed as a first approximation, if only to ensure that deviations from such policies are explicitly defended.

Finally, in the following section, we return to examine the effects of interventions that do not have direct budgetary implications. We will show that while such interventions may have no recorded budgetary impact, they may have identical real economic effects to policies with explicit effects on the budget. Certain regulations on private activity can be seen as equivalent to deficit-financed public spending, which can have significant implications for macroeconomic performance and intergenerational transfers.

A Brief Overview of Optimal Taxation

Taxes have three effects: first, they alter individuals' incentives by changing the prices they face; second, they alter the distribution of welfare; and third, they raise revenue. Suppose the government has decided which goods and services it should provide and that it has identified a certain set of taxes and subsidies designed to give individuals appropriate incentives—that is, that correct market failures induced by externalities, public goods, and merit goods. Note that these taxes and subsidies include the prices, if any, the government levies on publicly provided goods and services. The general rule for efficient allocation is that, absent externalities and merit-good arguments, the price charged should equal the marginal cost of production. Thus, for pure public goods, the price should be zero, while for goods with a positive marginal production cost, the price should be positive but not necessarily high enough to cover fixed costs.[15]

If the net revenue raised from taxes and subsidies to correct market failures (which may be negative), plus marginal-cost-pricing of publicly provided goods and services, is less than the cost of the publicly provided goods and services, additional taxes must be levied to finance the shortfall. In addition given the set of efficient taxes and subsidies, if the distribution of welfare is considered undesirable, redistribution of income may be called for, which requires that taxes be levied on some individuals to finance payments to others. Unless these financing and redistributing taxes are lump sum in nature—that is, unless they are not related to actions, such as the demand or

---

15. In the presence of capacity constraints, if price is set equal to marginal cost, demand may exceed supply. In this case, the efficient price is that which clears the market, subject to the supply constraint.

supply of goods or services, undertaken by individuals—they will inevitably introduce distortions into the allocation of resources. Optimal taxes trade off the size of these distortions against improvements in the distribution of income, subject to the requirement that the necessary revenue be raised.

A formal mathematical presentation of this problem will not be given here (see Diamond and Mirrlees 1971), but some simple qualitative analysis is possible. First, we know that to a first approximation, the economic cost of price distortions can be measured by the reduction in consumer surplus. Thus, if the price of a good is set above marginal social cost, individuals are worse-off to the extent of the reduction of their demand for the good, so that taxes on goods with high price elasticities impose larger distortionary costs than do equal-revenue taxes on goods with low price elasticities. This is the basis of the famous Ramsay (1927) rule, which says that optimal commodity taxes should be inversely proportional to the (compensated) elasticity of demand.

This rule may need to be modified, depending on the income elasticity of demand. For example, if goods with low price elasticities are consumed primarily by the poor, then while the Ramsay rule indicates that they should be taxed at a relatively high rate on efficiency grounds, the distributional consequences of such a policy may be unacceptable. The mix of commodity taxes may need to be shifted toward goods and services with somewhat higher price elasticities that are consumed more by the rich (see Diamond 1975).

Taxes on commodities are almost always proportional to the quantities purchased. However, it may be possible to levy nonuniform taxes on some revenue sources. The most common such tax is the income tax; the rate can be altered, depending on the income of the individual. When such differentiation is possible, some of the distributional concerns of the basic Ramsay rule may be reduced. But the income tax will still lead to distortions in labor supply, and some differential commodity taxes may be required. In the special case when individual preferences over leisure and commodities are separable, it can be shown that the income tax is sufficient to achieve the optimal distribution of income at lowest distortionary cost, so no commodity taxes need to be levied (see Atkinson and Stiglitz 1976). In this case, commodity taxes should correct market failures, and publicly provided goods and services should be priced at marginal cost. Any revenue shortfall is then financed with an income tax.

These largely theoretical arguments must obviously be placed in context before being applied. Especially in the setting of a developing country, the capacity of a government to design and implement optimal taxes is likely to be severely constrained, and it is probably better to use simple rules of thumb, such as the distribution-adjusted Ramsay rule, as a first indication of the desirability of a given tax. One very clear message of the analysis above, however, is that while taxes should be set to cover revenue requirements at rates with low distortionary costs, there is no sense in which the sectors that generate large revenue needs should also provide large revenue sources. Thus, if the public provision of expensive medical care makes the health sector responsible for relatively high expenditures, revenue-raising taxes on the sector should not necessarily be especially high. A specific corollary to this argument is that it is unlikely, within the framework of standard optimal tax models, that cost-recovery on a sector-by-sector basis is desirable. Taken further, it is very unlikely that requiring each separate health facility (hospital, clinic, and the like) to cover its costs is optimal.

An important aspect of the health sector that has not been included in the discussion so far is that consumption of medical services is a function of health needs, which are highly uncertain. Given an individual's current needs and income, it may be desirable to levy a particular charge on use of medical services. Such a policy, however, may expose the individual to a large amount of financial risk, and in the absence of well-functioning insurance markets, the optimal pricing and taxation rules may need to be modified. A full analysis of the treatment of insurance within the optimal tax framework is beyond to scope of this text, but it is clear that in the absence of perfect insurance markets (markets with no adverse selection or moral hazard), standard pricing and taxation rules will need to be modified. In this case, by adjusting the financial cost of certain medical services, the tax system can effectively provide insurance that the private market does not deliver. As with our discussion of market failures, it may be more appropriate for the government to address the cause of the failure of the insurance market directly, if possible.

Collection Incentives and Earmarked Funds

Based on the theory above, there appears to be little reason for the revenues derived from health care service charges to match the costs of provision of those services. Depending on demand conditions, the optimal tax-inclusive price might be such that the sector as a whole runs at a loss, or that it shows a profit. This is also true at the more disaggregated level—for example, the optimal provision and pricing of hospital meals may result in a profit for the service, which can be used to finance the loss incurred by an optimally priced immunization service.

In practice, however, many services are required to meet an externally imposed budget constraint that is not necessarily identifiable as the optimum. For example, the health ministry may receive a certain allocation of funds and be required to finance any additional expenditures from sources within its domain. Similarly, local clinics may be required to generate sufficient funds to finance their recurrent costs. Instead of having all revenues transferred to a central budget, at least some are retained at the level of the collection agency.

The main arguments in support of such financial arrangements rest on the important observation that tax rates and rules that are set by the central government usually must be implemented by individuals who may have objectives that are not in direct accordance with those of the center. Even if we are willing to take the central government's objective as a valid basis for making normative judgments—that is, even if we assume that the central government acts in the public interest—it is unreasonable to assume that individuals who implement its rules will do so without regard for their own personal goals.

This problem might be addressed in part by paying tax collectors sufficiently high wages and by linking these wages to performance. It is important to acknowledge that revenue collection involves both the tax collector and the taxpayer, and that it might be necessary to give taxpayers incentives to willingly surrender some portion of their income. One way to do this is to pay them to do so by reducing the tax rates they face, but this may be self-defeating if it leads to even lower revenue collection. A more efficient mechanism may be to effectively provide benefits in kind to taxpayers by allowing local decisionmakers to retain a portion of the revenues. While this may not be fully optimal in the theoretical framework above, it may induce sufficient tax compliance to be warranted.

Taxpayers may respond favorably to such incentives, but only if local government officials deliver public goods that are valued by the taxpayers. This, in turn, is a function of the political accountability of local officials, and it requires a degree of representative democracy that might be lacking in many societies. Such political arrangements need not necessarily be manifest in formal institutions, and they could instead represent a set of social norms and accepted behavior. Nonetheless, financial accountability is unlikely to improve the allocation of resources in the absence of political accountability.

At a more mundane level, technological constraints may influence both the choice of financing instruments and their assignment to different institutional bodies. For example, while charges for visits to health clinics might be warranted under an efficiency analysis, if the proceeds from such charges cannot be safely held, they could have a negative effect on the delivery of services (independent of the effect on demand). Thus, without secure banks or cash boxes, local collection and receipt of user fees may lead to increases in violent robberies, danger to clinic staff, and reduced provision of clinic services, even if the amount of money actually collected increases.

To the extent that local revenues are used to undertake capital expenditures, access to banking services is again required; otherwise, large quantities of funds will need to be accumulated before capital purchases can take place. Not only can this increase the incentive for theft, but it is intertemporally inefficient, and central financing of such expenditures may alleviate certain capital market imperfections. This said, the administrative costs involved in transferring funds from one institution to another, including the recording of receipts, deposits, transfers, and interest payments, and performance monitoring may be so high that local control of funds is favored.

User Fees

An important financing instrument that has received considerable attention in the health care literature is the user fee (see Mwabu 1997 for a review and Gertler and Hammer 1997 for a careful analysis). The usual focus is on publicly provided health care services, and whether fees for such services should be used to generate revenues, either to finance the services themselves or to pay for some other public expenditure.

ARGUMENTS IN FAVOR OF POSITIVE PRICES. A first point to note is that unless there is a fundamental objection to having consumers pay for medical care, the underlying pricing and taxation principles outlined in the earlier sections should guide our choices. Goods and services with price-inelastic demand that are consumed primarily by the rich should, other things being equal, be subject to higher fees than others (with the additional caveat with regard to insurance).

Some medical care services, such as immunizations, should probably be close to free both for externality and merit-good reasons. However, if all medical care services, including drugs, are free, it is likely that demand will be excessively high. Multiple-drug therapies will be used when a simple dose is sufficient, patients with mild health problems will be admitted to expensive curative hospitals, and highly paid physicians will perform tasks most appropriately performed by their assistants. In this case, no revenue will be raised, and costs will escalate, presenting a double problem for the budget. Charging some fees will both reduce the extent of overutilization and raise revenue.

It may be argued, of course, that demand is not so responsive to price, and that the effects of a zero price on total output are exaggerated. But if this is the case, then we know that, at least from an efficiency point of view, not only should such services bear a tax sufficiently high to cover their cost, but it probably should also be high enough to finance other publicly provided goods and services. Unless there is no scope for exempting the poor, or providing them with income supplements through the tax and transfer system, a zero price in this case seems quite inappropriate.

ARGUMENTS IN FAVOR OF LOW PRICES. Econometric estimates typically suggest that the demand for various kinds of medical care, while not entirely inelastic, is relatively fixed (elasticities of about 0.2 are common; see chapter 4). In itself, this would argue for relatively high rates of cost-recovery through the use of user fees. Probably the strongest arguments against such a policy include the insurance aspect and the special nature of health care. That is, if insurance markets do not exist, low prices may be required to protect individuals against financial risk. This can be thought of as an implicit government insurance program. Suppose, in the absence of risk considerations, the optimal public sector price of a particular medical service is 100 schillings, taking into account any market failures (such as externalities) and financing needs (such as optimal revenue-raising taxes). Now suppose that an individual can purchase private medical insurance, and that, with moral hazard constraints in mind, chooses a policy with a 20 percent coinsurance rate. Thus, in return for a premium payment up front, the policy ensures that the medical care service will cost only 20 schillings if and when it is used.

Now suppose that such an insurance market does not exist, either because of the administrative costs or for some other reason. The government can effectively replicate the insurance system by levying a lump-sum tax on the individual (equal to the premium she would have paid if private insurance were available), and setting the price equal to 20 schillings instead of 100. If it is not possible to levy such a premium tax, the government can finance the effective price subsidy out of general revenues. While not identical to the private insurance market outcome, the results of such a policy will be reasonably close.

This argument shows that user fees—at least large ones—may be inappropriate if private insurance markets do not work well, and low charges represent a means for the government to correct the insurance market failure. At the same time, just as insurance policies with zero co-insurance rates are uncommon, so too should public sector prices be set greater than zero. The only differences between the coinsurance rate that would emerge from a private insurance market and the optimal publicly set price stem from the possibility that the government may wish to subsidize the use of the service because of externalities and the like that may not be captured by private insurance companies.

The other argument against charging for medical care is that such services are different from normal consumer goods. There is a certain degree of merit to this proposition, and it certainly appears that societies in many parts of the world are willing to accept a much larger degree of inequality of income than of inequality of health (although measuring the equality of health and access to health care can be difficult; see Wagstaff and van Doorslaer forthcoming for a thorough survey). Again, however, it is important to distinguish between distributional arguments and pricing arguments.

Presumably the attainment of equal health will be more costly for those with higher health needs (worse health and general living conditions) and greater access costs (greater travel times and the like). If these effective cost differentials cannot be easily narrowed by improving living conditions or lowering the costs of travel and communication, for example, the first-best policy for ensuring equal health would be to grant income transfers to those with higher effective costs—the unhealthy, the poor, the remote. Those with high effective costs of health care, in particular, should, other things being equal, face them at the margin, but they should be given income transfers to improve their affordability. This ensures the joint objectives of efficient use (which depend on marginal costs) and equality of consumption and access (which depends on income). Even though first-best income transfers are unlikely to be feasible, attempting to ensure equality of access by setting prices equal to zero is likely to be quite inefficient, and not necessarily equitable, because access costs and nonpecuniary costs (such as inconvenience) remain unequalized. Second-best schemes, including possible discounts and exemptions for those with high needs (such as the elderly) or high access costs (rural residents, for example) are to be preferred to blanket zero prices.

QUALITY. It is sometimes argued that user fees are desirable, because they can increase the quality of services provided. This argument, however, is dangerously oversimplified and confuses the issues of raising revenue and providing service. True, if user fees are levied, and if they are retained by the service provider (such as a clinic), and if the workers in the clinic have appropriate incentives to spend the revenues on better facilities rather than consuming them themselves, an increase in fees may improve quality. But there are a number of holes in this argument.

First, if quality is "too low," this implies that social welfare would be increased by improving quality. The question of how to finance the necessary expenditure is the same as the general optimal tax problem, and its answer is unlikely to be solely with taxes on the good whose quality was increased. Second, the assumption that additional quality is desirable should be evaluated carefully. If such quality improvements are costly to implement, the net benefit may not be very high. This is particularly true when quality refers more to the aesthetic aspects of the surroundings than to the standard of medical treatment. While the former is important, there may be more pressing priorities for public expenditures. Third, additional financial resources retained by the service provider may not be useful in improving quality without complementary reforms at other stages of the production process. For example, if charges are levied for physician visits, but drug supplies continue to be disrupted by upstream bottlenecks and corruption, the productivity of the additional financial resources in improving quality may be limited. The idea that individuals will be better-off because they are paying higher prices certainly strikes one as disingenuous at best, and mildly nuts at worst. It is the use of these resources that is important, and there is no particular reason that they should be provided by users.

Financing Publicly Provided Insurance

In many countries, the provision of medical care is generally handled through the private market, with doctors, hospitals, and other providers charging for their services. At the same time, most countries provide some kind of public insurance to guard against the financial risks associated with unexpectedly high medical bills. Publicly provided insurance, which we will study in more detail in chapter 10, is often defended both on equity and efficiency grounds, providing all citizens with protection and avoiding some of the numerous market failures that characterize private insurance markets. Whatever the merits of public provision, it is interesting to investigate arguments relating to the desirability of possible financing mechanisms.

We might ask first whether taxes that finance publicly provided insurance should be related to the benefits that such insurance confers on individuals. If insurance is provided by the state because of the failure of an efficient private market to emerge, such a scheme could be seen as being equitable in some sense. Because the expected benefits from coverage are larger for higher-risk individuals than for those with lower risks, it would, however, require risk-based taxes. That is, higher-risk individuals would be required to pay larger contributions to financing than others.

If not all individuals are covered by the public system, the principle of benefit-related taxation would imply that only those covered would be required to make contributions. In practice, the causation may work in the opposite direction, with constraints on available tax instruments and revenue sources determining the eligible population. For example, if only workers in the public sector can be reliably taxed, and if it is thought desirable to somehow base contributions on benefits, then eligibility for coverage will need to be restricted to public sector employees.

Alternative public systems cover a restricted class of individuals based on demographic characteristics. For example, in the United States, the Medicare system caters primarily for the elderly (individuals over 65) and the disabled. Apart from relatively small, direct contributions from these individuals, however, most of their insurance coverage is financed by taxes on the uncovered population—that is, on current workers. While it is true that after such a system has been running for some time, the elderly will have contributed to the health insurance costs of their parents, there is a mismatch between the size of the contributions they make and the benefits they receive if the population and economy are growing. (The impact of these intergenerational transfers will be discussed in the next section.)

Public insurance schemes often include specific equity goals, frequently meant to ensure that higher-risk individuals do not pay more than others. The basis of this is simply that individuals with higher risks are effectively poorer, and if the government has an aversion to inequality they should be compensated. Because risk is difficult to observe, a rough way of achieving transfers from low- to high-risk individuals is to make contributions independent of risk. In this case, the net benefit of public insurance is greater for high-risks than it is for low-risks, and an effective in-kind transfer between the two types of individuals is implemented.

In principle, a sophisticated taxation system could implement transfers from low-risks to high-risks and transfers from rich to poor separately. Thus, a rich low-risk individual would make a relatively large tax payment, while a poor unhealthy person would receive a large subsidy. Sick but wealthy people and the healthy but poor would make smaller contributions to, or receive smaller net transfers from, the public purse. In the absence of such a system, uniform premium contributions coupled with progressive taxation might be considered a workable alternative. It should be clear, however, that the uniform (or any other) contribution to finance health insurance can be easily subsumed into the tax function, and separate taxes to finance health coverage are unnecessary.

In many countries that have public health insurance, however, there is a separate, earmarked tax to finance insurance (a notable exception is Australia, where health insurance is financed from general revenues). Often these take the form of payroll or other labor income taxes. The contributions for health insurance are positively related to an individual's wealth or income. To the extent that the benefits of public health insurance are generally independent of income, such financing not only redistributes welfare from low-risk to high-risk individuals, but also from the rich to the poor. While this may well be an intended and desirable outcome, it is not clear that such redistribution should occur through the health insurance–financing mechanism. Perhaps the main implication of this discussion is that while earmarked health insurance funds may formally exist, in practice, identical outcomes can be achieved with general tax financing.

One potential problem with earmarked funds is that they will typically rely on a single, or smaller number, of tax instruments, requiring relatively high tax rates on a small base. We know that the distortionary costs of taxation are related to the square of the tax rate, and thus the deadweight loss associated with financing health insurance can be reduced by broadening the tax base and lowering the rates. For example, high marginal rates of taxation on labor income could be reduced if other tax sources were employed (although it is an empirical question as to the relative welfare gains that would arise from such a policy shift).

Macroeconomic Effects of Mandatory Policies

The final issue in this chapter relates to the consequences of mandated health insurance coverage. We examine, in particular, the effects that such policies have on intergenerational transfers and their quasi-budgetary effects. While there may be no measured budgetary impact of the mandate, it will be shown that the real economic effects are similar to those that arise from any form of deficit spending. This may have important implications for macroeconomic performance and long-term growth and suggests that phased-in public insurance schemes may be desirable.

Suppose a government wishes to institute a community-rated universal health insurance system. That is, all individuals are required to be insured, and the premiums paid do not vary across the population. We assume that the policy is to be implemented through the public sector.[16] In this case, because the health care needs of the elderly are, on average, larger than those of the young, such a policy represents an implicit transfer of resources from the young to the old. That is, on average, the young pay more in premiums than they receive in benefits; the reverse is true for the old.

Note that as long as premiums are high enough to cover all benefits, the system will register no net deficit. If medical care expenditures relative to GDP are sufficiently high, however, there may be a significant impact on national savings. It is very likely that the young tend to save more than the elderly, precisely because one of the reasons for saving is to enable consumption when old. For example, consider the transfer of a dollar from the young to the old. Of this dollar, some fraction, σ, would have been saved by the young, but if the elderly do no saving at all, then the full dollar will be consumed. Even though public sector saving has not been affected by the transfer, private saving has fallen by σ. This reduction in saving feeds through into the size of the productive capital stock, labor productivity, and output growth of the economy.

It is useful to note that the macroeconomic impact of mandatory insurance as discussed above has little to do with the health sector. Any policy that transfers resources from the young to the old will have a similar effect. For example, the introduction of unfunded social security and increased government deficits to finance public consumption are both characterized by the same kind of intergenerational transfer, with similar macroeconomic impacts on savings and growth.[17] (For the interested reader, Auerbach and Kotlikoff 1987 provide a series of simulation results of such fiscal policies.)

These transition effects associated with the introduction of universal community-rated insurance suggest that it may be prudent to introduce such coverage gradually. A direct method would be to mandate insurance initially only for the young and to gradually increase the age limit of the

16. Alternatively, individuals may be mandated to purchase insurance from private insurance companies that are regulated to charge uniform premiums. The macroeconomic impact of such a policy is essentially the same.

17. Recall that in neoclassical growth theory, the long-run rate of growth is independent of fiscal policy. However, the intergenerational transfers identified in this section have short-run effects on the savings rate and capital accumulation, and thus on the steady-state level of output.

mandated group. This would reduce the size of the intergenerational transfer, depending on how the health care needs of the elderly were financed.

An alternative indirect mechanism for correcting the macroeconomic impact is to introduce contemporaneously an additional policy instrument that effectively transfers income from the elderly to the young. An explicit tax would probably be politically unworkable, but a broad-based consumption tax may be appropriate. Again, because the elderly consume relatively more of their income than the young, they pay relatively more tax under a consumption tax. The net effect of a well-designed health insurance–financing system and a broad-based consumption tax on national savings could thus be minimized.[18]

References

Arrow, Kenneth J. 1969. "Classificatory Notes on the Production and Transmission of Technological Knowledge." *American Economic Review* 59(2): 29–35.

Atkinson, Anthony B., and Joseph E. Stiglitz. 1976. "The Design of Tax Structure: Direct versus Indirect Taxation." *Journal of Public Economics* 6: 55–75.

Auerbach, Alan J., and Laurence J. Kotlikoff. 1987. *Dynamic Fiscal Policy.* Cambridge, U.K.: Cambridge University Press.

Baumol, William J., and Wallace E. Oates. 1988. *The Theory of Environmental Policy,* 2d ed. Cambridge, U.K.: Cambridge University Press.

Besley, Timothy J. 1988. "A Simple Model for Merit Good Arguments." *Journal of Public Economics* 35: 371–83.

Britto, Dagobert, Eytan Sheshinski, and Michael Intrilligator. 1991. "Externalities and Compulsory Vaccinations." *Journal of Public Economics* 45(1): 69–90.

Coase, Ronald. 1960. "The Problem of Social Cost." *Journal of Law and Economics* 3: 1–44.

Diamond, Peter. 1975. "A Many-Person Ramsey Tax Rule." *Journal of Public Economics* 4:335–42.

Diamond, Peter, and James Mirrlees. 1971. "Optimal Taxation and Public Production I: Production Efficiency and II: Tax Rules." *American Economic Review* 61: 8–27, 261–78.

---

18. Clearly we are abstracting from issues of intergenerational equity here. If the elderly are poor compared with the young, the transfer inherent in the introduction of universal insurance may be exactly what is desired by an egalitarian society, despite its impact on long-run output levels. However, because the reduction in long-run output is felt by many generations, the tradeoff in social welfare tends to favor restricting the size of the transfer.

Francis, Peter J. 1997. "Dynamic Epidemiology and the Market for Vaccinations." *Journal of Public Economics* 63)3: 383–406.

Geoffard, Pierre-Yves, and Tomas J. Philipson. 1996. "Rational Epidemics and Their Public Control." *International Economic Review* August: 603–24.

_____. 1997. "Disease Eradication: Private versus Public Vaccination." *American Economic Review* 87(1): 222–30.

Gertler, Paul J., and Jeffrey Hammer. 1997. "Strategies for Pricing Publicly Provided Health Services." Policy Research Working Paper 1762. World Bank, Washington, D.C.

Hart, Oliver, Andrei Shleifer, and Robert W. Vishny. 1997. "The Proper Scope of Government: Theory and an Application to Prisons." *Quarterly Journal of Economics* 112(4): 1127–61.

Hurwicz, Leonard. 1997. "On the Coase Theorems." Paper presented in the Economics Division, Research School of Social Sciences, Australian National University, July 8.

Mwabu, Germano. 1997. "User Charges for Health Care: A Review of the Underlying Theory and Assumptions." Working Paper 127. The United Nations University, World Institute for Development Economics Research, New York.

Philipson, Tomas J., and Richard A. Posner. 1993. *Private Choices and Public Health: The AIDS Epidemic in an Economic Perspective.* Cambridge, Massachusetts: Harvard University Press.

_____. 1995. "The Microeconomics of the AIDS Epidemic in Africa." *Population and Development Review* 21(4): 835–48.

Pigou, A. C. 1947. *A Study in Public Finance,* 3d ed. London: Macmillan.

Pitchford, Rohan, and Christopher M. Snyder. 1998. "Social Harm and Incomplete Contracts: An Analysis of Property Rights, Covenants and Land Ownership." Australian National University. Mimeo.

Ramsay, Frank. 1927. "A Contribution to the Theory of Taxation." *Economic Journal* 37: 41–61.

Sandmo, Agnar. 1983. "Ex post Welfare Economics and the Theory of Merit Goods." *Economica* 50: 19–33.

Siepert, E. 1997. "Ignorance, Hysteria, and Immunization: An Economic Perspective." Seminar presented at the Department of Economics, Australian National University, July 31.

Wagstaff, Adam, and Eddie van Doorslaer. Forthcoming. "Equity in Health Care Finance and Delivery." In A. J. Culyer and J. P. Newhouse, eds, *Handbook of Health Economics.* Amsterdam: North-Holland.

Weitzman, Martin L. 1974. "Prices vs. Quantities." *The Review of Economic Studies* 41(4): 477–91.

8

Welfare Economics and Project Appraisal

The previous four chapters have studied various aspects of the demand and supply of medical care and insurance and the efficiency of resource allocations mediated by the market. This chapter introduces the basic concepts of welfare economics that allow a more formal judgment about the social desirability of alternative resource allocations, incorporating both efficiency and equity concerns. The joint inclusion of both equity and efficiency objectives, by way of the social welfare function, allows one to move beyond the typical political debate that sees policy design as a choice between these alternatives without a means of quantifying the tradeoff. The analysis is particularly useful for quantifying the net social benefits of specific projects that the government might undertake, such as the building of rural hospitals, spraying for mosquito control, and the like. This chapter provides general theoretical background, and the following chapter examines the use of cost-benefit analysis (CBA) in the health sector in particular.

The next section of the chapter spends some time formalizing the way in which social choices might be made. This approach is founded in the "welfarist" tradition and views the social good as the combination of individual well-beings. In the area of health projects and policies, there are some fundamental problems of defining the outputs of projects in a way that is meaningful and useful for analysis, but standard welfare economics provides a solid basis on which to develop adjustments for health-specific issues. The standard approach is first addressed, followed by a discussion of an alternative approach which is often adopted when outputs are hard to measure and value—so-called cost-effectiveness analysis (CEA). A general discussion of this technique, as well as some criticisms, is presented. Its application to health sector projects is discussed at length in chapter 9.

Comparing Different Resource Allocations

When individuals make choices, one thinks of them as choosing between alternatives—for example, consumption, saving, and labor supply options—in a way that is consistent with some underlying preferences. These preferences are usually assumed to be representable in terms of utility functions, and certain assumptions are made that allow individual choices to be treated as if they were made to maximize utility. In particular, faced with two possible choices—for example "work hard and earn a lot, but have little leisure time," versus "work part-time and enjoy life,"—the individual calculates the utility that she would enjoy under each decision and chooses the option with the higher utility level.

When making social choices—that is, choices about the allocation of resources among a group of individuals—there are a number of alternative ways to compare different allocations, including (1) the Pareto criterion, (2) the compensation criterion, and (3) maximization of a social welfare function. The third of these is most closely akin to the utility-based theory of consumer behavior described above.

The Pareto Criterion

Suppose there are n individuals in a society or group and that there are m goods. We write $x_i = x_i^1, x_i^2, \ldots, x_i^m)$ as the vector of goods allocated to individual i. For each i, x_i is assumed to be in some set $X \subset \mathbb{R}^{m+}$.[1] We write $x = (x_1, x_2, \ldots, x_n)$ as the aggregate allocation of goods in the economy; x is an n-dimensional vector of m-dimensional vectors. Now consider two potential resource allocations, x and x', among a group of individuals. If all the members of the group prefer x to x', then x *Pareto-dominates* x', or x is *Pareto-preferred to* x'. It seems reasonable to require that any social choice rule between two alternatives should respect the Pareto criterion. That is, if everyone agrees on the choice between two alternatives, then it seems reasonable that a social choice should agree with this ordering. We say that a policy move from x' to x is a Pareto-improvement, because it makes everyone at least as well-off as before the change.

---

1. The restriction that the amount of each good allocated to an individual be nonnegative is sometimes dropped when considering production processes in which some goods are used as inputs. In the current example, however, there is no production.

Note that the Pareto criterion does not necessarily require that x_i is preferred to x'_i by individual i for all i. Thus, suppose there are two individuals, $n = 2$, and one good, $m = 1$. If people have altruistic tendencies, then the allocation (5, 5)—that is, five units of the single good to each person—might Pareto-dominate the allocation (8, 2)—that is, eight units to the first and two to the second—even though the first individual receives more resources in the second alternative. Usually, however, one makes the assumption that individuals are self-interested and care only (or at least primarily) about their own resource allocations. In this case, it would not be possible to rank the resource allocations in the example above based on the Pareto criterion, because (5, 5) is preferred by person 2, but (8, 2) is preferred by person 1.

Because rankings of alternative resource allocations using the Pareto criterion are based on individuals' preferences, it is useful to suppose that the preferences of each individual i can be represented by a utility index $u_i \in \mathbb{R}$, which is a function of x_i (or more generally, of x). We can then define a mapping $U: X^n \to \mathbb{R}^n$ that assigns to each vector of feasible resource allocations $x \in X^n$ a vector of utility indices $U(x) = [u_1(x_1), u_2(x_2), \dots , u_n(x_n)]$—or again, more generally, $U(x) = [u_1(x), u_2(x), \dots , u_n(x)]$. That is, each resource allocation is associated with a vector of utilities, and x is Pareto-preferred to x' if and only if $u_i(x_i) \geq u_i(x'_i)$ for all i, with strict inequality for at least one i.

For example, suppose two individuals must decide on the allocation of fixed quantities of m goods between themselves. We assume that when an individual receives none of each good, then her utility index is normalized to zero. If both individuals have decreasing marginal utility of each good, then the set of possible utility allocations between them—that is, the set of possible Us—is a convex set, S, as shown in figure 8.1. If we assume the individuals are permitted to dispose of the goods, then the utility possibility set contains all points along the frontier of S, as well as all points to the southwest of the frontier. All points on the frontier of S are Pareto-efficient, in the sense that neither individual can be made better-off without making the other worse-off. One would hope that the two individuals, when negotiating or bargaining over the allocation of the two goods, would ensure at least the agreed allocation left them on the frontier of S.[2]

---

2. Another useful example is that in which individuals have quasilinear preferences. In this case, utility is said to be "transferable" between individuals, and the frontier of the utility possibility set is linear. See Mas-Collel, Whinston, and Green (1995, p. 325).

Figure 8.1. *S is the Utility Possibility Set*

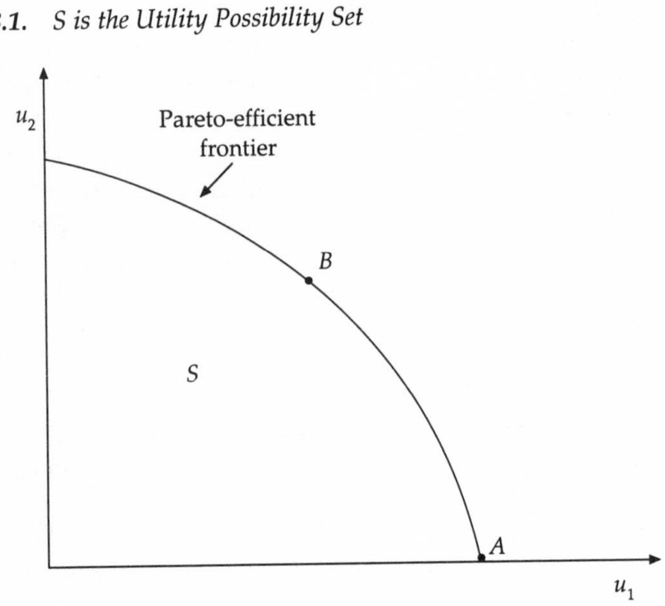

Note: A and B are both Pareto-efficient, but B is more egalitarian than A.
Source: Author.

The Pareto criterion is quite a weak condition on which to make social choices, and it seems to be a minimal requirement of any practical decision rule. For example, point *A* in figure 8.1 satisfies the Pareto criterion but allocates maximal utility to individual 1 and zero utility to individual 2. It is unlikely that such an allocation, in a social policy setting, would be considered acceptable in terms of some underlying concepts of justice or equity. Point *B*, in contrast, would appear more likely to satisfy such concerns. If the utility possibility set were not symmetric, however—say because individual 1 had greater capacity to enjoy consumption than individual 2—it is difficult to say which point on the frontier would appropriately satisfy equity concerns. The problem is that, as we saw above, there are many possible resource allocations that are not Pareto-comparable. Most policy decisions involve choices in which some individuals are made better-off, while others are made worse-off.

The Compensation Criterion

The compensation criterion tries to address some of the concerns expressed above by extending the notion of Pareto dominance. In particular, *x* is potentially Pareto-preferred to x' if there is some way to redistribute the resources entailed in the allocation x that Pareto-dominates x'. For example, suppose one wants to compare the following two allocations of a single good between two people: $x = (6, 2)$ and $x' = (3, 3)$. It is clear that x and x' are not Pareto-comparable, because individual 1 prefers x and individual 2 prefers x'. However, x is potentially Pareto-preferred to x', because the total resources of 8 in the first allocation can be distributed in such a way—say, (4, 4)—as to yield a Pareto improvement over the second allocation.

If we call an individual a "winner" if she prefers x to x' and a "loser" if she prefers the reverse, then the compensation test says that the society should prefer x to x' if the winners can compensate the losers without being made worse-off themselves. It seems reasonable that if the winners actually do compensate the losers, then the social preference rule is acceptable (in fact, it reverts to the Pareto criterion), but it is not necessarily clear that, just because the winners *could* compensate the losers (but do not), one allocation is socially more acceptable than the other. In a certain sense, then, the compensation principle ignores issues of income distribution.

There are some other fundamental problems with the compensation criterion. First, any two allocations that are part of the same Pareto-efficient frontier will remain noncomparable under the compensation criterion. For example, if there are fixed quantities of m goods to be distributed between 2 individuals as in figure 8.1, then no two allocations that lead to utility pairs on the Pareto-efficient frontier (for example, points A and B) are comparable using the compensation criterion. To see this, note that in moving from A to B, individual 1 is made worse-off and individual 2 better-off—that is, 2 is the winner. To compensate individual 1 for the loss she incurs, using a redistribution of the available goods, 2 must be made at least as badly off as she was at A. Thus the winner (individual 2) cannot compensate the loser (individual 1), and one cannot say that B is preferred to A on the basis of the compensation criterion. Similarly, it is not possible to say that A is preferred to B using the compensation test.

Second, it is possible that each of two alternative allocations is (inconsistently) preferred to the other. Thus, suppose that the alternative allocations consist of different aggregate quantities of goods, so that x and x' yield utility pairs U and U', respectively, that are located on the frontiers of *different* utility possibility sets, S and S' in figure 8.2. It is clear from the figure that x is potentially Pareto-preferred to x', because a reallocation of the resource bundle x can be used to attain the utility pair U'', which Pareto-dominates the utility pair U' derived from the allocation x'. But a similar argument can be used to establish that x' is potentially Pareto-preferred to

Figure 8.2.   *Inconsistent Comparisons of Alternative Resource Allocations under the Compensation Criterion*

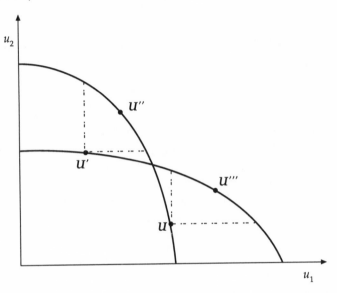

Source: Author.

x, because the bundle x' could be reallocated to attain the utility pair U''', which is Pareto-preferred to U. This is clearly inconsistent, unless one is somehow willing to argue that society should be indifferent between the allocations x and x'.

Using the Compensation Criterion: The National Income Test

Despite these shortcomings, the compensation test is often employed, sometimes implicitly, in applied welfare economics. One manifestation of the criterion is the so-called *national income test*, which states that if a project *reduces* national income, calculated at current prices, then it cannot be potentially Pareto-improving. This result may not seem particularly surprising, but it does require that the project concerns the production of private goods, and that existing prices properly measure social costs and benefits. Note that the converse is not true—that is, even if national income increases, it may not be possible for the winners to compensate the losers, even though the "size of the pie" has increased.

To see how the national income test works, consider again the case of two individuals and two goods ($n = m = 2$). There is initially a fixed supply of each good, $\bar{x}^1$ and $\bar{x}^2$, and these are allocated to the individuals in bundles $x_1 = (x_1^1, x_1^2)$ and $x_2 = (x_2^1, x_2^2)$ such that $\Sigma_{i=1}^2 x_i^j = \bar{x}^j$, for $j =$ 1 and 2. Bundles that satisfy this adding-up constraint are called feasible. Each point (u_1, u_2) on the Pareto-efficient frontier of the utility possibility set corresponds to a pair of feasible resource allocations (x_1, x_2), which can be represented as a point in an Edgeworth Box, shown in figure 8.3. Along the horizontal axis of the Edgeworth Box from the left is measured the quantity of good 1 allocated to individual 1 (so the length of the Box is $\bar{x}^1$, the maximum amount of good 1 that could be allocated to individual 1), and along the vertical axis from the bottom is measured the quantity of good 2 allocated to individual 1 (so the height of the Box is $\bar{x}^2$). Measured from the right and from the top are the quantities of goods 1 and 2 that are allocated to individual 2. The set of all

Figure 8.3. *The Edgeworth Box for the Two-Good, Two-Person Exchange Economy*

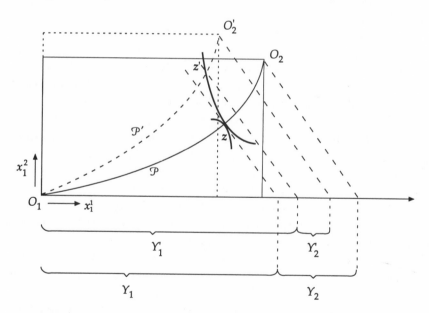

Note: The Pareto sets, $\mathcal{P}$ and $\mathcal{P}'$, denote all Pareto-efficient allocations of goods between the individuals.

Source: Author.

allocations of goods that corresponds to the Pareto possibility set is called the Pareto set, and it is marked $\mathcal{P}$ in the figure.

The individuals' indifference curves can also be drawn in the Edgeworth Box, and along the Pareto set $\mathcal{P}$ they are tangent, as shown. In particular, at any point on the Pareto set the slopes of the individuals' indifference curves are equal, and the common slope is identified with the relative price of the two goods, because it measures the marginal rate of substitution between them. Using these relative prices, the total value of goods (using good 1 as the numeraire) when the allocation is at point z, say, is equal to the distance $Y = Y_1 + Y_2$. Y then is a measure of "national income," being the value of goods consumed in this exchange economy. Note that the prices used to value the different goods correspond to their marginal rates of substitution.

Now suppose a project increases the net supply of good 2 by using up some of good 1, so that the new available resources are $\bar{x}^{1'} < \bar{x}^1$ and $\bar{x}^{2'} > \bar{x}^2$. (For example, good 1 might correspond to raw materials and good 2 to a produced good.) Because the available quantities of the goods have changed, so have the dimensions of the Edgeworth Box, which is now narrower and taller. The origin for individual 1 remains the same, O_1, but that for individual 2 moves from O_2 to O_2'. Similarly, the position of the Pareto set changes—to $\mathcal{P}'$, for example. Now consider the point on the new Pareto set z' at which the utility of individual 1 is the same as before the project. Using the original relative prices, we know that national income at the allocation z' has fallen to $Y' = Y_1' + Y_2' < Y$. In contrast, the value of goods allocated to individual 1 at z' has increased; that is, $Y_1' > Y_1$, so that it must be the case that individual 2's income (measured using the original prices) has fallen—that is, $Y_2' < Y_2$. This means that individual 2's budget set is strictly smaller after the project than before, so her attainable utility must have fallen. Thus, we have found a point z' on the Pareto set $\mathcal{P}'$ at which individual 1 has the same well-being as before the project, and individual 2's well-being has fallen. The project cannot therefore be potentially Pareto-improving.

The converse of the rule, however, is *not* true—that is, the fact that national income increases does not necessarily imply that the resulting resources can be distributed in a way that makes everyone better-off. This is easiest to see using figure 8.4, describing a similar situation as in figure 8.3, but in which the use of good 1 in the production of good 2 leads to an *increase* in national income from Y to Y''. The figure is drawn so that individual 1's indifference curve through the initial allocation z passes through the new origin for individual 2, O_2''. We assume that the new Pareto set $\mathcal{P}''$

Figure 8.4. *An Increase in National Income Does Not Necessarily Lead to a Potential Pareto Improvement*

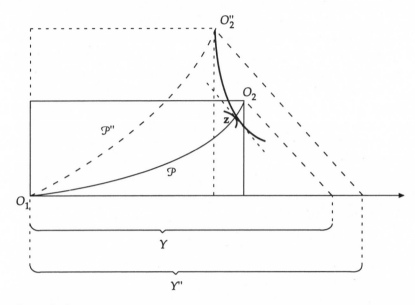

Source: Author.

passes through O_2''.[3] Clearly national income, measured at the original prices, has increased, but the project cannot be considered to yield a potential Pareto improvement because individual 2 has been made strictly worse-off (she now consumes nothing) while individual 1 is no better-off.

Welfare Functions

Individuals seem to have preferences over the distribution of income. It seems reasonable, then, to have a social choice rule that takes these distributional concerns, as well as efficiency issues, into consideration. The Pareto and compensation criteria essentially side-step the issue of distribution and assume that the appropriate distribution of society's resources can be achieved after

---

3. This is satisfied as long as the marginal utility of each good approaches infinity as the quantity becomes small for individual 2.

the size of the pie has been maximized. That is, the criteria pick out efficient allocations and then leave it up to a well-informed, benevolent social planner to make sure that reallocation takes place to address equity concerns.

There are two problems with this. First, such benevolent social planners are difficult to find. Second, there are certain constraints (relating to information asymmetries and dynamic choices) on the behavior of even the most well-intentioned governments that preclude costless redistribution of resources. It is necessary, then, to address efficiency and equity issues concurrently, and this is achieved by postulating the existence of a social welfare function. For a given population of n individuals, such a function maps vectors of utility levels of the individuals into the real numbers, and is represented by $W(u_1, u_2, \ldots, u_n)$.

There are a number of alternative welfare functions that may seem appropriate (see Atkinson and Stiglitz 1980). First, the utilitarian social welfare function is of the form

$$W(u_1, u_2, \ldots, u_n) = \sum_{i=1}^{n} u_i$$

which is simply the sum of individuals' utilities. It may appear that this welfare function has no distributional objective—indeed, the distribution of utility levels is irrelevant in its calculation. However, if each individual has the same utility function, and the marginal utility of income is declining, then the optimal allocation of income, and hence utility, is egalitarian.

Alternatively, the social welfare function suggested by Rawls (1974) is of the form

$$W(u_1, u_2, \ldots, u_n) = \min_i u_i$$

which says that social welfare is equal to the utility level of the least well-off individual in society. This function explicitly takes into account equity concerns by positing that if some individuals become better-off, while the poorest remain unaffected, then there is no increase in welfare. Only by improving the lot of the very poorest is social welfare increased.

An intermediate version of these two polar cases is the isoelastic welfare function employed by Atkinson (1970), of the form

$$W(u_1, u_2, \ldots, u_n) = \frac{1}{1-v} \sum_{i=1}^{n} [u_i^{1-v} - 1].$$

When $v = 0$, this function collapses to the utilitarian case (up to an additive constant), and as $v \to \infty$ it approaches the Rawlsian version. Then, v might be naturally identified with society's aversion to inequality.

In the case where $n = 2$, one can draw social indifference curves, as if W were a utility function and its arguments were consumption goods. Figure

8.5 shows social indifference curves for each of the above three cases. Given a social welfare function W, choosing between alternative resource allocations reduces to the problem of maximizing W subject to the constraints imposed by the utility possibility set. That is, x is preferred to x' if and only if $W[U(x)] > W[U(x')]$. The function W explicitly incorporates both equity and efficiency objectives simultaneously, allowing the choice over the size of the pie and its distribution to be made concurrently, not sequentially.

The main argument against the use of social welfare functions is that the utility index used to measure individual preferences is exactly that, an index. As such, it represents an ordinal measure of individual well-being and primarily serves as a tool for comparing the well-being of a given individual under different circumstances. Use of a social welfare function implicitly assumes that the utility index has *cardinal* significance as well, and that levels of utility can be compared across individuals. To alleviate this problem, it is necessary to reinterpret the individual utility indices, $u_i(x_i)$, as functions that assign socially agreed values of welfare to individuals. Typically it is assumed that the $u_i(.)$ functions are identical, although this can be relaxed to incorporate divergent abilities, capacities, and so on.

Good-Specific Equity

The discussion above has been phrased in terms of general allocations of consumption goods, the identity of which was of little concern. To the

Figure 8.5. *Social Indifference Curves for Alternative Social Welfare Functions: (a) Utilitarian, (b) Isoelastic, and (c) Rawlsian*

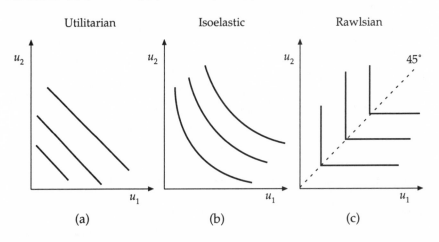

extent that equity concerns were incorporated into the discussion, they came via the construction of social welfare functions that exhibited varying degrees of inequality aversion. However, this aversion was to inequality of the *utilities* of individuals. In particular, there was no sense in which the government or social planner cared about *how* individuals attained their utility levels, just about their relative sizes.

In some cases, there is often expressed a preference for equity with respect to consumption of a particular good. For example, many countries try (at least in theory) to provide "equal access to education for children," or "equal treatment under the law." Similarly, equality of access to or consumption of health care is a frequent battle cry of those who wish to reform health care delivery and insurance systems. It seems that, although people may be prepared to put up with a certain degree of inequality of income, they are less prepared to accept such wide-ranging inequality of health care. These are difficult issues that pervade health policy debates in all countries, and, if not perfectly understood, they at least need to be acknowledged as reasonable additional criteria on which resource allocation decisions depend. (See Harberger 1984 for a thought-provoking discussion.)

Sometimes, concerns over equity in health care may actually stem from efficiency concerns. For example, if the distribution of vaccinations is inequitable, in the sense that some people are not vaccinated, then the effectiveness of the treatment for those who receive it may be severely limited. In this case, it may be better either to vaccinate everyone or to vaccinate no one (and use the money for something else), rather than waste the resources on ineffectual prevention. Here, equity of treatment is necessary for efficiency.

Project Appraisal in Practice

This section presents a brief review of the basic components of social cost-benefit analysis (CBA). For a fuller treatment, the reader is referred to the classic texts of Little and Mirrlees (1974) and Mishan (1994). This is the most widely used method of making decisions about the social value of projects and policy changes and can be based firmly on the conceptual material of the previous sections. In practice, some variants are used, depending on the nature of the particular project and the availability of information. Included in these alternatives, particularly in the appraisal of health sector projects, are so-called cost-effectiveness analysis (CEA) and cost-utility analysis (CUA). The main lesson to learn from the following analysis is that practitioners should be extremely careful in using the latter two methods of appraisal, because they can easily lead to sub-optimal choices.

Cost-Benefit Analysis of Generic Projects

If one is to accept the use of welfare functions as primitive representations of social preferences, then projects that increase the value of the chosen social welfare function should be undertaken, and those that reduce it should be avoided. In practice, the way the change in the value of the social welfare function is calculated is to examine the change in net supplies of goods in the economy and to calculate the value using appropriate prices. For example, when the supply of some goods (like foreign exchange, labor, raw materials, and the like) is reduced, the value of the reduction is measured as a cost, C. Similarly, the value of those goods that see an increase in net supply (for example, clean water, health clinic visits, electric power) is measured as a benefit, B, and the difference between the two is the net social benefit of the project, $B - C$.

THE EFFECTS OF SIZE. A first point to note is that this method of calculating the net increase in social welfare is appropriate only for *small* projects—that is, projects that have relatively small effects on net supplies of the relevant goods and services. This can most easily be seen by considering an economy in which all individuals are identical and receive the same allocations of goods. In this case, the economy can be treated as if it consisted of a single representative consumer. Suppose there are two goods in the economy, 1 and 2, and the initial net supply vector (per capita) is at point $x = (x^1, x^2)$ in figure 8.6. Also drawn is the individual's indifference curve through x, which coincides with the social indifference curve. All net supply vectors above this curve represent per capita allocations of the two goods that can be used to increase social welfare.

Now, suppose a proposed project uses good 2 to produce more of good 1 and will have the effect of moving the net per capita supply vector to point y. Clearly this project increases social welfare, because y is above the social indifference curve through x. As before, let us identify the slope of the individual's indifference curve at x, which reflects her marginal rate of substitution between the two goods, with relative prices. Valuing costs (reductions in good 2) and benefits (increases in good 1) at these prices results in the calculation of a positive net benefit, because y lies to the right of the tangent line through x. In this case, positive net benefits as calculated correspond to an increase in social welfare.

Figure 8.6. *Large Projects Might Increase National Income but Reduce Welfare*

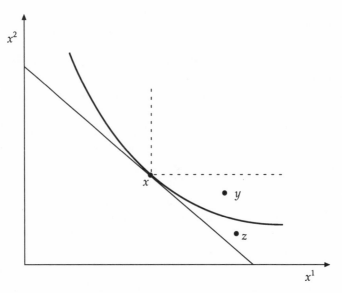

Note: From a starting point x, projects that result in net supply vectors y and z both increase national income at initial prices, but only y increases social welfare.
Source: Author.

Consider, however, a project that results in a somewhat larger change in the per capita net supply vector to point z. Because this point lies below the social indifference curve, the project should not be accepted. However, calculating the value of the project using existing prices yields positive net benefits, and a standard CBA would suggest acceptance of the project. Because individuals are identical, this disagreement between the direction of change of the value of consumption and that of the value of social welfare is not related to the Pareto comparability issues discussed earlier. Indeed, all distributional issues have been ignored. When the project is small enough, there will be no disagreement, and a positive net benefit calculation will be indicative of an increase in social welfare. However, for large projects this may not be the case. The reason is essentially that, when chosen properly, prices measure *marginal* social benefits, but these marginal social benefits can change as the quantities of the corresponding goods change.

CHOOSING THE RIGHT PRICES. In figure 8.6, we argued that as long as the price vector was tangent to the social indifference curve, the net benefit of a small project calculated using these prices would be a good indicator of the associated change in social welfare. Even under the assumption that the change in the value of output is a good measure of the change in social welfare (that is, even when the project is small), there are two fundamental reasons that market prices may not be equal to shadow prices—that is, those prices that provide the appropriate weights to use in aggregating across goods in order to make welfare judgments. The first reason is distributional and arises when individuals are not identical, as was assumed above. The second reason is that relative market prices may not reflect marginal rates of substitution, and therefore they may not provide a good first approximation to the slope of the social indifference curve. Relative market prices are likely to diverge from marginal rates of substitution whenever there are significant market failures, which may arise owing to (1) externalities in consumption or production; (2) public goods; (3) the presence of distortionary taxation; (4) market nonclearing, such as the existence of involuntary unemployment; and (5) nonprice market interventions such as import quotas and many other examples.

Suppose there are n individuals and m goods, and that one wants to decide whether a project that changes the allocation of goods from $x = (x_1, x_2, \ldots, x_n)$ to $x' = (x'_1, x'_2, \ldots, x'_n)$ should go ahead. (Recall that $x_i = (x_i^1, x_i^2, \ldots, x_i^m)$ is the vector of goods allocated to individual i.) Given a welfare function $W(\ldots)$, the level of social well-being changes from $W_0 = W[u(x_1), u(x_2), \ldots, u(x_n)]$ to $W'_0 = W[u(x'_1), u(x'_2), \ldots, u(x'_n)]$. For small changes in the allocation of goods, $dx_i^j = x_i^{j\prime} - x_i^j$, the change in welfare can be written

$$dW = W'_0 - W_0$$
$$= \sum_{i=1}^{n} \frac{\partial W}{\partial u_i} du_i$$
$$= \sum_{i=1}^{n} \frac{\partial W}{\partial u_i} \left(\sum_{j=1}^{m} \frac{\partial u_i}{\partial x_i^j} dx_i^j \right)$$
$$= \sum_{j=1}^{m} \sum_{i=1}^{n} \left(\frac{\partial W}{\partial u_i} \frac{\partial u_i}{\partial x_i^j} \right) dx_i^j$$
$$= \sum_{j=1}^{m} \sum_{i=1}^{n} p_i^{j*} dx_i^j$$

where $p_i^{j*} = (\partial W/\partial u_i)(\partial u_i/\partial x_i^j)$ defines the shadow price of consumption of good j by individual i and comprises the joint effect of an increase in consumption of the good on individual utility and the effect of the increase in utility on social welfare. This decomposition makes it clear, that for making welfare judgments, simple aggregation of goods across individuals using uniform prices is not justified, and that personalized shadow prices are in general required.

If there are no market failures, then relative market prices p^j/p^k will be equated with the marginal rate of substitution between goods i and k, so that actual market prices p^j will be proportional to each individual's marginal utility of consumption of good j, $\partial u_i / \partial x_i^j$. In this case, the change in welfare is

$$dW = \sum_{j=1}^{m} \sum_{i=1}^{n} \left(\frac{\partial W}{\partial u_i} \frac{\partial u_i}{\partial x_i^j} \right) dx_i^j$$

$$= \sum_{j=1}^{m} p^j \sum_{i=1}^{n} \frac{\partial W}{\partial u_i} dx_i^j$$

$$= \sum_{j=1}^{m} p^j \, \hat{dx}^j$$

where $\hat{dx}^j = \sum_{i=1}^{n} \omega_i \, dx_i^j$ is the weighted sum of the quantity changes. The weighting factors, $\omega_i = \partial W / \partial u_i$, are referred to as distributional weights. Note that if W is quasi-concave (as one would expect for a social planner with some degree of inequality aversion), then the weights are larger for individuals with lower initial utility levels. That is, an increase in the consumption of a good by a poor person receives a larger weight than that of a rich person. These weighted aggregates of consumption changes are then valued using market prices.

Note that if all individuals are identical and receive identical allocations, then the individual shadow prices p_i^{j*} are independent of i, and the change in welfare can be written

$$dW = W_0' - W_0$$

$$= \sum_{j=1}^{m} \sum_{i=1}^{n} p^{j*} \, dx_i^j$$

(8.1)

$$= \sum_{j=1}^{m} p^{j*} \left(\sum_{i=1}^{n} dx_i^j \right)$$

$$= \sum_{j=1}^{m} p^{j*} \, dx^j$$

where $dx^j = \sum_{i=1}^{n} dx_i^j$ is the unweighted change in the net supply of good j. If in addition there are no market failures, then $p^{j*} = p^j$, and social welfare increases as long as the market value of output does (for small enough projects).

A possibly surprising implication of this discussion is that, absent distributional concerns and market failures, the change in social welfare from a public project *must* be either zero or negative. One way to see this is to note that when $p^{j*} = p^j$, the final term in equation (8.1) is equal to the change in profits from the change in the resource allocation. But in a competitive economy with profit maximizing firms, this must be at most zero.

Alternatively, recall the first fundamental theorem of welfare economics, which states that, absent market failures, the competitive equilibrium allocation of resources is Pareto-efficient. Now, in the absence of distributional concerns, different Pareto-efficient allocations cannot be ranked in terms of social welfare, so it must be the case that a public project either leaves welfare unchanged (if it results in another Pareto-efficient allocation) or reduces welfare (if the new allocation is Pareto-inefficient).[4] Thus, as a matter of principle, to justify undertaking a public project, we require either distributional concerns or market failures. While some authors shun the idea that distributional concerns should be allowed to influence the choice of projects, they often invoke market failures as a rationale. The market failure is usually identified by asking the question "Why is the project not being undertaken by the private sector?"[5]

In practice, distributional adjustments are made, if at all, in an ad hoc way when costs and benefits have been calculated using standard shadow prices—say, by giving extra weight to recipients in rural or remote areas. An argument against incorporating distributional weights directly into project appraisal is that the government should act to address such concerns directly through the tax system and should not rely on the blunt instrument of project selection and design to redistribute income. While this is true, the project analyst is often not in a position to influence general government tax and transfer policies and must take them as given.

We saw above that the appropriate relative weights with which to aggregate goods in order to make welfare judgments are marginal rates of substitution in consumption. Even if all individuals are identical, market failures can mean that individuals are constrained from equating their marginal rates of substitution with relative market prices, so market prices will not yield the required aggregation.

The general principle can be illustrated most easily in the case of an economy with involuntary unemployment. In this situation, at the existing wage rate, there are some individuals who are willing but unable to work—say, due to the existence of a minimum wage. If the government employs some of this surplus labor in the proposed project, then it incurs a financial cost (equal to the wage rate times the number of workers

---

4. It is important to note that this argument has nothing to do with the relative efficiency of production in the public and private sectors. In fact, it implicitly assumes that they are equal.

5. See Devarajan, Squire, and Suthiwart-Narueput (1997).

employed). However, the social cost of this employment is likely to be much less than the financial cost and could be close to zero. What one really wants to measure is the opportunity cost of the (previously unemployed) worker's time, which may be very low. That the government must pay the worker is not central to the calculation of economic cost, or more precisely, of the reduction in social welfare arising from the use of the worker's time.[6]

Two other important shadow prices are the social rate of discount—the price at which future benefits and costs are valued—and the value of foreign exchange. The former is often unlikely to be equal to the market rate of interest, especially when intergenerational issues are considered. The latter is of particular importance in countries considering projects with large import or export components that maintain misaligned exchange rates.

SHADOW COST OF PUBLIC FUNDS. An important price that requires separate attention is that of public revenue. It may seem that a schilling is a schilling is a schilling, as far as the government is concerned. However, if the government must make large financial transfers to pay for the project, and if these transfers must be funded by distortionary taxation, then the cost of financing must be included. Consider, for example, a project costing 10 percent of the annual budget. The government must find these resources, through either taxation or borrowing. If taxes are increased, then the distortions they impose on the economy represent real economic costs and should be taken into account in evaluating costs. If external borrowing is used to finance the project, however, future taxes must be raised, and interest charges must be financed. While the appropriate mix of debt and taxes is nontrivial, it is clear that the requirement that at some stage costs are financed through taxation implies that, other things being equal, the economic cost of inputs generally exceeds the financial cost. As a general rule, the shadow price of one unit of government revenue is greater than one. It has been estimated by Browning (1987) for the United States at between 1.1 and 1.5 and at a much higher level for some developing countries. Thus, if the shadow cost of public funds is 1.4, a project that just broke

---

6. Note that employment used in production represents an economic *cost*, and that even though the particular individual concerned is probably happy to get the job, the use of her labor still represents a reduction in net supply of a good (leisure). The value of this cost may be very low, but it is unlikely to be negative (except for considerations of the important social effects of unemployment, particularly among youth).

even using shadow prices unadjusted for the distortionary costs of taxation would need to have benefits at least 40 percent higher to pass a rigorous CBA.

ALTERNATIVE PROJECTS. When projects are small and mutually exclusive, the general rule of accepting all those that have positive net social benefits and rejecting the others is appropriate. But project evaluations also include choices among projects that are mutually exclusive. Such choices include the technique of production (a malaria control project using bed netting is different from one using vector control spraying), timing decisions (a project started today is different from one deferred until tomorrow when its effects will be better known), and size (a proposal to build a 100 MW generator is different from one to build a 1,000 MW station).

The two implications of these observations are that the analyst should be careful to establish the counterfactual—what would have happened in the absence of the project—and to calculate net benefits relative to that scenario; and that the use of some common alternative net benefit measures can be misleading. For example, a common measure of net benefit is the benefit-cost ratio, B/C. If this is larger than one, the project should go ahead, and if it is smaller than one it should be rejected. However, in comparing two mutually exclusive projects, it is *not* the case that the one with the larger benefit-cost ratio should be preferred. An obvious example is of two projects of different sizes. If the first costs 100 with benefits of 200, and the second costs 1,000 with benefits of 1,500, then the net benefits of the second (500) are larger than those of the first (100), and the second should be chosen. However, the benefit-cost ratio of the first (2.0) is higher than that of the second (1.5).

Similarly, when evaluating an investment project with future costs and benefits, the internal rate of return (IRR) is often used as a measure of the project's desirability. Technically, the IRR is that interest rate that makes the net present value of the project equal to zero. If the IRR is greater than the social discount rate (or the social cost of capital), then the project should go ahead. But again, in comparing two mutually exclusive projects, it is not possible to infer that the one with the higher IRR has a larger net social benefit. For example, suppose the social rate of discount is zero, and consider two projects with costs incurred in the first year and benefits that accrue in the second. The first project has costs of 20 and benefits of 40 and so has an IRR of 100 percent, while the second project has costs of 10 and benefits of 25 and has a higher IRR of 150 percent. However, the net social benefit of the first project is 20 and that of the second is 15, so the first is preferable.

Cost-Effectiveness Analysis

CEA has been described by Mishan (1994, p. 110) as "a truncated form of cost-benefit analysis and draws guidance only from the cost side—or alternatively, only from the benefit side—of a cost-benefit format." It is best thought of as a tool for ordering proposed projects in terms of their social desirability, given some exogenous budget or other constraint. In most cases of CEA that are relevant to health projects, project outputs are quantified but not evaluated. CEA then provides a basis on which to choose those projects that either yield the largest output for a given dollar budget or minimize the cost of producing a required output level. However, the extent to which normative judgments can be made with such information is limited, and according to some authors (Hammer 1997; Hammer and Berman 1995), cost-effectiveness measures are essentially useless. Given its wide use in the health evaluation sphere, it is clearly important to understand the limitations of the technique.

The principle of efficient use of resources is close to economists' hearts, so on the face of it the use of the cost-effectiveness criterion is appealing. However, economists are generally concerned with allocative efficiency, as well as productive efficiency, and it is only the second of these that CEA addresses. In particular, CEA may provide guidance on the best way to spend a given health budget in order to attain some exogenous goal (for example, to maximize the number of children vaccinated), but it provides no information on whether the attainment of such a goal is worth the resources spent. Alternatively, it can suggest the cheapest way of attaining a particular outcome (for example, a 95 percent vaccination rate among children), but it does not help the analyst decide on what that outcome should be (why is 95 percent preferred to 100 percent, or to 50 percent?).

CEAs generally value costs in terms of dollars or some other monetary measure. However, the measurement of output is usually in terms of some quantity or effectiveness index E, such as tons of steel or lives saved. One reason for adopting this differential treatment of costs and benefits is that in some cases—particularly projects with direct effects on health—analysts feel uneasy about placing a monetary value on outputs (such as lives saved). Typically it is assumed that the outputs of steel projects, for example, can be more defensibly valued than can outputs of projects that affect health and life directly.

Given the choice of output measure (and this choice is often not beyond contention), the main tool of CEA is the cost-effectiveness ratio, C/E. Project analyses often report average C/E ratios (that is, total cost divided by total output), but it is also possible, and more useful, to calculate marginal or incremental C/E ratios, dC/dE. These two measures correspond directly with the concepts of average and marginal costs of production in standard production theory.

It is uncontroversial that, under suitable regularity conditions, efficient production of a given quantity of a particular good requires that marginal costs be equated across different inputs and techniques. Similarly, the same marginal conditions characterize the production of a maximal level of output given a particular resource constraint.[7] Thus, a necessary (but not sufficient) condition for optimal project choice is that incremental C/E ratios are equated across different projects.

For example, if the budget of the department of health is fixed, and the stated objective is to maximize health in terms of lives saved, then a certain combination of drug treatment, preventive care, and emergency services may be optimal, assuming that each of these production techniques (techniques of producing saved lives) has sufficiently increasing marginal costs that devotion of all of the health budget to one of them is inefficient. In contrast, if the objective of the ministry of health is to reduce the infant mortality rate to x percent, and this requires saving the lives of 1,000 children a year, then the optimal choice of projects to effect this outcome is that which minimizes total costs, and thus equates marginal cost of an extra child saved across projects. In both cases, CEA can be used to implement this efficiency rule by requiring that incremental C/E ratios are equated across projects.

In practice, projects tend to be less than infinitely divisible, so equality of marginal costs is unlikely to be feasible at a given output. In this case, CEAs are used to choose between projects with different C/E ratios, those projects with the smaller ratios being chosen either until the budget is exhausted or until the quantity goal is achieved. However, CEA itself provides no basis on which to decide the optimal size of the budget or the optimal quantity target, because benefits are not measured in a way that makes them comparable with costs.

By contrast, CBAs that base acceptance of projects on the basis of (discounted) net benefits assume neither that the budget available for financing,

---

7. Usually in production theory one does not consider the firm to face a fixed budget. However, there is a direct correspondence between both the problem of efficient production of a given output and efficient use of a given budget in consumer theory. These are the standard utility maximization and expenditure minimization problems, respectively.

nor the output targets, of potential projects are fixed. All projects with positive net benefits are accepted, and all those with negative net benefits are
rejected. In an operational sense, CBA may appear closely related to CEA
when project choice is made on the basis of IRR calculations. In this case, all
projects with IRRs greater than a given cutoff rate—the social discount rate—
are accepted. This cutoff rate is common to all projects, be they in the agriculture, industry, health, education, or other sectors, and its use is equivalent to
the requirement that the social net present value of the project is positive. A
corresponding choice rule in CEA is to accept all projects with a C/E ratio
less than a certain cutoff rate. However, the appropriate cutoff rate will generally differ among different kinds of projects because the measure of effectiveness or output is different—tons of steel versus lives saved—and because the social value of the output will differ across projects with different
outputs. The only way in which to calculate appropriate cutoff rates for
projects with different outputs is to calculate social benefits as well as costs,
but this means effectively reverting to CBA.[8]

Other Issues in Generic Project Evaluation

Let us deal briefly with three further issues in the appraisal of investment
projects. These turn out to be important for various kinds of health projects.

DIRECT AND INDIRECT COSTS AND BENEFITS. Most of the general discussion
has implicitly dealt with the appraisal of projects in terms of their effects
on net supplies of consumption goods and services (because these are the
arguments of utility functions). However, the direct outputs of projects are
often intermediate inputs into subsequent production processes and therefore have indirect effects on consumption and hence welfare. It is necessary to be careful, then, in evaluating the net impact of such projects: such
care can be particularly important in the analysis of health projects.

Let us start with a nonhealth example. Suppose a project under consideration produces 100 units of cement as a direct output. One way of valuing

---

8. In the next chapter an attempt is made to make health projects with qualitatively different outcomes comparable using cost-effectiveness criteria. This method,
known as CUA (cost-utility analysis), converts different types of health outcomes
into a common unit—most often quality adjusted life years (QALYs)—and com-
pares different projects using standard cost-effectiveness techniques. Clearly, however, these projects remain incomparable with nonhealth projects, such as the construction of steel mills and dams.

this output is at the international price (possibly calculated using a shadow exchange rate different from the official exchange rate), net of transportation costs, assuming that cement is tradable. Alternatively, the value of the cement could be calculated on the basis of the consumption services provided by construction made possible by the cement-generating project. Suppose these services have a gross value S. Clearly, if other inputs such as labor and steel are required at the construction stage at a cost C, the net value of the cement is $S - C$. Also, if the services are rendered over time but can only persist if maintenance is carried out, the effective depreciation costs must also be deducted in arriving at a valuation of the cement.[9]

This example illustrates that in evaluating projects it is sometimes necessary to incorporate apparently unrelated costs and benefits (especially if the output of the project is used to produce an input into yet another production process). Essentially, if benefits cannot be calculated on a net basis directly (perhaps because there is no market for the good as an input), then they must be calculated indirectly as the appropriate algebraic combination of gross valuations of other goods and services (S and C above). It turns out that this is of central concern in the evaluation of certain health projects that extend the length of life. Such projects effectively increase the supply of time (which is a necessary input into virtually all consumption processes). The question becomes, Should additional costs (such as future medical care costs) that result from the extension of life be included in the appraisal of the original project? A more complete discussion of this issue is deferred until chapter 9.

DISCOUNTING. As touched on previously, it is usually necessary to value costs and benefits that arise in the future in a way that makes them directly comparable with each other, and with costs and benefits that arise in the first year of a project. Usually future streams are discounted at a rate that should represent a social discount rate. The appropriate value of this rate is not clear. In a world of infinitely lived individuals and perfect capital markets with no market failures, the appropriate rate would be the market rate of interest, which accurately measures individuals' time preferences.

---

9. The two methods of calculating the value of the cement are qualitatively the same. Each calculates the net value of the cement in the production of consumption by using different production processes. The first uses exports of cement to produce imports, while the second uses the cement (and other inputs) to directly produce services domestically.

Market failures, which may be ubiquitous in markets for intertemporal trades, naturally lead to adjustments to the discount rate away from the market interest rate, just like any shadow price.

However, the other important issue concerns the fact that individuals are not infinitely lived, and benefits and costs that arise in the future may well affect *different people* from those affected early in the project's life. Only if currently living generations fully take into account the well-being of future generations in making their consumption and saving decisions will the market interest rate properly reflect the value of forgone consumption. This is unlikely to be the case, because future generations are not party to any transaction involving the interest rate (because they are not alive yet). In general, it is questionable whether the costs and benefits to future generations should be discounted at all. In practice, standard CBA uses a discount rate of around 10 percent, but many health-related analyses assume a much smaller one of 3 percent. If the temporal patterns of costs and benefits are sufficiently different (for example, large up-front costs with deferred future benefits), then the choice of the discount rate can make a large difference in whether the project is accepted or not.

RISK AND IRREVERSIBILITY. The outcomes of projects are nearly always uncertain, either because of the possibilities of cost overruns, delays, or other production glitches, or because of uncertain demand for the produced good or uncertain takeup rates for certain interventions. Should the analyst adjust calculations of net benefits to account for this risk? In general, for small projects the answer to this question is no, because the government is in a position to fully diversify the risks across the population. (This result is often referred to as the Arrow-Lind Theorem; see Arrow and Lind 1970.)

However, when projects involve irreversible investments—that is, investments that cannot easily be converted to other uses once sunk—then the presence of uncertainty may well alter the analyst's appraisal of the project. This is not so much due to risk aversion on the part of the government as to the fact that, if one waits, new information may become available that will alter the optimal decision regarding a project. When the investment is reversible, the value of waiting is limited, because the government can always alter course midstream. But in the large majority of cases this is not true, and waiting has a positive value, known as an option value. In general, the higher is this option value, the greater the net benefits need to be in order to justify the project.

References

Arrow, Kenneth, and R. C. Lind. 1970. "Uncertainty and the Evaluation of Public Investment Decisions." *American Economic Review* 60: 364–78.

Atkinson, Anthony B. 1970. "On the Measurement of Inequality." *Journal of Economic Theory* 2: 244–63.

Atkinson, Anthony, and Joseph Stiglitz. 1980. *Lectures on Public Economics.* New York: McGraw-Hill.

Berman, Peter. 1995. *Health Sector Reform in Developing Countries: Making Health Development Sustainable.* Cambridge, Massachusetts: Harvard School of Public Health, Department of Population and International Health.

Browning, Edgar. 1987. "On the Marginal Welfare Cost of Taxation." *American Economic Review* 77(1): 11–23.

Devarajan, Shantayanan, Lyn Squire, and Sethaput Suthiwart-Narueput. 1997. "Beyond Rate of Return: Reorienting Project Appraisal." *World Bank Research Observer* 12(1): 35–46.

Hammer, Jeffrey. 1997. "Prices and Protocols in Public Health Care." *World Bank Economic Review* 11(3): 409–32.

Hammer, Jeffrey, and Peter Berman. 1995. "Ends and Means in Public Health Policy in Developing Countries." In Peter Berman, ed., *Health Sector Reform in Developing Countries: Making Health Development Sustainable.* Cambridge, Massachusetts: Harvard School of Public Health, Department of Population and International Health.

Harberger, Arnold. 1984. "Basic Needs versus Distributional Weights in Social Cost-Benefit Analysis." *Economic Development and Cultural Change* 32: 455–74.

Little, I. M. D., and James Mirrlees. 1974. *Project Appraisal and Planning for Developing Countries.* London: Heinemann.

Mas-Collel, Andrew, Michael D. Whinston, and Jerry R. Green. 1995. *Microeconomic Theory.* New York: Oxford University Press.

Mishan E. J. 1994. *Cost Benefit Analysis,* 4th ed. London and New York: Routledge.

Rawls, John. 1974. "Concepts of Distributional Equity: Some Reasons for the Maximin Criterion." *American Economic Review,* papers and proceedings, 64: 141–46.

9

Health Projects and the Burden of Disease

After the fairly lengthy and detailed introduction to the general theory of project appraisal of the previous chapter, the analysis of health care projects more specifically can be considered. Examples of such projects include direct health care interventions (for example, immunization programs and screening for breast cancer), behavioral interventions (AIDS awareness campaigns, anti-smoking campaigns, general education regarding sanitation, and so on), infrastructure projects (sanitation and water supply, mosquito spraying), health care provision projects, (such as hospital and clinic construction and training of medical care providers), and drug policies (research and development policies, choice of drugs, and so forth).

A natural question to ask is whether, and why, it is necessary to devote an additional chapter to specific issues in health project evaluation. Are the techniques and principles of the general theory not sufficient? Essentially, the answer is that the benefits of health projects can be difficult to measure directly, and that special approaches have been developed for their estimation.

To highlight this point, it is perhaps useful to summarize Johannesson's (1996, chapter 1) historical review of the development of health policy and project evaluation. Rice (1967) was one of the first to attempt to implement cost-benefit analysis in the health sector by estimating the monetary value of health improvement on the basis of the costs of illness averted (see below). This approach is based on human capital theory (Becker 1964), and effectively identifies the value of healthy life with the labor earnings (wages) it makes possible.

Mishan (1971) was a strong critic of the human capital approach to measuring benefits. Recognizing that health might be valued in its own right, somewhat divergent approaches to measuring project benefits were adopted.

Within the realm of orthodox cost-benefit analysis, various methods for calculating measures of willingness to pay were developed. These were based either on direct elicitation of valuations (the contingent valuation approach) or on estimating demand curves and inferring consumer surplus measures.

One way to understand the reason that both these approaches to benefit estimation can be useful is to recall from our discussion in chapter 4 that we think of inputs to the health production process (physician services, immunizations, drugs, improved environmental quality, and so forth) as being valued because of their impact on health. Now for some projects, the link between the inputs and health outcomes may be tenuous at best and not well understood by individuals. In this case, their demand for the inputs into the project may not be good indicators of the value they place on the final output. Eliciting preferences for health improvement directly may then be preferred to estimating an implicit demand curve for project inputs and using this to measure consumer surplus. We might think of these projects as being public health type projects, like AIDS awareness campaigns. This approach, of valuing health improvements that derive from these types of projects directly, is adopted, for example, by Tolley, Kenkel, and Fabian (1994).

By contrast, the benefits of the introduction of a new drug, whose effects are well understood, might be elicited directly. Johansson (1995) and Johannesson (1996) adopt this approach, using various methods such as contingent value estimates for the health goods themselves (as opposed to the health outcomes, as above). If, in addition, the demand curve can be estimated for such goods, direct measures of consumer surplus are possible. Because of limited price variability in health goods markets, travel cost methods (see Clarke 1998 and Gertler and van der Gaag 1990) or other synthetic approaches are required. This estimation method has the advantage of basing valuation measures on the actions of individuals and not their stated intentions.

An alternative approach to benefit estimation that arose was to quantify, but not value, the health outcomes of projects and interventions. These quantities were then used to construct cost-effectiveness measures (for example , Klarman, Francis, and Rosenthal 1968) that, it was claimed, could be used to provide a useful mechanism for choosing between alternative projects. To allow comparison of projects with qualitatively different health outcomes, this approach was expanded to what is referred to as cost-utility analysis (CUA). Like the public health approach mentioned above, these techniques focus on health outcomes and not the valuation by consumers of inputs into health production. However, an important distinction is that cost-effectiveness analysis (CEA) and CUA measures of outcomes are not valued in a way that is comparable with costs (that is, in monetary terms).

Cost-Benefit Analysis of Health Projects

We saw in the previous chapter that the operational method of calculating the increase in social welfare produced by a project is to measure its benefits and costs (using suitably chosen prices) and to take the difference between them. The most significant problem faced in evaluating the net impact on social welfare of health projects is the valuation of benefits. Because the general goal of health projects is to increase the quality and length of life, these particular outcomes must be valued in a full cost-benefit analysis (CBA), but this can be difficult. Possible health outcomes that need to be addressed include increased life expectancy, decreased morbidity, reduced disability, improved quality of life, averted future medical costs, and increased productivity.

There will also be nonhealth benefits associated with the health effects, including improved environmental quality; higher property values; and reduced waiting times at, and travel costs to, hospitals and clinics. It is difficult to draw distinct lines between some of the health benefits and the nonhealth benefits (for example, productivity increases and reduced waiting times).

Valuation of Costs

There are no specific problems associated with the valuation of costs that are more severe in the analysis of health projects than in other projects. Care should be taken to include all these items, including nonpecuniary costs, such as travel times to clinics and the like. These can be included either as costs or as negative benefits (so that reductions in costs show up on the benefit side). This choice has no impact on the calculation of net benefits, but it can alter reported benefit-cost ratios significantly. As long as the net benefit is positive, the benefit-cost ratio can be made arbitrarily high by labeling enough of the costs as negative benefits. This is another argument against the use of benefit-cost ratios as the primary tool of analysis.

One type of cost associated with health projects that deserves special mention is that of future medical care. This is a particularly striking example of the treatment of apparently unrelated costs (see chapter 8). Suppose the result of a particular health intervention is a reduction in deaths from AIDS. Because this disease strikes mainly individuals between the ages of 20 and 40, the increase in life expectancy for affected individuals may be relatively large. With such an increase in life expectancy, individuals can expect to incur additional future health care costs during these added years of life (such as treatment for unrelated heart disease). Similarly, suppose a medical intervention increases life expectancy, but it requires continued palliative use of expensive drugs to maintain a tolerable quality of life. Should the costs of these drugs be included in the appraisal of the original project? These questions are best addressed in conjunction with the measurement of benefits, to which we now turn.

Valuation of Benefits

There are three main candidates for valuing the benefits of health projects: the cost of illness approach, the willingness to pay approach, and the "do nothing" approach.

COST OF ILLNESS. Under this method of valuing the benefits of health projects, the analyst first estimates the costs of continuing the existing treatment strategy without the project and the value of forgone production because of the illness. These are direct economic costs of the illness, and they may represent a lower bound on the benefits of a project that removes the necessity of continuing the current treatment and restores the individuals to full working capacity. However, there are a number of reasons that this approach, while workable, is not fully satisfactory.

- First, the project may not be fully effective in removing the need for existing medical treatment and cost. It can easily increase the costs of treatment, in which case the benefits would be negative.
- Second, while the value of new production arising from the effects of the project on individuals' health and productivity is certainly a benefit, these benefits are not restricted to market production. This may be particularly important in some developing countries where home and informal sector production make up a large share of domestic economic activity. Analyses based on market production would tend to inappropriately bias project analysis toward interventions that improved the health of working-age men.
- Third, this method does not attribute any positive value to individuals' just *feeling better* because of the project. That is, to the extent that individuals are more than just production units, improvements in health have beneficial effects on general quality of life concerns beyond the savings in medical care costs and increases in productivity.

As an example of a case when the cost of illness method of valuing the benefits of health care projects can backfire, consider a project aimed at improving the health of children with chronic respiratory illness. Suppose they receive no treatment initially, and that the project delivers a weekly dose of a drug that removes all symptoms of the illness. There is clearly no saving of medical costs because of the project, and because the subjects are children, there is no increase in productivity, so the value of benefits is zero.

This example illustrates that there is no necessary relationship between the social value of a project and the costs avoided because of the program. Or, as Mishan (1994, p. 8) has observed, "Only a moment's reflection is needed to perceive that the sum a community is ready to pay for eradicating a particular disease has no necessary relation to the costs incidental to its current treatment." Indeed, it is only possible to use avoided costs to measure benefits when dealing with small changes in undistorted competitive markets, when individuals are operating on their demand curves.

The example also highlights the need to carefully establish the counterfactual in project appraisal. That is, it is important to know what would have happened in the absence of the project. It would be somewhat misleading for a government to claim that the benefits of the drug project example above were very high—in the absence of the project, it was willing to send all the children to Switzerland for expensive treatment! This shows that, by varying the counterfactual, interested parties can enhance or reduce the measured benefits of a project, and the analyst must have a good idea of what *really* would have occurred without it.

Cost of illness measures can sometimes be useful in establishing the magnitude, if not the exact size, of potential benefits from disease prevention or control. Studies of the direct medical costs and indirect economic costs (mainly in lost or reduced labor productivity) of disease reveal that the latter can sometimes far outweigh the former. For example, the direct medical costs of avoiding a death caused by suicide are virtually zero, because there is no medical treatment for the condition.[1] However, the indirect costs can be enormous, mainly because individuals who commit suicide are usually young, and they have potentially long working lives ahead of them. Heart disease, in contrast, has large direct medical care costs associated with treatment in the last few months of life (usually after a heart attack), and relatively lower indirect economic costs, because those who die from coronary disease are generally older. Care must be taken in making inferences from these figures,

---

1. There may, of course, be costs involved in outreach programs and the like that provide ongoing counseling for potentially suicidal individuals.

however, for a number of reasons. First, the rate of discount used to aggregate over time is clearly important. And second, it may be the case that the productivity of individuals who die of different causes would have differed markedly if they had remained alive for a longer period. For example, suicidal youths may have little education, poor social support, and so forth, and they may face the prospect of very low future wages. Those who suffer heart attacks, however, may be more likely to be (overweight) businessmen, with prospectively high future labor earnings. Assuming the same foregone productivity levels in each case may produce quite misleading results.

WILLINGNESS TO PAY. Suppose we know the likely effects of a project on health status outcomes (life expectancy, morbidity, and the like). Consider giving each affected individual i the following choice: continue with the status quo, or implement the project, with the predicted effects on health status, with some amount of money, Δm_i, being taken from the individual. We can imagine starting from a low value of Δm_i, at which individual i is very willing to accept the project minus Δm_i in favor of the status quo, and then increasing Δm_i, asking the individual to choose each time, until we reach a value Δm_i^* at which the individual is indifferent between the two choices. This maximal amount of money that the individual would be willing to give up to ensure the project proceeded is called the individual's *willingness to pay* for the project. Δm_i^* is a monetary measure of the benefits that the individual receives from the project.

If the effect of the project is to change the supply of some good or service that enters each individual's utility function directly, then a simple graphic representation of willingness to pay is possible. Suppose the supply of good x available to a given individual is to be increased from x_0 to x_1 as a result of the project. Suppose also that the inverse demand function for the good is $p(x)$. Then the gross willingness to pay is

$$\int_{x_0}^{x_1} p(x)dx$$

which is just the area $A + B$ under the demand curve between x_0 and x_1, shown in figure 9.1.[2]

---

2. This is only an approximation to the true change in the individual's welfare as a result of the change in quantity. Ideally, the welfare change is estimated by either the compensating variation (the willingness to pay) or the equivalent variation (the willingness to accept), which are represented by areas to the left of the relevant Hicksian demand curves. When the share of expenditure on good x is small enough, the approximation is reasonably accurate.

Figure 9.1. *Willingness to Pay*

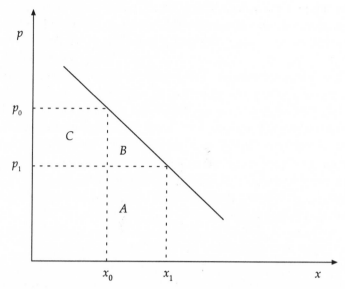

Note: The willingness to pay, or consumer surplus, from an increase in quantity of good x from x_0 to x_1, is equal to area $A + B$. The consumer surplus resulting from a price decrease from p_0 to p_1 is $B + C$.
Source: Author.

Alternatively, suppose the consumer is initially purchasing the amount x_0 at a price p_0, and that the "project" is a policy to subsidize the price so it falls to p_1. The total change in consumer surplus is now the area $B + C$ in figure 9.1.[3]

A significant problem with this approach is that for health-related services, and other similar social sector projects, it is difficult to estimate the inverse demand curve $p(x)$. Because medical care services are often provided at zero or small monetary prices, other measures of privately incurred cost—such as travel costs—need to be used to estimate the demand curve (see chapter 4).

---

3. The effect of both projects is to increase consumption from x_0 to x_1, but the consumer surplus measures are, in general, different. This is because in the case of a direct increase in consumption, the individual does not pay for the increment, *and* the project has no effect on the amount paid for the initial quantity. However, with a price decrease, the consumer pays an amount $A = p_1(x_1 - x_0)$ for the increment, and saves an amount $C = (p_0 - p_1)x_0$ on her initial purchase. Thus, the difference between the two measures is $A - C$.

The total willingness to pay for a project, equal to the aggregation of each Δm_i^* over the affected population, is

$$WTP = \sum_{i=1}^{n} \Delta m_i^*$$

where there are n individuals. This is often used as a measure of the benefits of a project. One problem with willingness to pay is that rich people will be more *willing* to pay for a project than poor people, because they are more *able* to pay for it. Each individual faces the budget constraint $\Delta m_i^* \leq m_i$, where m_i is i's total income. Thus if benefits are measured by willingness to pay, we are likely to see projects that benefit the rich being measured as having greater social returns than those benefiting the poor.

However, what we are really interested in is the increase in social welfare produced by the project, which can be written as

$$\Delta W^* = \sum_{i=1}^{n} \frac{\partial W}{\partial u_i} \frac{\partial u_i}{\partial m_i} \Delta m_i^*.$$

If it is reasonable to assume that the marginal utility of income falls with income, and the social welfare function entails some aversion to inequality, then values of Δm_i^* reported by those with high m_i will receive relatively little weight in the calculation of ΔW^*, because both $\partial u / \partial m_i$ and $\partial W / \partial u_i$ are likely to be relatively small. If we assume a utilitarian social welfare function, then $\partial W / \partial u_i = 1$ for all i, and ΔW^* differs from aggregate willingness to pay to the extent that individuals' marginal utilities of income differ. In practice, these distributional weights are usually not included, and, if anything, a more qualitative distributional analysis is conducted separately.

ESTIMATING WILLINGNESS TO PAY. Two standard ways of calculating willingness to pay are to conduct surveys of individuals and to use existing market and nonmarket data to make estimates. The first approach is known as contingent valuation, and the second essentially tries to estimate the consumer surplus of figure 9.1 directly from observable data.

The contingent valuation approach is based on surveys of individuals, in which their willingness to pay for a project is elicited directly. The approach has been used most widely in the valuation of recreational facilities (such as parks) and other environmental amenities.[4,5] There are at

---

4. For general treatments of the contingent valuation approach, see Hausman (1993), Johansson (1987), and Mitchell and Carson (1989).

5. Contingent valuation analysis has also been used to estimate individuals' so-called "nonuse" valuations. For example, even though most people will never

least two problems with this method. First, unless the individuals are actually required to pay what they report as their valuations, they may have a large incentive to strategically manipulate their reported willingness to pay. For example, if they are confident that the amount they are required to contribute to the financing of the project is not related to their expressed willingness to pay, they can increase the chances of the project going ahead by overreporting, while not necessarily bearing the costs. If they are required to make a contribution that is positively related to their valuation, however, then they may underreport their willingness to pay, assuming that such a strategy will not greatly reduce the chance of the project being undertaken.[6]

The second problem is that the contingent valuation approach is based on what people *say* and not on what they *do*. Even though they might feel strongly when presented with a hypothetical choice, they may change their minds when they actually have to make such decisions in practice. A related problem is that the analyst, by framing questions differently, may be in a position to bias the outcome of the survey.

The basic task of calculating consumer surplus measures is to estimate underlying demand curves. In the absence of reliable information on demand functions, it is possible to make rough estimates on the basis of relative prices in related markets. For example, the "required compensation" method is used to estimate the willingness to pay for additional safety of workers in dangerous occupations by comparing their wages with those of similar individuals in less dangerous jobs (see Viscusi 1978). There are many econometric problems for such analyses, and adjustments may need to be made for factors such as employee ignorance (for example, when employees are unaware of the negative health effects of particular behaviors or environments), self-selection (when individuals who enjoy taking risks enter more dangerous jobs), and inflexible labor markets (wherein individuals in dangerous jobs may be willing to changes jobs, despite the extra pay they receive in their current position, but are unable to do so).[7]

In place of such limited analyses, one may try to estimate a demand curve directly for the relevant good. This can be problematic if the good in question is difficult to define (such as higher quality of life) or does not

---

see (or otherwise use) remote wilderness areas, they may place large values on maintaining them, free of development and exploration.

6. For a thorough analysis of information revelation issues in the provision of public goods, see Green and Laffont (1979).

7. Regarding the factor of employee ignorance, it is unclear how the preferences of uninformed individuals should be weighted in social evaluations.

have a natural market interpretation (for example, greater life expectancy). In these cases, selected intermediary goods (such as clinic visits) can be used as the object of analysis, and various methods, such as those of chapter 4, can be used to estimate demand curves.

TREATMENT OF FUTURE MEDICAL AND NONMEDICAL COSTS. The issue of the treatment of future medical and nonmedical costs in project evaluation can now be addressed. Recall the earlier examples of health interventions increasing future health care costs, either solely through the extension of life (with the accompanying vulnerability to future disease and illness), or as a consequence of the ongoing nature of the treatment. On the face of it, one is tempted to argue that the first kind of unrelated costs should not be included in the calculation of project costs, but that the second should be. However, there is little economic rationale for this choice.

There is a direct analogy here with the example (see chapter 8) of the project that produces cement, which can be valued by its productive use. In the current example, we can think of additional life years gained as an input into the production of future consumption. The other inputs would include, in addition to time, the physical goods themselves, including future medical treatments, but also such things as movies and shoes.[8] If individuals are required to pay directly for future medical costs (as they are for future consumption goods), and if benefits are estimated on the basis of willingness to pay, then future medical costs need not be included. If individuals are not required to pay for future medical costs under the projects, however, willingness to pay will measure gross benefits, and future medical costs should be included in the calculation of costs. A similar procedure would be required for any future costs, medical or otherwise, related or unrelated. If benefits are estimated on the basis of willingness to pay, but individuals are not required to incur the future costs themselves, such costs should be included on the cost side of the CBA.

The fact that the treatment of future costs depends crucially on the way in which future benefits are estimated suggests that their appropriate treatment in project appraisal methods that do not include benefit calculations (for example, cost-effectiveness analysis) will be difficult to establish.

---

8. One difference is that in this instance, time can be directly consumed (cement could not be), so it has both a consumption and production use. In addition, these uses may not be mutually exclusive.

Sensitivity Analysis for CBA of Health Projects

Even the most rigorous cost-benefit analysis requires that assumptions be made. To check that these assumptions do not affect the results of the analysis too much, it is useful to undertake the estimation of net social benefits for a range of such assumptions. Useful parameters that might be varied include compliance and acceptance rates (in estimating the effectiveness of drug therapies, for example); the discount rate; the direct costs of the project, including cost and time overruns; and various aspects of the value of benefits.

CEA and CUA of Health Projects

As mentioned previously, when project outcomes are difficult to quantify or evaluate, alternative methods of appraisal, based primarily on the cost side, are sometimes employed in place of cost-benefit analysis. Cost-effectiveness analysis should be used when the analyst is choosing between alternative production techniques that result in the same qualitative, quantitative, and distributional level of output. Cost-utility analysis can be used when the qualitative nature of the output may differ between projects (for example, one produces vaccinations, and the other reduces road accidents), but it still requires fixed quantity and distributional allocation of the output. For example, the number of years of healthy life gained under alternative projects, and the people who enjoy those additional years, should be the same.

Cost-Effectiveness Analysis of Health Projects

The underlying principles and shortcomings of cost-effectiveness analysis (CEA) were presented earlier (see chapter 8), but some examples of the approach in health project appraisal are of use. First, note that the unit of output must be the same when comparing two different projects. In CEA of health projects, the unit is often something like "number of lives saved," "reduction in infant mortality rate," and the like.

MISLEADING CEAs OF HEALTH PROJECTS. Two related examples help illustrate the short-comings of CEA in health project appraisal. The first, from Mishan (1994, chapter 16), regards the analysis of a screening program, and the second, from Hammer (1993) considers the CEA of a drug project.

Suppose there are three tests that can detect lung cancer, and that once detected, the cancer is curable. Each test costs $1,000 per person to administer. There is a population of 10,000 people, and full screening with the first test costs a total of $10 million, and it will detect 100 cases. But some individuals with lung cancer will not be detected, so the second test can be performed. This costs an additional $9.9 million but will only detect 10 cases. Finally, a third test costing a total of $9.89 million is available, and of the remaining 9,890 individuals, it will detect just a single case.

The cost per life saved (or, at least, per case detected) with the first test is $100,000, that of the second is about $1 million, and that of the third test is close to $10 million. This might suggest that the first test is "worth it," the second one is "marginal," and the third is "a waste." Indeed, the project with the lowest C/E ratio is the first test. Now assume that the individuals are told that they can undertake "a series of three tests" to detect lung cancer, and that they are asked to value the opportunity to take those tests. The tests reduce the risk of death from lung cancer from $111/10,000 \approx 1$ percent, to zero, at a total personal cost of $3,000. Now, it is not unreasonable (in a rich country) to expect that the average valuation of removing the risk of death from lung cancer is greater than this figure, in which case the benefits of the three tests outweigh the costs, and all three tests should be administered.

At the same time, the three tests cost about $270,000 per life saved, which is greater than the cost-effectiveness of implementing just the first test.[9] In this case, a CEA would mistakenly suggest the adoption of a single-test screening program against a multiple-test approach.

Alternatively, consider the example of Hammer (1993, p. 20),

> Consider a situation in which two drugs are available to treat a particular disease. Drug 1 changes the probability of avoiding death from 0.2 to 0.3 and costs $5 per treatment. Drug 2 changes the probability from 0.2 to 0.25 and costs $2 per treatment. The cost per life saved by drug 1 is $50 ($5 ÷ [0.3–0.2]), while lives saved by drug 2 cost $40 ($2 ÷ [0.25–0.2]), making drug 2 more cost-effective.
>
> Most people probably would opt for drug 1, though, provided they are willing to pay more than $60 to save their life. For any imputed value of life greater than $60, the value of the increased

---

9. The total cost is $10 million + $9.9 million + $9.89 million = $29.79 million, and the number of lives saved is 111. So the cost-effectiveness ratio is $268,380 per life saved.

probability of recovery outweighs the extra cost of the drug...Cost-effectiveness ratios, while seeming to avoid the contentious issue of deciding on a monetary value of life, merely disguise an implicit valuation that may not reflect people's preferences.

In both of these examples, the level of output (increase in probability of recovery) is not fixed under the alternative projects. Thus, while average costs may be minimized by choosing the less expensive screening technique or drug, aggregate net benefits are higher if an alternative is adopted.

SOME APPROPRIATE USES OF CEA. The preceding examples suggest that one should be careful in using cost-effectiveness analysis in evaluating alternative health projects. It is possible, however, to define a restricted class of examples in which CEA can be applied. Such examples might include:

- The choice between free distribution of condoms and AIDS education programs aimed at reducing the HIV infection rate. The C/E ratio may be of the form "dollars per infection prevented." Distributional issues aside, CEA is appropriate only if the reduction in the infection rate is similar under the two schemes (for example, 50 percent), in which case the cheaper alternative is chosen, or if the cost of the two programs is the same, in which case the more effective one is chosen.[10]
- The choice between two drugs that cure sleeping sickness, assuming that both drugs have the same success rates and similar side effects (if any). The C/E ratio would be of the form "dollars per case cured."
- The choice between an anti-smoking campaign targeted at children and a tax on cigarettes, assuming that the tax rate is set at a level that has the same effect on the number of children smoking. The C/E ratio upon which the choice might be made could be "dollars per person who gave up, or who was dissuaded from taking up, smoking."

These examples illustrate the narrow range of settings in which CEA is satisfactory. They also suggest an additional criticism, which is that the units of measurement chosen for the denominator of the C/E ratio may not provide a useful normative indicator for the purposes of decisionmaking. For instance, in the smoking example, should we be concerned about the number

---

10. Notice, however, that either success rate targets or costs have presumably been set at an earlier date, and that choice could not have been made on the basis of CEA.

of people who give up, or the improvement in their quality of life because they give up? If giving up increases the irritability of some people but not others, we would want to measure these outcomes differently. This is essentially a distributional issue highlighting the need for the distributional allocations of the outputs of a pair of projects compared using CEA to be identical.

Cost-Utility Analysis

To address this and other problems, cost-utility analysis (CUA) attempts to measure outcomes in a way that, while not comparable to input costs, allows comparison of qualitatively and sometimes distributionally different outputs. In CBA, outcomes are measured in a common unit (usually money), which allows them to be compared not only with each other but also with costs. CUA stops short of this, but tries to improve the applicability of CEA.

The unit of analysis is most often some measure of life saved, adjusted for the health and other conditions of that life—that is, the quality of life. A popular unit of analysis is thus the quality adjusted life year, or QALY. Some authors interpret the QALY as a measure of the *utility* of the outcomes of a project (hence the name cost-utility analysis, although this can create confusion). The CUA ratio used for making decisions is thus a measure of dollars per QALY. Because it remains an average cost concept, it suffers from the same problems regarding project size as the standard cost-effectiveness ratio. Nevertheless, it has the advantage that more alternative projects can be compared, as long as they produce the same number of QALYs.

Notice also that there is some scope to include distributional concerns in CUA. Differences in income across individuals are generally not used to adjust QALY measures, but other adjustments, based on the ages of the individuals concerned, their sexes, and other characteristics, can be made. These adjustments are not always made in the direction one might expect, based on distributional justice—for example, the value of QALYs gained by an unskilled worker may be less than those gained by a rich man if the rich man can afford a higher quality of life—but they can be used in ways that reflect distributional goals.

MEASURING QALYs. The main conceptual issue in calculating QALYs surrounds the comparison and aggregation of years of life in different health states. How do we measure a year spent with a broken leg, compared with one spent with fully working limbs? Are two years spent in fear of infection with a disease, but without contraction, equal to two years or to one without such fear? These comparisons can only be made by somehow measuring the strength (and direction) of individuals' preferences over different health states. Thus, in relation to some comparator state of health (usually defined as *full health*), quality adjustments are numbers between 0 and 1, where 0 represents death and 1 represents the comparator state.[11]

There are four basic methods (with many variants) aimed at calculating QALYs—the standard gamble, time tradeoffs, rating scales, and attribute-based techniques. The first three methods involve direct elicitation of preferences, either by offering the individual a choice over artificially constructed alternatives, or by asking for scaled rankings of alternatives. The last provides a more objective measure of quality of life based on defined functional capabilities of individuals in particular health states.

Suppose one wishes to elicit the relative value of a year of life spent with a given health status—caused by a chronic disease, for example—compared with a year of full health. In the standard gamble method, an individual is offered a choice between living with the disease and taking a gamble that offers the possibility of full health, but with some probability p of death. For example, the choice might be between continuing with the status quo, or undergoing some kind of corrective surgery that has a probability p of being fatal. This choice is shown in figure 9.2.

The lower is the probability at which the individual would be willing to accept the gamble, the higher her quality of life must be in the chronic illness state. Thus, the probability p provides a ranking of the desirability of alternative health states, so that if p is the minimum probability at which the gamble would be taken, the value of a year of life with the illness is assumed to be p times the value of a year of life in full health.

Notice that an individual's attitude toward risk may well influence the choice, and so it will affect the cutoff probability that is used to weight illness states. Thus, two individuals who find life in a particular disease state equally distressing may be allocated different weights if one is more risk-averse than the other. This is a potential shortcoming of this approach. Also, the use of death as the opposite of full health may present some problems. It is possible to imagine an individual with a debilitating disease

---

11. It is easy to imagine that the quality adjustment figure may be negative if a disease or condition is sufficiently distressing. Support for the legalization of euthanasia in some countries suggests that such values are by no means unlikely to exist. We assume for now, however, that the adjustment is always nonnegative.

Figure 9.2.   *Standard Gamble for Elicitation of Relative Weights of Chronic Illness versus Full Health*

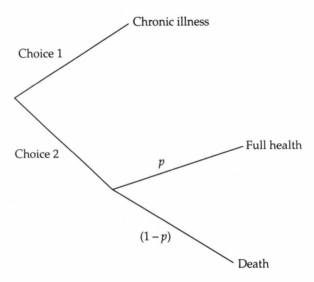

Source: Author.

demanding a very high probability of full health to agree to the gamble, if that person is sufficiently averse to death itself. Another person (perhaps one who believes in reincarnation) may not find death particularly unpalatable and would thus be willing to lower p somewhat more.

In the time tradeoff method, instead of choosing a probability of full health less than the given probability of a chronic condition (which is one), individuals are asked to report a length of life in full health, t_h, that is less than the projected length of life in the chronic unhealthy condition, t_u. The ratio t_h/t_u is assigned as the relative weight of life with the chronic condition to life in full health. Geometrically, this can be interpreted as a conversion of unhealthy life of a given length into healthy life of a shorter length, as in figure 9.3.

This method appears to avoid the problem of risk aversion, but it introduces the problem that life lived at different ages may not be of the same value to different individuals. Thus, if an individual has a very high discount rate, then life lived after the age of 50, for example, may be of very little value to that person at age 30. If the individual had a life expectancy greater than 50 with two different chronic diseases, she would likely rank

Figure 9.3. *Time Tradeoff Method of Calculating the Relative Weight, w, of Life with a Chronic Illness to Life in Full Health*

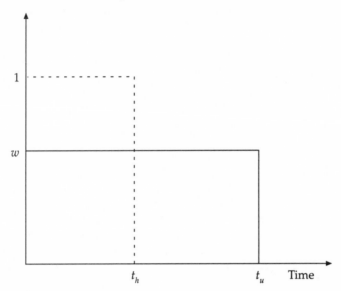

Source: Author.

the two diseases very closely using the time tradeoff approach, despite finding life with one much less distressing than life with the other.[12]

The rating-scale method directly elicits an individual's relative weighting of different health states by asking that a numerical value be assigned between 0 and 1 (or 0 and 100) corresponding to each alternative. There is no risk involved, and there are no time preference issues, although it is difficult to interpret the weights. It is tempting to suggest that a value of 0.5 would imply that the individual would be indifferent between living in the particular health state and living with full health, but with half the income (or wealth). In this sense, the rating-scale method might provide a kind of "willingness to pay relative to income," but the conceptual foundations of such an interpretation are questionable, because the individual is not explicitly given such a choice.

Attribute-based techniques of QALY calculation rely less on measuring individual preferences and more on identifying objective functional

---

12. In addition, of course, her life expectancy with the condition is risky, so the issue of risk aversion is not entirely avoided.

capabilities. Selected dimensions of function are defined, such as physical function, role function, social-emotional function, and other coexisting health problems (see Torrance, Boyle, and Horwood 1982). For a given health state or condition, various weights are assigned to measure the degree to which it reduces function in each dimension. These weights may be derived from direct elicitation from individuals, using methods similar to the three methods above, but where the choices are between states of full health and with the selected functional incapacities identified. These weighted dimensions are then aggregated together to form a so-called "multiattribute utility (MAU) model," which allows the effects of diseases on functional capacity to be compared, and a QALY measure to be derived.

USING QALYS IN A COST-UTILITY ANALYSIS. This subsection presents a simple example of the use of QALYs to perform cost-utility analysis. Subsequent sections will look in more detail at issues that need to be addressed when QALYs are used to measure the burden of disease, although the underlying principles remain valid.

In calculating the number of QALYs gained from a particular project, there are four main steps to be undertaken in a CUA:

- First, identify the alternatives: for example, the premise may be excellent health from birth with the project, versus a chronic health condition from birth, which deteriorates after age 15.
- Second, assign utility weights to the different states: 1 for excellent health, 0.7 for the chronic condition until age 15, and 0.3 thereafter.
- Third, estimate life expectancies in the different states: for example, 75 in the case of full health, and 25 with the condition.
- Fourth, calculate the total QALYs in each state, and the difference: with the project, the individual has 75 QALYs, and without it, 13.5 (= 0.7 times 15 + 0.3 times 10) QALYs. The difference is 61.5 QALYs.

This calculation is represented graphically in figure 9.4. There are many additional factors that need to be incorporated, including the proper choice of life expectancy, discounting, and the treatment of individual attributes (including sex, income, and so on).

The Burden of Disease—International Comparisons and Aggregation

This section presents a review of methods used in calculating the burden of disease as developed by the World Bank and the World Health Organization

Figure 9.4.   *Calculating QALYs*

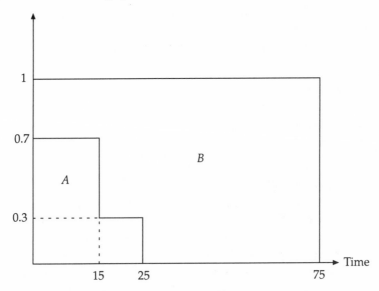

Note: A CUA for a project that produces excellent health with a life expectancy of 75 years, compared with a chronic disease that leads to poor and deteriorating health until death at age 25.
Source: Author.

(see Murray and Lopez 1994; World Bank 1993). Much of the technical analysis is drawn from Murray (1994). The exercise may be best thought of as one input into a large-scale application of CUA. That is, the burden of disease as calculated represents a measure of the *utility* (weakly defined) that could be gained by eradicating all disease. It should be noted, however, that measures disaggregated by country or disease (or both) are potentially more important for policy design and project appraisal, because the utility measures developed are only useful to the extent that they are used for comparative analyses. Only if the global measure could be compared with costs (which can only be done within a CBA framework) would it serve a rigorous analytical purpose.

In place of the defining tool of CUA—the QALY—the World Health Organization (WHO) and the World Bank estimates of the burden of disease use the DALY—the disability adjusted life year. The DALY differs in some respects from the QALY, because it attempts to inch toward a more economic measure of the benefits of improvements in health status—for example, by introducing productivity weights, age weights, and discounting. However, many of these attempts to adjust the QALY without undertaking a full calculation of benefits are based on arbitrary assumptions with little basis in welfare economic theory. Anand and Hanson (1995) present a thorough analysis of the potential pitfalls of the approach. Here we present the technique accompanied by some critical commentary.

General Conceptual Issues

The burden of disease calculations aim at being comprehensive, comparable, and consistent. To this end, the following principles are followed (Murray and Lopez 1994):

a. The effects of all health-related outcomes that represent a loss in human welfare are included. Thus, the calculation attempts to estimate the *total* burden of disease from all sources, in contrast to narrower measures such as infant mortality rates, life expectancy rates, and so forth. This implies that the standard against which health outcomes are measured—the *full health* standard—is quite high.

b. The calculation methodology attempts to treat individuals more or less identically, but only in some areas. For example, the effects of a health state experienced by a poor person are given the same weight as those experienced by a rich person. Women's welfare in a particular health state, however, is weighted slightly less than that of men, and health states experienced by individuals of different ages are weighted differently, which renders the attempt at anonymity incomplete.

c. As a special case of treating individuals identically, the method attempts to allow international comparisons by treating health states similarly across countries. The example given in Murray and Lopez (1994) is that the death of a 40-year-old woman in Bogota should be treated the same as the death of a 40-year-old woman in Boston, despite potentially large differences in local income-earning opportunities, life expectancies, and quality of life.

d. Finally, the unit of analysis, that is, the unit in which welfare losses from premature mortality and morbidity are measured, is time. This is meant to be an improvement on more case-specific units, such as deaths per population (used in the case of infant mortality studies, for example) or the incidence of certain diseases. It does conform to the requirement of output measures in CUAs by allowing comparison of qualitatively different health outcomes, but again, it does not allow comparison with costs.

Measuring the Burden of Disease

Within these guiding principles, the WHO/World Bank method attempts to measure the burden of disease by calculating the number of years of healthy life lost because of the health condition. If the health condition is death, then the number of years lost is equal to the difference between the age of the person at death and his or her life expectancy. If the health condition results in disability of some kind, then the measure of welfare loss is the difference between normal life expectancy and the equivalent number of healthy years the individual has to live (using, for example, the QALY-based measures discussed earlier to establish the equivalence).

MEASURING LIFE EXPECTANCY. The first problem that arises is the choice of *life expectancy L* without the health condition. A number of alternative choices for L can be made, including:

i. L equals the maximum possible attainable age, usually set between 60 and 85, depending on the country. But because individuals can live to 100 or more, by choosing some arbitrary cutoff, one implicitly assumes that deaths occurring at ages greater than the cutoff impose no burden.

ii. L equals the "period expected years of life." This is defined as the expected length of life, given the age of the individual and her location. Thus, the burden associated with the death of an individual older than the population life expectancy would be negative under this measure. However, because life expectancies can change across and within countries, this measure would contravene the requirement that individuals be treated identically (as in b, above).

iii. L equals the "cohort expected years of life." This cohort measure of life expectancy is an adjusted version of the period measure in ii. It estimates life expectancy, given age and location, under the assumption that long-term trends in life expectancy will be in effect, abstracting from possible short-term deviations. Classic examples arise during periods of war when the life expectancy of men in their twenties plummets (see chapter 2). The period life expectancy of such individuals is temporarily low, but the cohort measure abstracts from this effect and results in higher life expectancies consistent with long-term trends. Also, the measure assumes continuing improvements in life expectancy consistent with past changes, so even in peace time, the cohort value is greater than the

period value. By making the estimate location-specific, this measure still contravenes b, above.
iv. L equals "standard expected life years." If b is to be satisfied, some measure of life expectancy independent of location must be used, but it remains desirable that the measure chosen reflects some empirically based notion of the length of a *normal* life. The standard chosen is that of Japan, the country with the highest life expectancy, with $L = 82.5$ for women and $L = 80$ for men.

There is clearly some inconsistency in the choices made, because the method differentiates between men and women (because they have different life expectancies), but not between rich and poor, rural and urban, and so forth, who also have different life expectancies. One way to justify this choice is to imagine the burden of disease calculation as constituting the benefit calculation of an extremely ambitious project that aims not only to *improve* the health of the world's people, but also to increase their life expectancies *up to the level of Japan*, while at the same time increasing the quality of life of all individuals to the same level. In a sense, the burden of disease might be better thought of as a measure of the burden of underdevelopment.

AGE-WEIGHTED VALUATION OF LIFE YEARS. The second choice that needs to be made in calculating the burden of disease is *how to measure the social value of a year of life lived at different ages*. The underlying question here is: Should the burden attributed to the loss of 60 years of healthy life from the death of a young person be considered 6 times as large as the burden associated with the loss of 10 years of healthy life from the death of an elderly person? That is, should the value of a year of life depend on the age at which it is lived?

From an ethical point of view, it seems reasonable to value years of life at different ages equally, especially when comparing different people. But a given individual may well express preferences that suggest unequal valuation.[13] It should be noted that the issue of valuation of years of life at different ages is conceptually separate from the issue of discounting, which examines the value of years of life lived at different calendar periods.

---

13. It is difficult, however, to imagine offering an individual the choice of living a year at age 30 versus living a year at age 60, because to do the latter she must do the former!

Unequal weights for years lived at different ages might be justified on the basis of some notion of productivity. If individuals are seen solely as productive units, then their value, like that of a machine, depends on their productivity. This *human capital* approach suggests that young children, who are not yet educated (that is, who have not yet "invested" in human capital) are relatively unproductive, and similarly that the elderly (whose human capital has "depreciated," possibly by becoming redundant) also have low productivity. Individuals in their early- to mid-adult lives are considered to be relatively more productive, suggesting an age profile of the social value of a year of life as shown in figure 9.5.

While the human capital approach may have some intuitive appeal, it should be noted that in standard welfare economics we measure individuals' well-being on the basis of their *consumption* and not their *income*. In fact, in orthodox life-cycle models, it is assumed that individuals save and invest in a manner that smoothes their consumption stream relative to their income stream, which means that the utility of a year of life at each age would be equal. Certainly it seems a bit unreasonable to suggest that a year of life for a 40-year-old coal miner who spends most of the year down

Figure 9.5.   *Social Value of a Year of Healthy Life Lived at Each Age*

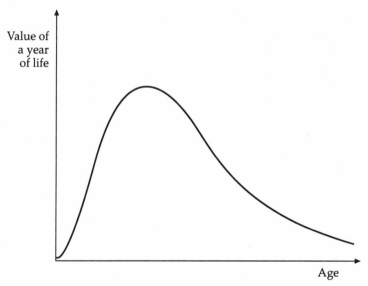

Source: Author.

a mine shaft should be valued more highly than a year of life after his retirement, when he can enjoy the fruits of his labor.

A further problem with this approach is that, if it is based solely on formal sector productivity, it will underrepresent the output of informal and home sector production. The value of women's lives, in particular, is likely to be undervalued, as is that of rural sector workers (who consume a portion of their output instead of selling it on the market).

An alternative justification for the bell-shaped weighting profile in figure 9.5 is that the social roles of individuals may change over their lives, and their contributions to social welfare will change accordingly. Thus, the young and the elderly are considered more dependent on society than those of working age, and a year of life lived at these outer ages should be valued less. This is really just a modification to the human capital argument, couched in terms of *net* productivity, and it is open to the same criticisms. It also suffers from a high dependency on cultural norms. In some societies the social costs of caring for the elderly are relatively low because of traditions of family care and support, while in others, with more formal arrangements, the dependency of the elderly may be somewhat higher.

These justifications for valuing years of life lived at different ages are clearly based on an *individual's* (net or gross) productivity profile. Because such profiles differ among individuals and across countries, separate profiles would ideally be constructed for each individual. This approach, however, would contravene the notion of treating individuals identically, because the productivity profile of a 40-year-old woman in Bogota is very likely to differ from that of a similarly aged woman in Boston. To avoid this problem, while maintaining the capacity to assign age-varying weights, the methodology applies the same profile to all individuals. While it is fair enough to weight years of life lived at different ages *by the same individual* differently if such a weighting conforms with the individual's preferences, the use of a single profile for all individuals remains questionable.

TIME PREFERENCE. Just like the consumption of different goods that must be aggregated using relative prices, aggregation of consumption at different times requires the use of some kind of price. When consumption at different dates is traded on the market, we can use the observed price— that is, the interest rate—to construct a shadow price of future consumption relative to current consumption. This price might be an adjusted version of the market price if there are significant market failures.

If years of life have value because of the consumption they permit, then years lived at different times should be valued using a discount rate. In valuing the years of life lived by a particular individual, this seems a reasonable approach. But often we will be aggregating years of life lived by different individuals, and particularly by individuals currently not alive. The critical characteristic of such future generations is that they are not party to the transactions that determine the observed market interest rate, so it is not at all clear that their consumption (or their lives lived) should be valued using the associated discount rate. Just as we should not arbitrarily discount the value of the life of one individual currently alive relative to that of another, it seems inappropriate to discount the value of the life of a member of a future generation solely on the basis of membership in that generation. This would suggest using a zero discount rate for valuing intergenerational allocations.

There may be some equity arguments in favor of discounting the value of life lived by future generations, if it is assumed that living standards will increase over time. In this case, future generations are richer, and therefore, if we are adjusting for income distributional concerns, should receive lower weight in any aggregation exercise. But, one could argue that, being richer, the value of a year of life is higher, so that the value of life of current, and not future, generations should be discounted.

AGGREGATING ACROSS INDIVIDUALS. Even abstracting from the issue of intertemporal weights, we must examine the validity of aggregating years of healthy life across individuals. It is perhaps useful to begin by recalling why it is meaningful to add up individuals' consumption of goods to arrive at a measure of GDP. First we add up quantities of different goods by weighting them by their prices, under the assumption that the marginal rate of substitution between any two goods is equal to their relative prices (that is, assuming that individuals are consuming optimally). Second, we add up the consumption of different individuals to arrive at total GDP, either because we are not concerned with distribution, or because we want to measure the envelope of resources available for redistribution. In other words, as long as resources are transferable among individuals, aggregate GDP provides a measure, admittedly an imperfect one, of potential social welfare. In particular, a dollar taken from one individual yields a dollar available to another—that is, the marginal rate of transformation between the income of one individual and that of another is one.[14]

---

14. This statement abstracts from issues of information asymmetries that will tend to constrain the efficacy of redistribution (see Roberts 1984). However, these problems exist equally when redistributing QALYs.

Adding up years of life saved across individuals creates a problem: it is difficult to imagine how a year of life can be directly transferred from one individual to another. To put it bluntly, killing Peter to save Paul does not sound feasible, although allowing Peter to die by withholding certain resources (such as food) in order to save Paul's life might be. The important point is that the marginal rate of transformation between QALYs of one individual and those of another is not necessarily one.

For example, consider a rural community of 1,000 identical peasants that lacks a health clinic. Suppose that by delaying the construction of a clinic, each peasant's estimated QALYs are reduced by 10. Total QALYs foregone are 10,000. The resources that are made available by the delay are deployed in an urban area to provide milk for 500 schoolchildren. This project is estimated to increase the QALYs of each child by 2, so that the total increase in QALYs is 1,000. The marginal rate of transformation between QALYs of different individuals is not one, but one-tenth. That is, a reduction of a rural peasant's QALYs by one permits an increase of an urban schoolchild's QALYs by one-tenth.

Thus, adding up a particular distribution of QALYs across individuals does not give a useful measure of the total number of QALYs available. An alternative distribution of resources will yield a different QALY total, but there is no way that we can say a higher total number of QALYs is better. To see this more explicitly, consider an economy with two individuals, A and B. We can think of individual A as a peasant in the example above, and individual B as an urban schoolchild. Let us suppose that with a rural health clinic in place, individual A has a stock of n_A QALYs, and individual B has a stock of n_B QALYs. This allocation is marked as the point x in figure 9.6, in which A's QALYs are measured on the horizontal axis, and B's on the vertical axis. Without the health clinic, but with the school milk project, the QALY allocations are n_A' and n_B', respectively, marked as point x' in the figure. Total QALYs are greater at point x', as displayed by line L', which has a slope of -1 and passes through x', to the right of the line L, which has the same slope and passes through x. However, the points to the southeast of x' along L' are not attainable through the redistribution of resources from point x'. Only points along the line $L^{*\prime}$, which has slope -10, are available to the economy. It is clear that weighting QALYs of the two individuals in this way makes the allocation x appear to be on line L^*, which defines a larger "budget set" than the allocation x'. This suggests that x should be preferred to x', especially when considering small changes (see chapter 8).

Figure 9.6.   *Aggregation of QALYs*

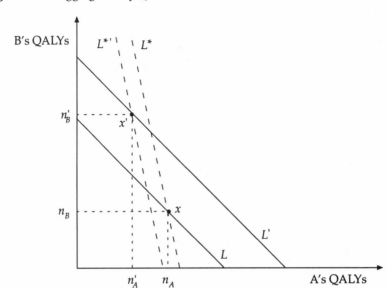

Note: Aggregating QALYs across individuals using equal weights ignores that the marginal rate of transformation between QALYs of different individuals is not necessarily equal to one.
Source: Author.

VALUATION OF NONFATAL HEALTH CONDITIONS. Some time was spent earlier discussing the estimation of QALYs that measure the value of a year of life lived with a particular medical condition relative to full health. Because the WHO/World Bank methodology attempts to include the burden of all health-related conditions, it is necessary to choose a method of making this valuation.

The approach adopted is closest in spirit to the attribute-based methods discussed earlier. Six classes of varying disability are identified that relate to various functions and capabilities, and each class is assigned a weight between zero and one. The classification and weights are shown in table 9.1 (drawn from Murray and Lopez 1994). These weights are used to calculate the number of DALYs associated with particular conditions.

The assignment of weights in the table is clearly somewhat arbitrary, and sensitivity analysis would be highly desirable in estimating aggregate burdens. At a more conceptual level, it might be asked whether the weights should be constant or vary, depending on the expected duration

Table 9.1.   *Adjusting for Disability Based on Functional Analysis*

Class	Description	Weight
Class 1	Limited ability to perform at least one activity in one of the following areas: recreation, education, procreation, or occupation	0.096
Class 2	Limited ability to perform most activities in one of the following areas: recreation, education, procreation, or occupation	0.220
Class 3	Limited ability to perform activities in two or more of the following areas: recreation, education, procreation, or occupation	0.400
Class 4	Limited ability to perform most activities in all of the following areas: recreation, education, procreation, or occupation	0.600
Class 5	Needs assistance with instrumental activities of daily living, such as meal preparation, shopping, or housework	0.810
Class 6	Needs assistance with activities of daily living, such as eating, personal hygiene, or toilet use	0.920

Source: Murray and Lopez (1994).

of the disease of condition. Essentially we are asking whether the marginal cost of the condition is constant, or whether it might vary with the length of time the individual suffers. A good example is a condition that makes procreation impossible. If the condition is temporary, then the affected individual, while inconvenienced, may not feel too badly, because having a family may become possible at some point. If the condition is permanent, however, the impact on the individual's well-being may be more than proportionately worse. By assuming a constant weight, it is possible to aggregate DALYs across individuals (that is, 10 DALYs for one person is equal to 1 DALY each for 10 people).

THE DALY FORMULA AND SOME CALCULATIONS. Pulling all these strands together, the calculation of DALYs lost because of a health condition encountered at age a is given by

$$\int_{x=a}^{x=a+L} D(x)\omega(x)e^{-r(x-a)}dx$$

where x ranges over future ages; $D(x)$ is the disability factor from the table, which can vary by age (if the extent of the disability changes—for example, if the individual recovers or dies); $\omega(x)$ is the productivity weighting factor for different ages; r is the discount rate, and L is the assumed life expectancy measure (which can depend on sex). The WHO/World Bank study assumes that $\omega(x)$ has the form

$$\omega(x) = Ce^{-\beta x}$$

for constants C and β. The general pattern of DALYs lost through death at each age is thus shown in figure 9.7.

Using this formula, the World Bank's *World Development Report 1993* calculated DALYs lost through poor health according to a range of factors, including geographic region and cause of illness and death. Table 9.2 reproduces box table 1.3 of the *Report*, which provides a summary of the distribution of DALYs lost according to these two factors.

References

Anand, Sudhir, and Kara Hanson. 1995. "Disability-Adjusted Life Years: A Critical Review." Applied Economic Discussion Paper 174. Oxford, U.K.: Institute of Economics and Statistics.

Figure 9.7. *DALYs Lost due to Death at Each Age*

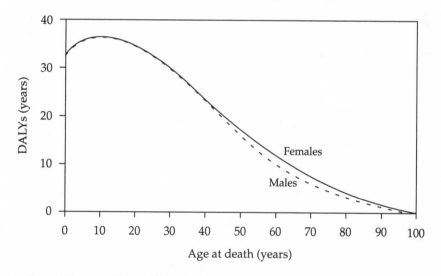

Source: Murray and Lopez (figure 5, 1994. p. 15).

Table 9.2. *Distribution of DALY Loss by Cause and Demographic Region, 1990* (percent)

Category	World	SSA	India	China	Asia[a]	LAC	MEC	FSEE	EME
Population (millions)	5,267	510	850	1,134	683	444	503	346	798
Communicable diseases	45.8	71.3	50.5	25.3	48.5	42.2	51.0	8.6	9.7
Tuberculosis	3.4	4.7	3.7	2.9	5.1	2.5	2.8	0.6	0.2
STDs and HIV	3.8	8.8	2.7	1.7	1.5	6.6	0.7	1.2	3.4
Diarrhea	7.3	10.4	9.6	2.1	8.3	5.7	10.7	0.4	0.3
Vaccine-preventable childhood infections	5.0	9.6	6.7	0.9	4.5	1.6	6.0	0.1	0.1
Malaria	2.6	10.8	0.3	*	1.4	0.4	0.2	*	*
Worm infections	1.8	1.8	0.9	3.4	3.4	2.5	0.4	*	*
Respiratory infections	9.0	10.8	10.9	6.4	11.1	6.2	11.5	2.6	2.6
Maternal causes	2.2	2.7	2.7	1.2	2.5	1.7	2.9	0.8	0.6
Perinatal causes	7.3	7.1	9.1	5.2	7.4	9.1	10.9	2.4	2.2
Other	3.5	4.6	4.0	1.4	3.3	5.8	4.9	0.6	0.5
Noncommunicable diseases	42.2	19.4	40.4	58.0	40.1	42.8	36.0	74.8	78.4
Cancer	5.8	1.5	4.1	9.2	4.4	5.2	3.4	14.8	19.1
Nutrition deficiencies	3.9	2.8	6.2	3.3	4.6	4.6	3.7	1.4	1.7
Neuropsychiatric disease	6.8	3.3	6.1	8.0	7.0	8.0	5.6	11.1	15.0
Cerebrovascular disease	3.2	1.5	2.1	6.3	2.1	2.6	2.4	8.9	5.3

(table continues on following page)

266

(Table 9.2 continued)

Category	World	SSA	India	China	Asia[a]	LAC	MEC	FSEE	EME
Ischemic heart disease	3.1	0.4	2.8	2.1	3.5	2.7	1.8	13.7	10.0
Pulmonary obstruction	1.3	0.2	0.6	5.5	0.5	0.7	0.5	1.6	1.7
Other	18.0	9.7	18.5	23.6	17.9	19.1	18.7	23.4	25.6
Injuries	11.9	9.3	9.1	16.7	11.3	15.0	13.0	16.6	11.9
Motor vehicle	2.3	1.3	1.1	2.3	2.3	5.7	3.3	3.7	3.5
Intentional	3.7	4.2	1.2	5.1	3.2	4.3	5.2	4.8	4.0
Other	5.9	3.9	6.8	9.3	5.8	5.0	4.6	8.1	4.3
Total	100.0	100.0	100.0	100.0	100.0	100.0	100.0	100.0	100.0
Millions of DALYs	1,362	293	292	201	177	103	144	58	94
Equivalent infant deaths (millions)	42.0	9.0	9.0	6.2	5.5	3.2	4.4	1.8	2.9
DALYs per 1,000 population	259	575	344	178	260	233	286	168	117

SSA Sub-Saharan Africa.
LAC Latin America and the Caribbean.
MEC Middle Eastern Crescent.
FSEE Former socialist economies of Europe.
EME Established market economies.
* Less than 0.05 percent.
a. Includes other Asian economies and islands other than China and India.
Note: DALY, disability adjusted life year; STD, sexually transmitted disease; HIV, human immunodeficiency virus.
Source: World Bank (1993, table 1.3, p. 27).

Becker, Gary S. 1964. *Human Capital.* Chicago, Illinois: University of Chicago Press.

Clarke, Philip M. 1998. "Cost-Benefit Analysis and Mammographic Screening: A Travel Cost Approach." *Journal of Health Economics* 17(6): 767–88.

Gertler, Paul, and Jaques van der Gaag. 1990. *The Willingness to Pay for Medical Care: Evidence from Two Developing Countries.* Washington, D.C.: World Bank.

Green, Jerry, and Jean-Jaques Laffont. 1979. *Individual Incentives in Public Decision Making.* Amsterdam: North-Holland.

Hammer, Jeffrey. 1993. "The Economics of Malaria Control." *World Bank Research Observer* 8(1):1–22.

Hausman, Jerry A. 1993. *Contingent Valuation: A Critical Assessment.* Amsterdam: North-Holland.

Johannesson, Magnus. 1996. *Theory and Methods of Economic Evaluation of Health Care,* vol.4, *Developments in Health Economics and Public Policy.* Dordrecht, Netherlands: Kluwer Academic Publishers.

Johansson, Per-Olaf. 1987. *The Economic Theory and Measurement of Environmental Benefits.* Cambridge, U.K.: Cambridge University Press.

_____. 1995. *Evaluating Health Risks: An Economic Approach.* Cambridge, U.K.: Cambridge University Press.

Klarman, H. E., J. O. Francis, and G. Rosenthal. 1968. "Cost-Effectiveness Analysis Applied to the Treatment of Chronic Renal Disease." *Medical Care* 6: 48–54.

Mishan, E. J. 1971. "Evaluation of Life and Limb: A Theoretical Approach." *Journal of Political Economy* 79(4): 687–705.

_____. 1994. *Cost Benefit Analysis,* 4th ed. London and New York: Routledge.

Mitchell, Cameron, and Richard T. Carson. 1989. *Using Surveys to Value Public Goods: The Contingent Valuation Method.* Washington, D.C.: Resources for the Future.

Murray, C. J. L. 1994. "Quantifying the Burden of Disease: The Technical Basis for Disability-Adjusted Life Years." In C. J. L. Murray and A. D. Lopez, eds., *Global Comparative Assessments in the Health Sector: Disease Burden, Expenditures, and Intervention Packages.* Geneva: World Health Organization.

Murray, C. J. L., and A. D. Lopez, eds. 1994. *Global Comparative Assessments in the Health Sector: Disease Burden, Expenditures, and Intervention Packages.* Geneva: World Health Organization.

Rice, Dorothy. 1967. "Estimating the Cost of Illness." *American Journal of Public Health* 57: 424–40.

Roberts, Kevin. 1984. "The Theoretical Limits of Redistribution." *Review of Economic Studies* 51(2): 177–95.

Tolley, George, Donal Kenkel, and Robert Fabian, eds. 1994. *Valuing Health for Policy: An Economic Approach*. Chicago and London: University of Chicago Press.

Torrance, G. W., M. H. Boyle, and S. P. Horwood. 1982. "Application of Multi-Attribute Utility Theory to Measure Social Preferences for Health States." *Operations Research* 30(6): 1043–69.

Viscusi, W. K. 1978. "Labor Market Valuations of Life and Limb: Empirical Estimates and Policy Implications." *Public Policy* 26: 359–86.

World Bank. 1993. *World Development Report 1993: Investing in Health*. New York: Oxford University Press.

10

Integrated Health Systems

In this chapter we use the theory and evidence of the preceding chapters to address issues that directly concern policymakers in ministries of health and finance. As should be clear by now, while on ethical or moral grounds there may well be reason to consider health to be "different," delivery of health care services does use scarce resources. In developing countries, these resources are especially scarce, and their alternative uses—for education, infrastructure, industry, agriculture, and the like—are abundant. This places a particular responsibility on planners and bureaucrats in such countries to use the available resources both compassionately and sensibly.

The orthodox approach of economists to policy analysis is to first ask, "What is the market failure?" That is, why are resources not being allocated in a socially desirable fashion by the market? (Hammer 1996 is a good example). Once the basis for public sector involvement is identified, suitable instruments are considered and a choice of intervention made. This kind of analysis was the subject of chapter 6, where we considered mainly the use of public intervention to improve the efficiency of an economy's resource allocation. We will argue below that in the health sector, there are relatively few pure public goods, and that based on the efficiency analysis, intervention would primarily be concerned with "getting the prices right." In practice, however, governments are observed in most countries, rich and poor, to intervene in the health sector much more actively and to a greater extent than this would imply, so our first challenge is to understand the possible normative and political-economic reasons for this.

Given these additional rationales for and means of government intervention, we examine in some depth the issues of implementation that are likely to arise. These include choices between a focus on health care and on health insurance, means of controlling incentives of consumers and providers of both types of service, and the integration of public and private means of production and resource allocation. We shall also examine the use of prices or other rationing mechanisms, both on the demand and supply sides, and the extent to which prices, when used, are determined by market forces or by the government. Finally, given these potential choices facing policymakers, we shall investigate the special circumstances facing developing countries—their relatively low incomes, sometimes poor administrative structures and capacity, and the existence of other high priorities for public spending—and the implications these might have for policymaking in the health sector.

The Extent of Government Intervention: Theory and Practice

The pure public goods identified in chapter 6 included services that affected the physical environment in which individuals live and work, as well as services that generate information that is useful to individuals in making health—more specifically, health care—decisions. Examples of the first type include spraying for mosquito control, purification of nonexcludable water resources (such as lakes), and control of ambient pollution. Accreditation procedures for licensing physicians and other medical personnel, regulation of drug quality, and information campaigns detailing the effects of cigarette use and AIDS risks are examples of information-based public goods.

In addition, we might include the provision of certain excludable resources, such as clean water, as goods that should be publicly provided, not because they will fail to be provided by the private sector, but because they may be underprovided, given the large fixed costs (and small marginal costs) of production.

The other market failures, characterized by situations in which individuals face the wrong prices, can, in principle, be corrected by the use of a set of budget-neutral taxes and subsidies. Thus, some merit goods may be subsidized, while others with negative externalities may be taxed, and as long as the tax system has a sufficient array of instruments, relative prices can be adjusted to ensure efficient resource allocation without requiring high levels of public spending.

But governments typically devote sizable quantities of resources to the health sector, and commentators often call for increases in these budget allocations (see, for example, United Nations Development Programme 1991). While the size of the resource allocation is sometimes high, it is often not used to deliver the public goods identified above. Thus, particularly in developing countries, there might be little effective control of those practicing medicine, much uncertainty about the quality of drugs, large geographical areas where malaria continues to be prevalent, and woefully inadequate public infrastructure. At the same time, however, there are large and expensive public hospitals, mainly in urban areas. The services provided by such institutions have primarily private benefits, and they are easily excludable, suggesting that there is little in the way of standard externality or public good reasons for their public provision.

Table 10.1 reports the distribution of global health expenditures in 1990 by region and the share of these expenditures financed by the public sector. By far the most spending on health is carried out in the rich countries, precisely because the distribution of world income is so skewed (column 1). Of the expenditures that are made in developing countries, an average of 50 percent is implemented through the public sector, compared with 60 percent in the established market economies, and more than 70 percent in former socialist economies (column 2). Excluding India, where the share of private sector spending in total health expenditure is nearly 80 percent, and Southeast Asia, the share of the public sector in health is reasonably

Table 10.1.   *Health Expenditures by Region*

Region	Health expenditure as a percentage of world total	Public sector expenditure as a percentage of regional total	Percentage of GDP spent on health
Established market economies	87	60	9.2
Former socialist economies of Europe	3	71	3.6
Latin America	3	60	4.0
Middle Eastern Crescent	2	58	4.1
Other Asian economies and islands	2	39	4.5
India	1	22	6.0
China	1	59	3.5
Sub-Saharan Africa	1	55	4.5
Demographically developing countries	10	50	4.7
World	100	60	8.0

Source: World Bank (1993, table 3.1).

constant across countries. Of course, the size of public sector spending relative to total health spending does not represent a full picture of the importance of government in the health care sector, because the share of GDP devoted to health varies considerably across countries (column 3). For example, while governments in both the established market economies and China contribute about 60 percent of health expenditures, in the market economies this public contribution represents 5.5 percent of GDP, while in China it makes up just 2.1 percent.

Even the failures of insurance markets—particularly as a consequence of adverse selection and hidden information and hidden action moral hazard—do not necessarily represent efficiency reasons for the government to actively provide health insurance for large segments of the population. The essential reason for this is that the insurance market failures arise from information asymmetries between insurer and consumer, and it is very unlikely that the government will have superior information (at comparable cost) that would enable it to deliver insurance more effectively than private insurance companies. Probably the strongest efficiency-based arguments in favor of public provision of insurance rely on comparative administrative costs. These cost advantages are likely to be greatest when all individuals are mandated to have insurance coverage, and insurance companies must charge the same price to all consumers. This set of conditions provides insurers with the incentive to devote extensive resources to discovering the risk characteristics of potential clients before providing insurance—so-called "medical underwriting"—which feed directly into larger premiums. The government would have no such incentive to select good risks, and it would therefore avoid these underwriting costs. Of course, there are likely to be certain economies of scale in recordkeeping, claim settlement, and other administrative functions as well. See Diamond (1992) for a discussion of these points (and others).

Equity and Public Provision as an Instrument of Redistribution

In popular policy debate, efficiency arguments based on the analyses of market failures do not command a prominent position. A somewhat more important justification for public intervention is the proposed positive impact on the distribution of well-being in the community. As discussed in chapter 7, equity can mean different things to different people. It may mean that individuals have similar money incomes, similar opportunities, similar health statuses, and so forth. Whatever the precise definition (and, in policy debate, the definition is often imprecise), equity concerns are either implicitly or explicitly behind many public interventions in the health care and health insurance sectors.

The implication of this observation is that those who favor public intervention must be of the opinion that the distribution of welfare without government action is not satisfactory. In practice, this is almost certainly the case, but a question that immediately arises in this context is whether the government should not implement the desired redistribution of resources through more direct income transfers. Such instruments are preferred as a matter of principle by some economists, and the arguments against in-kind transfers can be found in any elementary undergraduate text. Essentially, giving a certain amount of money to the poor allows them to choose among a range of alternative consumption increments, one of which might have been provided in kind by the government. This extra choice means that cash transfers (weakly) dominate in-kind redistribution.

There are, however, a number of possible arguments for the public provision of services in order to effect an in-kind transfer to those in need. These can be considered to generally reflect differences in production costs and the need to target transfers to contain their budgetary impact. In addition, there are arguments in favor of universal public provision—that is, nontargeted, in-kind transfers—that are also based on equity considerations. These issues will be discussed below with the help of a simple characterization of how individuals differ in relation to income and health.

Those who are relatively badly off, in their use of and access to health care, are likely to have low money incomes, to have high health care needs, or to face high costs of consuming health care services (if they must travel a long way to visit a clinic, for example). A useful way to represent these differences is in terms of budget constraints. Recall the simple description of consumer preferences in chapter 3, where utility was represented as a function $u(h,c)$, of health, h, and other consumption, c. The budget constraint for such an individual was written $m = c + \theta h$, where m was money income and θ was the *price* of health. It was argued there that θ would be higher for individuals with higher health care needs, and that they would consequently have a relatively small budget set available to them. Similarly, individuals with relatively high access costs—interpreted as travel costs—face a higher effective price for health, not because they need to consume more health care services in order to attain a given health improvement, but because they need to forego more nonhealth consumption (in the form of travel costs) for a given number of doctor visits. Finally, individuals may differ in the amount of money income, m, that they have available to allocate between health and other consumption.

These three factors—income, health needs, and access costs—combine to determine an individual's effective budget constraint; some examples are shown in figure 10.1. Assuming that the government can identify an individual's income without distorting his behavior, differences in money incomes can be eradicated by use of lump-sum income transfers from the wealthy to the poor. Such a policy ensures that all budget sets intersect the horizontal axis at the same point, such as m_0. But it remains the case that individuals with different health needs and access costs face different budget sets.

To achieve full equality, starting from our already heroic assumption regarding the possibility of equalizing money incomes, the government can select from two alternative strategies. The first is to take the effective prices that individuals face (the slopes of their budget sets), which reflect their health needs and access costs, as given, and to transfer additional money to those who face high prices. Thus, additional transfers would be made to those with relatively high health needs and to those who live in areas that were not well served by medical care facilities. This is the standard public finance response to situations where individuals differ with respect to the prices they face; the most notable example is the income tax problem, where individuals are assumed to face different prices for their labor—that is, different wage rates (see Mirrlees 1971). This theory suggests that, if possible, lump-sum income transfers based on prices (wages

Figure 10.1. *Income, Health Needs, and Access Costs Combine to Determine an Individual's Effective Budget Set*

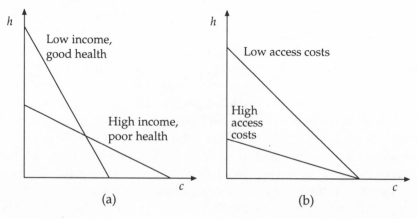

Source: Author.

in the income tax model) should be used, instead of altering the prices by the use of proportional subsidies and taxes. There would be no special role for public provision of services in such a model. Note that optimal lump-sum transfers do not result in all individuals facing the same budget constraint, but they can be chosen to equalize individuals' utility levels. This is shown for the case of two individuals in figure 10.2.

The assumption that health needs and access costs are exogenous, however, is clearly unrealistic. By providing more physicians per capita in remote areas, access costs for peasants can be reduced, and by improving roads, travel costs can be reduced. Similarly, by controlling pollution, the health status of a particular population can be improved. Thus, the government can alter the prices individuals face in ways that are not necessarily distortionary, and it can effectively redistribute real income by providing certain services to selected groups of individuals.

In general, the optimal method of redistributing real income toward those with relatively high health needs and access costs depends on the nature of the costs of providing services. For example, suppose there are increasing returns to scale, and the government intends to improve the

Figure 10.2. *Optimal Lump-Sum Redistribution*

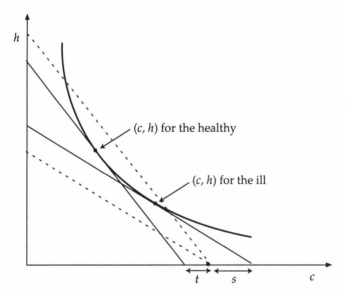

Note: A lump-sum tax t on the healthy finances a subsidy s to the ill that allows each to reach the same utility level. (The dashed lines represent pretransfer budget sets.)
Source: Author.

accessibility of peasants in a remote village to medical services. The two options are to provide income transfers that compensate villagers for their high transport costs, or to build and run a local clinic. If very few individuals are served by the clinic, it may be cheaper to subsidize their travel costs, but with a sufficiently high number of users, a local clinic may be preferred (because of the scale economies).

Sometimes, however, direct provision is far less economical than subsidizing access to existing suppliers. A telling example comes from New York City, where, to improve the access costs of individuals who found it difficult to get on and off buses, the city government modified buses to allow them to "kneel"—that is, the front of the bus can be lowered—to facilitate boarding. This technical modification turned out to be so expensive that it would have been cheaper to provide free taxi fares (to subsidize taxi prices at a rate of 100 percent) to all affected individuals.

This last example helps illustrate the importance of targeting transfers to the needy. If the government had offered taxi fare subsidies to those who had difficulty boarding buses, we can be sure that many people would have found themselves having trouble mounting the steps. That is, the analysis above assumed that the government faced no problem in determining the health needs and access costs of individuals. But this is clearly another heroic assumption (to add to our first implausible contention that money incomes can be equalized). Public in-kind provision may then prove to be an effective means of targeting benefits to those who "really" need them. The essential features of such in-kind benefits, if they are to be well targeted, are that they be valued by those who need them, but not by those who do not need them, and that they be nontradable. Thus, providing free medical care as a means of subsidizing those with either low incomes or high health needs will be expensive if other less-needy individuals also value such care. Similarly, it is likely that free immunizations would be used by both rich and poor (and possibly more by the former, if they are better educated), while public clinics staffed by adequately trained personnel but without fancy equipment might be used more by the poor. We clearly face an unpleasant tradeoff in such circumstances—reducing the overall quality of public provision to lessen its attractiveness to the nonneedy. To illustrate the second requirement of a well-targeted publicly provided good, note that if the government issues tradable vouchers for "adequate but plain" medical care, the nonneedy may acquire the vouchers for future sale. They may not value the service the vouchers represent, but if there is a market for them, this does not reduce their demand for the publicly provided good.

Redistribution through in-kind transfers may also be preferred when the government is concerned with intra- as well as interhousehold distribution, and when within-family resource allocations are not considered optimal. Thus, if income transfers are effected through income tax rebates, they will accrue in large part to primary earners. If such individuals do not use these additional resources in the interests of the family as a whole, then an in-kind transfer that is not tradable (and therefore potentially of little use to primary earners) may well increase the welfare of disadvantaged families relatively more. For example, if fathers tend to spend some fixed fraction of their income on personal consumption, then cash transfers to encourage child immunization will have a smaller impact than direct provision of immunization services. Note that vouchers for immunization would not be desirable in this case as long as they are potentially tradable.

This discussion of targeting is brief, not because it is unimportant, but because a complete survey of the issues is beyond the scope of this text. However, the central feature of the analysis is that when the government has less than complete information about the needs and incomes of individuals—which is certainly true in all countries—it cannot target delivery of income or in-kind transfers perfectly. It must rely on designing transfer mechanisms that induce those in need to take up the assistance, while ensuring that most of those who are not considered in need do not. To affect such so-called "self-selection," the transfers offered must be of sufficiently low quality, but this, of course, reduces their ability to improve the well-being of the needy.

Recent literature has addressed the desirability of universal versus targeted benefits in a political economy context. Realizing that policy is made in a political environment in which decisionmakers act in their own interests, some authors have suggested that public support for a narrow, targeted system may be lower than for a more universal system that offers the expectation of benefits to most of the population. These discussions and models then predict that targeted systems will be of low quality, while universal systems will be of higher quality and benefit the needy relatively more. By making the size of the budget endogenous, such analyses can turn the orthodox targeting argument on its head. (See Pritchett and Gelbach 1997.)

A final equity argument for public provision concerns the use of public insurance within the context of a redistributive income tax system. Suppose individuals can differ with respect to their wage rates and their probabilities of falling ill. As above, we would like to redistribute income to those with low wages (because they are poor) and high-risks (because they have to pay a lot for insurance), but suppose also that the government cannot accurately discern these characteristics. Rochet (1991) has shown that as long as there is a negative correlation between an individual's wage rate and probability of falling ill—that is, as long as generally high-risk individuals have lower wages—universal public insurance is optimal. (See also Blomqvist and Horn 1984.)

Specific Issues in the Provision of Public Insurance

In this section we address issues in the public provision of medical insurance. First we discuss the distinction between insurance and medical care, and why public provision of the first may be more important than that of the second. Acknowledging that, just as with private insurance, there will be moral hazard problems in any public insurance scheme that tend to lead to overuse of free services, we examine demand- and supply-side controls, with particular emphasis on the latter. We then examine the role of the private sector within a public system, and the potential rationing mechanisms that a government may use, including the price system.

Insurance versus Medical Care

Medical insurance may be unaffordable to the poor or those with high health risks, and even minimal coverage may not be offered if adverse selection causes the insurance market to fail.[1] If the government provides universal insurance, it is likely that the demand for medical care from these populations will be sufficient to make private provision of such care profitable. That is, except for certain medical care services with externalities or public good features, the provision of care might well be left to the (regulated) private market if insurance is available to all.

Instead of providing insurance, the government may prefer to mandate that all individuals purchase their own. Concerned with the ability of high-risks to afford coverage, the authorities may impose a "community rating" requirement on insurance companies, requiring them to charge the same price to all individuals, regardless of risk. Low-risk individuals will then

---

1. Jalan and Ravallion (1997) report evidence that, in general, poorer households are more exposed to income risks than are wealthier households. It seems reasonable to expect that such a pattern of exposure is also found with regard to health risks.

pay a price that, on average, is higher than the value of the insurance to them, while the price paid by high-risks will be lower than its value. This cross-subsidy will tend to force low-risks out of the market (this is exactly the problem of adverse selection), and to restrain such behavior, it will be necessary to compel all individuals to be insured.

Such a compulsory private scheme of insurance redistributes income from low- to high-risks, but not from rich to poor. Those on low incomes will tend to find it difficult to comply with the mandate, and targeted income trans- fers or premium subsidies may be required. Then, of course, we return to the issue of targeting and the imperfect nature of available mechanisms.

Note that a mandate to purchase insurance can be considered identical to a publicly provided insurance scheme with a particular financing mecha- nism. For example, suppose that all individuals have the same income, but differ by risk. Then a mandated scheme with community rating, which results in a cross-subsidy from low- to high-risks, has similar effects to a public scheme financed by a uniform poll tax on all individuals. As under any poll tax, those who benefit most from the goods and services financed by the tax revenue (here, the high-risks) gain at the expense of those who benefit least from such goods and services (here, the low-risks).

Alternatively, the mandated purchase of community-rated insurance can be seen as the product of an income transfer from low-risks to high-risks, combined with the purchase of insurance at actuarially fair rates (that is, at prices that are higher for high-risks than for low-risks). This characterization clarifies the need for compulsion: without it, low-risks would not be willing to pay the taxes required to finance the subsidies to the high-risks.

A further undesirable incentive introduced into the health insurance market when community-rated coverage is mandated is for insurance companies to try to attract predominantly low-risk individuals. Recall- ing that they must charge the same price to both types of individuals, it is clearly in the interests of an insurer to cover as many low-risks and as few high-risks as possible in order to maximize profits. Such selection activities, however, may be considered socially wasteful—after all, with mandated coverage, all individuals will purchase insurance from some insurer, so it is only a matter of which insurer they choose. The govern- ment may choose to remove the incentive to select the good-risks by as- signing individuals to insurance companies on a geographic basis, for example. Such a policy would have desirable effects on selection—insur- ers would not be able to affect the mix of individuals they cover and would not spend any money trying to do so—but could significantly constrain the incentives of insurers to perform. Guaranteed a captive market of consumers, the insurer would have no incentive to maintain or improve quality (through faster claim payment, and the like) or to lower premiums, because demand would be entirely inelastic.

Demand-Side Controls

A public insurance scheme or a mandated private scheme must specify which services are covered, what kinds of treatments are acceptable in different circumstances, which patients receive priority over others, and what kinds of contributions covered individuals are required to make when they consume medical care. In the absence of both hidden-action and hidden-information moral hazard, these issues would be dealt with on the basis of perceived (social) benefits relative to costs. Thus, services that yield net increases in welfare would be provided, which, in principle, would allow a priority list to be compiled. In the presence of moral hazard, however, service use is likely to be higher than is socially optimal, depending on the price elasticity of demand. To control this overuse, especially elastic services may require relatively large coinsurance rates or deductibles, although this clearly puts low-income individuals at a disadvantage.

Although positive coinsurance rates are effective means of restraining demand, other mechanisms are available. For example, the government may require that use of specialist services (which are typically expensive) be permitted only after a consultation with a general practitioner has confirmed that such a treatment strategy is appropriate. Such a "gatekeeper" model would be effective as long as the net savings of deterring some individuals from using specialist services outweigh the additional costs associated with the requirement that individuals who do use such services visit a general practitioner. Note that such a system is similar to the HMO-type models described in chapter 5, in which nonprice instruments are used to counter the moral hazard problem.

Alternatively, the government might try to restrict the degree of "shopping around" by consumers for additional services. Thus, faced with a low monetary price of consumption, an individual who does not agree with the advice of his doctor that further treatment is unwarranted may seek additional consultations until he finds a physician who will perform the sought-after service. It is not entirely clear that the government should try to control this sort of behavior, although casual reflection would suggest that excessive shopping around is socially inefficient, particularly if physician quality is generally uniform. One approach is to use the price mechanism and to increase copayment rates for second opinions, although this clearly has negative effects as well, because second opinions are often used to ensure that unwarranted expensive procedures are minimized (so that second opinions should be cheap for the consumer). Another mechanism that is used is to prohibit such shopping around, or at least to make it costly in other ways. Thus, in the United Kingdom, individuals are assigned to a general practitioner's practice, and their ability to switch general practitioners is constrained by law. The obvious negative effect of this practice is that general practitioners have very little incentive to respond to the demands of their patients, because they perceive—correctly—a captive market.

Supply-Side Controls

In addition to controlling individuals' incentives to consume insured medical care services through price and other demand-side instruments, the government may control the level of provision through supply-side intervention. Such policies have been strongly supported by Ellis and McGuire (1993), for example. Recognizing that patients' decisions to consume medical care are often a function of the advice they receive from doctors, there is scope for so-called "supplier-induced demand" (see chapter 6). If left unconstrained, this may lead to excessive resource use. Thus, if providers are reimbursed for the costs of provision, they will have very little incentive to economize on treatment or to engage in cost-reducing strategies that are inconvenient or personally costly. In the markets of textbook economics, these incentives to oversupply and to be inefficient are constrained by consumer demand, but when consumers have little information or expertise with regard to the appropriateness of treatments or costs, they are not very effective in constraining the behavior of suppliers.

In order to restrain resource use and to induce efficient production, supply-side interventions operate by altering the way providers are paid. Four methods of payment will be presented below, with their strengths and weaknesses identified.

FEE FOR SERVICE. In the reimbursement model, mentioned above, providers send the government a bill for services provided to insured individuals. The government does not question the appropriateness of services provided (although it does check to ensure that the correct charges are claimed and that the service was delivered), but leaves that decision to the patient and doctor. Some copayments might be required of the individual, but otherwise the constraints on provision are limited to the physical quantities available (for example, the physician's time) and ethical factors (such as not providing services that will harm the patient).

Under such an arrangement, doctors have few incentives to be efficient, because any costs of inefficiency are borne by the government. In general, however, they will provide care of good (perhaps excessive) quality, and they will not have a preference for treating "cheap" cases over "expensive" ones. Thus, providers would not be expected to actively discriminate against individuals requiring difficult and expensive treatments.

DIAGNOSIS-BASED PROSPECTIVE PAYMENT. To improve incentives for providers to be cost-conscious, it is necessary that they bear at least some of the cost of inefficiency. For example, if a hospital employs highly trained personnel to perform rudimentary tasks, it may be held responsible for the costs above those that would be incurred if appropriately trained lower-level technicians had performed the tasks. Having to bear the burden of this inefficiency would presumably lead to some alteration of production techniques—that is, a change in the input mix.

One way to implement a strategy to make providers responsible for inefficiencies is to have some benchmark indicator of the "appropriate" cost of treating a particular illness, and to reimburse the provider only for that amount. If the provider succeeds in holding costs below the benchmark level, it receives the difference as profit, but if actual costs exceed the benchmark, it makes a loss. Thus, the provider would be paid not on the basis of the actual costs incurred, but prospectively, on the basis of the diagnosis of the patient when first entering the medical care establishment.

The definition of "diagnosis" in this context is clearly important. Too coarse a partitioning of the possible illness types either means that the provider is exposed to large variations in net income from patients, or that it has large incentives to discriminate between patients with the same diagnosis, but with observationally different expected costs of treatment. But too fine a partitioning would entail large administrative costs and give providers additional margins on which to improperly diagnose patients. Thus, a patient with a given ailment might be reported as suffering from a more severe condition, with a higher prospective payment rate. If it is difficult for the government to monitor the veracity of admissions data, this incentive may lead to increased costs.

The other important negative incentive effect that prospective payment systems introduce relates to quality of care. Although a provider may not report an incorrect diagnosis, it may have every incentive to economize on the quality of care provided in order to take advantage of any cost savings. Thus, a problem with prospective payment systems is that they allow providers to keep all cost savings, whether these originate from efficient use of inputs or from a reduction in effective output, as measured by the improvement in the health of patients (which is affected by the quality of care). (See Ellis and McGuire1986.)[2]

A final effect of prospective payment mechanisms, identified by Dranove (1987), is that the diagnosis-based payment may induce hospitals to efficiently specialize. If hospitals can direct resources toward certain diagnoses, an efficient allocation of cases among hospitals may emerge. Of course, for this kind of specialization to be socially beneficial, there must be enough hospitals engaging in the practice to cover all diagnoses. Dranove notes, however, that instead of efficiently specializing with respect to diagnoses, hospitals may instead specialize in the kinds of patients they treat *within* all diagnoses—that is, hospitals may discriminate against high-cost patients, as discussed above.

CAPITATION. The capitation method is sometimes used to pay general practitioners (as in the United Kingdom), and it is similar in some respects to an HMO arrangement. A general practitioner is paid a lump sum yearly (or for any time period stipulated), based on the number of individuals on the physician's patient list. The amount paid for each patient may depend on some risk-related criteria, such as the age and sex, and may vary by region, for such reasons as variations in local costs or health status (for example, brought about by environmental factors). Under this arrangement, general practitioners have every incentive to be efficient in the care they provide, but again they face strong incentives to include only healthy individuals on their patient lists. One way to reduce the number of expensive patients is to refer them to higher-level care facilities instead of treating them locally. This may well impose large costs on the patient as well as on the health budget. Of course, the more closely the capitation payment is related to each patient's health status, the less incentive a general practitioner has to discriminate among patients on the basis of risk.

---

2. This is a good example of the problems that arise when paying a provider on the basis of inputs used instead of outputs delivered. In the health care context, however, it is very difficult to measure outputs, and even if output could be measured, payments based on such output may expose providers to a large degree of risk because of the uncertainty associated with many treatment strategies.

As in the case of prospective payment schemes, there will also be incentives to skimp on the quality of care. The underprovision of quality can be controlled to some degree through regulation—for example, requiring general practitioners' surgeries to be open at certain hours, to be staffed and equipped with suitable resources, and so forth—but such regulation might not be perfect.

SALARY PAYMENTS. In response to supply-side incentive problems, the government may choose to incorporate medical practitioners into the public sector directly and to make them salaried public servants. At least in the short run, general practitioners' rewards are then only tenuously related to performance and costs, and there is little financial incentive to be either efficient or innovative in the provision of care, but neither is there an incentive to be selective in the type of patient treated. The essential feature of salary contracts is that duties are often left implicit, or at best described in vague terms, based on established norms and practices. Depending on the physician's view of social responsibilities—reflected in her willingness to work additional hours for no extra financial remuneration—a salary system can leave substantial room for outside labor supply. Such moonlighting activities may be significant if salaries are low and monitoring of performance (attendance at clinics, and the like) is poor. (See chapter 6 for a fuller discussion of moonlighting.) Of course, from a purely economic viewpoint, a higher salary will have little negative effect on the incentive a physician faces to moonlight (it may strengthen the incentive if the price for moonlighting services increases), although there are two mechanisms that may lead higher salaries to improve unmonitored performance. First, if the physician does have some degree of altruism, higher salaries may increase her willingness to engage in altruistic activities (not moonlighting). Second, even if monitoring is infrequent and imperfect but does occur with some probability, increasing the salary increases the potential loss incurred if the moonlighting physician is detected and punished (by being struck off the register of licensed physicians, for example). This second argument is essentially an efficiency-wage argument in favor of higher salaries, not only for physicians, but also for other salaried staff whose duties elude explicit description in contractual form and whose actions are difficult to monitor.

Private-Public Mix

Many countries combine a system of mandatory publicly provided insurance with optional private insurance coverage. For there to be any incentive for individuals to choose to purchase additional insurance coverage, the publicly provided component must be incomplete in some sense. For example, suppose the public insurance scheme covered 80 percent of all medical costs. Individuals may wish to purchase additional insurance to cover the residual risk presented by the 20 percent coinsurance rate they would be required to pay if they had no private coverage. We can think of this "topping-up" of coverage as occurring at the intensive margin, in the sense that the types of services covered are not extended, but the financial consequences of consuming them are altered. (It is also referred to as "gap insurance"—insurance that covers the gap between the total cost and that covered by the public scheme.)

Alternatively, suppose public insurance provides coverage against some medical treatments, but not others. For example, use of experimental drugs may not be reimbursable under the public plan, and some kinds of cosmetic surgery may not be permitted. In this case, additional insurance may be purchased on the extensive margin, whereby the types of services covered are expanded. The cost-sharing components—coinsurance rates, deductibles, and the like—might be the same as under the public plan, but in general these financial arrangements will depend on demand elasticities and risk aversion.

A special case of expansion of coverage on the extensive margin relates to a consumer's control of the inputs used in the delivery of services. Thus, a public scheme may cover a wide range of medical treatments, but problems of moral hazard may cause these services to be offered only through public hospitals and clinics (see the preceding discussion), institutions that permit the individual consumers little control. If they wish to be able to choose their own doctor and possibly to make other decisions regarding their treatment, they may need to be treated outside the public system. Unless they are willing to face large risks, they will need to be insured against the financial costs involved, and some private coverage will be required.

Two policy issues with regard to supplementary insurance coverage immediately emerge. First, should extensions be allowed, and second, what should be the tax implications? The social desirability of expanded private coverage depends on the type of expansion. For example, intensive expansion, which reduces the copayments required of individuals at the point of care provision, may impose negative externalities on other taxpayers if the public scheme is not financed with premiums that are actuarially fair on a person-by-person basis. To see this, suppose the public system pays for 80 percent of the cost of medical treatment, and that this public expenditure is financed by an income tax. If an individual purchases insurance from a private insurer to cover the 20 percent copayment, she will face a money price equal to zero, and her demand for services will increase. The private insurance company will be able to charge a premium equal to (or greater than, depending on the degree of competition) 20 percent of the expected value of expenditures based on demand generated by a zero price, and will make a nonnegative profit. Public expenditures will increase proportionately with the increase in demand, and they will need to be financed through increases in the income tax. To the extent that this increase is borne by individuals other than the person taking out the private coverage, there is a negative externality. The response may be to prohibit expansion on the intensive margin—that is, to prohibit gap insurance.

Expansions at the extensive margin are less likely to directly impose additional costs on the public system, and thus taxpayers. To the extent that they result in a substitution of privately provided care for public care, the burden on the public system is reduced. Thus, if individuals purchase private insurance to ensure that they can choose their own doctor, their use of public hospital facilities will likely fall. In such cases, individuals essentially replace their public coverage with private insurance. To the extent that their tax liability does not fall because of this replacement (it could actually rise if there is a value added tax that includes insurance services, for example), the burden on the public system is reduced.

It is reasonable to expect that private insurance that effectively replaces public coverage will be chosen primarily by the better-off. Such an arrangement appears at first to be quite attractive—public health care is provided to the less-well-off, while being financed by the better-off. But recall that the better-off are likely to opt out of the public system only if they perceive high enough relative benefits from choosing private coverage. This requires that the public system be of a lower standard than the private system. Particularly in developing countries where resource constraints limit the potential quality of private as well as public care, the implication may well be that the quality of publicly provided care must be quite low to induce significant numbers of individuals to opt out. Thus the issue of targeting again emerges, and it is the basis for the argument that "services for the poor are poor services." It may be preferable, on equity grounds, to provide reasonably high-quality care through the public system, financed with progressive taxation, and to constrain individuals' ability to opt out. This may be particularly important if we consider the political process for allocating public health care resources. If the public system only serves the poor, it is likely that it will be underfunded and of poor quality, not only because of the imperatives of targeting constraints, but also because of the ability of the politically powerful to allocate public resources toward themselves.

Price Setting and Other Rationing Mechanisms

In our discussion of the public provision of insurance and medical care services, we have spoken often of how to charge consumers and how to pay providers, keeping both efficiency issues (such as moral hazard, adverse selection, and production efficiency) and equity issues in mind. Most of the discussion has assumed, however, at least implicitly, that such charges and payments are based on existing prices. For example, we have investigated the conditions under which the price charged to the consumer should be perhaps 20 or 50 percent of the "cost" of the service, but the underlying price is taken as given. Similarly, we have examined the conditions that would permit providers to be paid on the basis of incurred costs, number of patients, diagnosis of the patient, and the like, but have taken the underlying resource costs of provision as given.

One interpretation is that underlying prices are determined endogenously by market forces, taking into account the effective taxes and subsidies that characterize the government's choice of consumer charges and provider payments. If this interpretation were valid, markets would always clear—that is, demand at the consumer price (including the effects of subsidies, taxes, and insurance copayments) would equal supply at the producer price (including the effects of provider payment mechanisms). However, a major issue facing many public delivery systems revolves around the existence and size of waiting lists—individuals who would like to consume certain medical services at the existing consumer price but are restrained from doing so by a lack of supply. This disequilibrium, which is similar in nature to those characterizing labor markets that exhibit involuntary unemployment, arises when consumer prices and provider payments are set independently. Thus, if the government chooses to charge consumers a low price or to provide them with insurance, but it also pays providers a low price in order to keep budgetary costs under control, demand is very likely to exceed supply. This is shown simply in figure 10.3, where the demand and supply schedules for a particular service are drawn.

In the diagram, the initial equilibrium is characterized by a price p_0 and quantity q_0. Suppose the government wishes to provide some insurance against medical costs by reducing the price of the service under consideration by an amount s. With this subsidy, the demand curve shifts up in the usual way by an amount s. If producer prices are allowed to vary, the new

Figure 10.3.   *Effects of Setting Consumer and Producer Prices Independently*

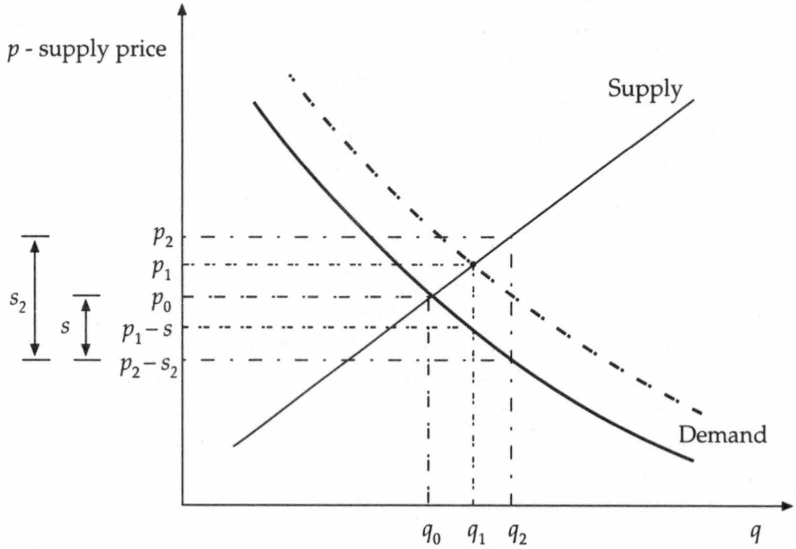

equilibrium price p_1 and quantity q, will be higher. However, the price faced by the consumer is $p_1 - s$, which provides an effective reduction in the price of services of $\Delta p = p_0 - (p_1 - s) < s$. In order to reduce the equilibrium price by an amount s, the nominal subsidy would need to be significantly higher. In the diagram, the subsidy is s_2, which is determined by the condition that demand at the consumer price $p_2 - s_2$ equals supply at the producer price p_2, and that $p_2 - s_2 = p_0 - s$. In the particular case of linear demand and supply curves, with slopes equal to minus and plus one, respectively, prices received by providers increase by as much as those paid by consumers decrease. The cost of the subsidy borne by the government is equal to the area $s_2.q_2$, which is much larger than $s.q_0$.

This example highlights the constraints that the market imposes on government actions. More precisely, it shows the effect of price-based equilibrating mechanisms on the budgetary costs of public insurance schemes and other subsidies. If the supply curve is completely inelastic (vertical) and prices are freely variable, it will be impossible for the government to lower the consumer price by means of a subsidy. In these cases, to contain budgetary costs, the government may choose to directly control both the consumer price and the producer price. For example, in the figure, if a subsidy of s is provided to consumers, but the price paid to providers is fixed at p_0, then the desired impact on the consumer price will be affected. However, because the producer price is not permitted to increase, supply will remain at the level q_0, and it will not be sufficiently high to clear the market.

It is important to understand the inefficiency that results from the excess of demand over supply. Recall that the primary motivation for providing the subsidy to consumers is to protect them from the financial risks associated with uncertain medical expenditures. In the absence of risk and other externality, public good, merit good, or distributional considerations, the demand curve provides an appropriate measure of social marginal benefits of consumption. Assuming a competitive market, the supply curve also accurately represents marginal social costs, so the socially desirable level of consumption is q_0. Ideally, insurance would provide income support to those individuals who find themselves with a high valuation of the medical service in question (those at the top of the demand curve, with valuations above p_0), and consumption would remain at q_0. The budgetary cost of the subsidy would then be equal to the area $s.q_0$. The actual allocation of the subsidy, if it is implemented through the price system, keeping producer prices fixed, depends on the method of allocation of supply q_0 among individuals who demand q_2. If there is some mechanism to identify those with the highest valuation, on the basis of diagnosis, for example (ignoring differences in willingness to pay based on income, and the like), and to whom the limited supply can be directed, there is no efficiency loss from market nonclearing. To allow the market to clear through producer price increases would be inefficient, because aggregate consumption of the service (q_1) would be too high, and the amount of subsidy received by individuals with high needs would be too low ($p_0 - (p_1 - s)$).

Clearly, the inefficiency of nonmarket clearing arises if the wrong people receive the limited supply. Thus, if individuals with marginal benefit less than p_0 but greater than ($p_2 - s$) receive the service (because they live near to the clinic, know the doctor, or the good is allocated randomly to anyone with a valuation above p_2) at the expense of someone with a valuation above p_0, then an inefficiency arises. The cost of these allocative inefficiencies must be weighed against the cost of alternative mechanisms that would provide the desired subsidy, s. In particular, allowing producer prices to increase so that supply and demand (at the subsidized price) are equated will entail service use well in excess of the level q_0, and impose significant financing requirements on the tax system. The distortionary costs of higher tax rates, as well as the inefficiency of overconsumption, may well support the use of nonprice rationing mechanisms in the provision of public insurance.

References

Blomqvist, Ake, and H. Horn. 1984. "Public Health Insurance and Optimal Income Taxation." *Journal of Public Economics* 24: 353–71.

Diamond, Peter. 1992. "Organizing the Health Insurance Market." *Econometrica* 60(6): 1233–54.

Dranove, David. 1987. "Rate-Setting by Diagnosis Related Groups and Hospital Specialization." *Rand Journal of Economics* 18(3): 417–27.

Ellis, Randall, and Thomas McGuire. 1986 "Provider Behavior under Prospective Reimbursement: Cost Sharing and Supply." *Journal of Health Economics* 5: 129–51.

_____. 1993. "Supply-Side and Demand-Side Cost Sharing in Health Care." *Journal of Economic Perspectives* 7(4): 135–51.

Hammer, Jeffrey. 1996. "Economic Analysis for Health Projects." Policy Research Working Paper 1611. World Bank, Washington, D.C.

Jalan, Jyotsna, and Martin Ravallion. 1997. "Are the Poor Less Well-Insured? Evidence on Vulnerability to Income Risk in Rural China?" Policy Research Working Paper 1863. World Bank, Washington, D.C.

Mirrlees, James. 1971. "An Exploration in the Theory of Optimum Income Taxation." *Review of Economic Studies* 38: 175–208.

Pritchett, Lant, and Jonah Gelbach. 1997. "More for the Poor Is Less for the Poor: The Politics of Targeting." Policy Research Working Paper 1799. World Bank, Washington, D.C.

Rochet, Jean-Charles. 1991. "Incentives, Redistribution and Social Insurance." *The Geneva Papers on Risk and Insurance Theory* 16(2):143–65.

United Nations Development Programme (UNDP). 1991. *Human Development Report.*

World Bank. 1993. *World Development Report 1993: Investing in Health.* New York: Oxford University Press.

Index

(*Page numbers in italics indicate material in tables or figures.*)